THE MENSTRUAL CYCLE

THE MENSTRUAL CYCLE

Physiology,
Reproductive Disorders,
and Infertility

Michel Ferin
Raphael Jewelewicz
Michelle Warren

New York   Oxford
OXFORD UNIVERSITY PRESS
1993

Oxford University Press

Oxford   New York   Toronto
Delhi   Bombay   Calcutta   Madras   Karachi
Kuala Lumpur   Singapore   Hong Kong   Tokyo
Nairobi   Dar es Salaam   Cape Town
Melbourne   Auckland   Madrid
and associated companies in
Berlin   Ibadan

Copyright © 1993 by Oxford University Press, Inc.

Published by Oxford University Press, Inc.,
200 Madison Avenue, New York, New York 10016

Oxford is a registered trademark of Oxford University Press

Library of Congress Cataloging-in-Publication Data
Ferin, Michel
The menstrual cycle: physiology, reproductive disorders,
and infertility / Michel Ferin, Raphael
Jewelewicz, Michelle Warren.
p. cm.   ISBN 0-19-506193-4
1. Menstruation disorders.
2. Menstruation.
3. Infertility, Female—Endocrine aspects.
I. Jewelewicz, Raphael, 1932–   .
II. Warren, Michelle P.   III. Title.
[DNLM: 1. Menstrual Cycle. 2. Menstruation Disorders.
WP 540   F356m]   RG161.F37
1992   618.1'72—dc20   DNLM/DLC
for Library of Congress   92-1058

1 3 5 7 9 6 4 2
Printed in the United States of America
on acid-free paper

This book is dedicated
to the memory of
Dr. Raymond Vande Wiele,
our teacher

Preface

This book represents our effort to outline in a logical and didactic fashion the critical events that characterize the menstrual cycle. Each chapter is the result of a thorough review of the literature and a critical distillation of the pertinent data. The book encompasses fundamental cellular processes, physiological events within each of the organ entities critical to the cycle, and cyclic endocrine feedback relationships between organs. It covers the major pathology of the menstrual cycle and relates abnormalities to the physiological process as it is understood today. The book also includes a review of the general endocrine therapeutic approaches presently available to restore a normal menstrual cycle. References to other reviews and articles of specific interest are provided at the end of the book; the reader is encouraged to examine these for a broader or more detailed overview of the subject of interest.

We would like to thank Ms. Bambi Aharon and Jacqueline Zengotita for their expert dedication in helping us bring this manuscript together, and acknowledge the critical help of Thomas Wong in the graphical design.

M.F.
R.J.
M.W.

Contents

THE MENSTRUAL CYCLE

1

The Reproductive Cycle: An Overview

The major function of the ovary is to produce mature and fertilizable ova. The dynamic relationships between the different components of the reproductive axis in the adult female are such that this reproductive process occurs in a cyclic fashion, in an orderly sequence of events. This sequence involves a remarkable coordination between hormonal secretion and morphologic changes in various organs and will be described in the first chapters.

The reproductive cycle of the female primate can be divided into three stages: (1) the *follicular phase,* the time for follicular growth; (2) the *ovulatory period,* when final maturation of the oocyte and its release into the reproductive tract occur; and (3) the *luteal phase,* when a newly formed corpus luteum secretes hormones in preparation for implantation. If the egg is not fertilized and implantation does not occur, a new cycle is initiated (the phenomenon of *cyclicity*) as soon as the activity of the corpus luteum wanes. If the fertilized egg implants into the uterus, the luteal phase is prolonged and becomes the progestational phase of the pregnancy that follows.

Ovulation is induced by the sudden release of large amounts of gonadotropins from the pituitary gland (the gonadotropin surge). Species can be differentiated as to whether the trigger to the surge of gonadotropins is external or internal. Species in which the trigger to the surge is external, such as the rabbit, cat, mink, and ferret, are termed *reflex ovulators.* The ovulatory surge is induced by mating and the genital stimuli, transmitted via neural pathways connecting the copuloreceptive area to the hypothalamus, stimulate luteinizing hormone (LH) and follicle-stimulating hormone (FSH) release. In these species, the ovarian steroids merely act to promote sexual receptivity. Species in which the trigger to the surge is internal, such as the rat, guinea pig, sheep, cow, and primate including the human, are termed *spontaneous ovulators.* The ovulatory surge is triggered by the changing endogenous ovarian steroid titers that accompany follicular maturation. In these species, the ovarian steroids also promote sexual receptivity.

Corpus luteum development, which follows ovulation and the expulsion of the egg, may be *induced* or *spontaneous,* depending on the species. The rat, mouse, and hamster lack a spontaneous luteal phase: after ovulation, the corpus luteum regresses within 2 or 3 days, unless stimulation of the cervix occurs, in which

3

case a full-length secretory luteal phase can be observed. In contrast, the sheep, cow, and primate have a full-length luteal phase that spontaneously follows each ovulatory period.

THE ENVIRONMENT AND CYCLICITY

In many species, the environment undoubtedly influences normal cyclicity, and photoperiod is the primary environmental cue that controls seasonal breeding. In the ewe, for example, exposure to short daylight periods initiates estrous cycles, while long daylight periods induce anestrus and anovulation. Some species, such as the laboratory rat, seem to have escaped these seasonal variations in cyclicity and cycle year round, perhaps because they have been removed from environmental cues such as the seasonal changes in the relative length of light and dark periods. Even in the laboratory rat, however, the spontaneous gonadotropin surge will not occur unless a proper diurnal light–dark regimen is in place. For example, the proestrous ovulatory surge of gonadotropins, while primarily induced by estradiol, will be timed to occur about 8 hours after the lights are turned on; it will fail to occur if the light stimulus is absent or if the neural pathways that transmit this information are interfered with. The primate, and especially the human, is most removed from environmental influences. Thus, women can give birth throughout the year, while most other mammals have distinct breeding seasons, and the ovulatory gonadotropin surge can occur at any time of the day or night.

MENSTRUAL CYCLE LENGTH

In the majority of women, the menstrual cycle lasts between 25 and 30 days, with the distribution within this range skewed toward cycles with a 28–30 day length. The normal cycle starts with the follicular phase. By convention, the day of menstruation is labeled day 1 of the menstrual cycle. Yet, although the onset of menstruation clearly delineates the termination of an endometrial cycle and the beginning of a new one, it is important to recognize that the use of menstruation as a marker for the initiation of the follicular phase may sometimes be incorrect; indeed, an early hormonal marker for the follicular phase, the early follicular phase FSH rise (see later), may appropriately encompass a period that includes 1 or 2 days before the onset of menstruation.

Although in a "typical" cycle the follicular phase lasts approximately 14 days, its length can be variable; in contrast, the luteal phase is remarkably constant in duration and lasts 12–15 days.

PRINCIPAL HORMONAL MARKERS OF THE MENSTRUAL CYCLE

There are four major hormonal markers that characterize the menstrual cycle: two are of pituitary origin—*LH* and *FSH*—and two are of ovarian origin— *estradiol* and *progesterone.* These four hormones are easily monitored in the peripheral circulation by modern assay methods. When mean daily patterns of these four hormones are determined throughout the menstrual cycle in large groups of women, and therefore individual variations and pulsatile activity are masked, characteristic patterns such as those illustrated in Figure 1–1 can be observed.

1. In regard to *LH* secretion, the most striking event is a spectacular and abrupt rise in concentrations at the end of the follicular phase: the *preovulatory LH surge* (3 in Fig. 1–1). Mean duration of the gonadotropin surge is 48 hours. By careful comparative evaluation of hormonal measurements and ultrasound observations of ovarian folliculogenesis, it is estimated that ovulation occurs about 18 hours after the LH peak or 36 hours after the initiation of the LH surge. Mean daily changes in LH secretion at other times of the menstrual cycle are modest.

2. *FSH* also rises at the end of the follicular phase as part of the preovulatory gonadotropin surge (3) but this increase is more modest than that for LH. Of importance to FSH secretion is the slight but physiologically very significant (about twofold) rise in FSH on the day(s) preceding or on the day of menstruation; peak FSH values at this time are reached about 24 hours after menstrual flow has started: *the early follicular phase FSH rise* (1). This is the only time in the menstrual cycle at which the FSH:LH ratio favors FSH.

3. *Estradiol* (E2) secretion remains low during the early follicular phase period, but increases 1 week prior to the midcycle gonadotropin surge, first at a slow, then at a very rapid, quasi-exponential rate to reach a peak at the time of the onset of the LH surge: the *late follicular phase estradiol peak* (2). Within a few hours after the initiation of the midcycle gonadotropin surge, estradiol concentrations fall abruptly. They rise again with the appearance of the corpus luteum.

4. *Progesterone* (P) secretion remains insignificant throughout the follicular phase, rises suddenly and modestly about 12 hours prior to the onset of the LH surge, then remains at a plateau for about 12 hours: the *preovulatory progesterone rise* (4). Progesterone rises again 36 hours after the onset of the LH surge. During the luteal phase, levels of both progesterone and estradiol rise, to reach a maximum about 6–9 days after the midcycle gonadotropin surge: *the luteal phase estradiol and progesterone secretory curve* (5).

In addition to these daily hormonal rhythms that form the basis for the 28-day menstrual cycle, there are also very important *ultradian* (shorter than a day) rhythms that shape the hormonal signals: plasma levels of all four hormones undergo episodic fluctuations of variable amplitude and frequency, referred to as secretory *pulses,* or *episodes.* For a given hormone, pulse frequency may vary between species, and within each species, pulse patterns usually change with the endocrine milieu. Thus, the circulating levels of most major reproductive hormones have been shown to fluctuate, often quite dramatically. This accounts for the large variations (from the norms of Fig. 1–1) shown by individual cycles, even among successive menstrual cycles in the same woman.

As the reader readily realizes from a cursory look at Figure 1–1, the menstrual cycle is the result of the precise coordination of events that take place in geo-

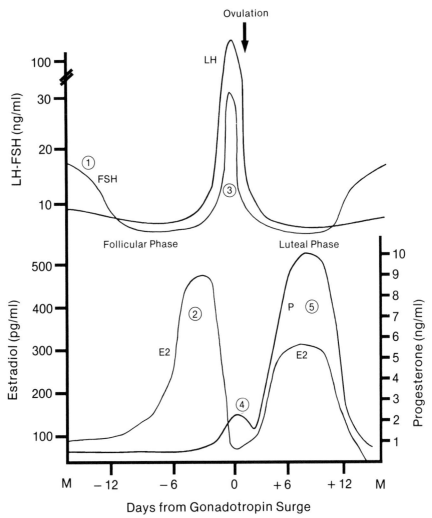

Fig. 1-1. Four hormonal markers of the menstrual cycle. Mean daily hormonal levels throughout a "typical" 28-day ovulatory menstrual cycle. (Because of variations in length of the follicular phase, it is useful in graphic representations of mean daily values to synchronize mean hormonal changes around the day of the gonadotropin surge [day 0]; follicular phase days are then characterized as occurring before the surge [days −], and luteal phase days as occurring after the surge [days +]. *1*, the *early follicular phase follicle-stimulating hormone (FSH) rise* initiates the follicular phase; *2*, the *late follicular phase estradiol-17β (E2) peak* signifies maturation of the dominant follicle; *3*, the *preovulatory gonadotropin surge* luteinizing hormone ([LH] + FSH) is the signal for ovulation; *4*, the *preovulatory progesterone (P) rise* is triggered by the gonadotropin surge; *5*, the *luteal phase E2 and P secretory curve* reflects the lifetime of the corpus luteum.

6

graphically disparate organs of the body, such as the brain, the pituitary gland, the ovaries, and the reproductive tract. In order to review the mechanisms of control of the menstrual cycle, it is first necessary to understand the sequence of events in each component. Thus, in the first chapters, we will review the hypothalamic-pituitary unit (the neuroendocrine component), the ovaries, and the genital tract during the menstrual cycle. In later chapters, we will review pituitary-ovarian communications and the feedback signals that coordinate hormonal and morphologic changes in the different organs.

While modern techniques, such as radioimmunoassay and ultrasound, have allowed significant gathering of data on the human menstrual cycle, a large amount of our knowledge of basic mechanisms of control of the reproductive cycle derives from studies in animals. When relevant to our concerns, some of this information will be included. Particular emphasis will be placed on research in nonhuman primates, for example the rhesus monkey and other related species, since they demonstrate a menstrual cycle that resembles that of the human both in its length and cyclic hormonal patterns.

2

The Neuroendocrine Component: The Hypothalamic-Pituitary Unit

There is overwhelming evidence in all mammals that pituitary gonadotropin secretion is driven by the hypothalamus, and that hypothalamic control is exerted via the release of a neurohormone, *gonadotropin-releasing hormone* (GnRH, also referred to as LH-RH). Thus, when discussing the menstrual cycle and its control, it is necessary to first talk about the hypothalamic component and to elaborate on neuroendocrine aspects. In this chapter, we will review normal GnRH function, which is crucial to cyclicity; the function of the pituitary gland and how it responds to particular GnRH signals; and the role of neuropeptides, such as the endogenous opioid peptides, and how they modulate the GnRH system.

THE HYPOTHALAMIC GnRH SYSTEM

GnRH: STRUCTURE

GnRH is a small peptide consisting of 10 amino acids (decapeptide). As many other neuropeptides, it is synthesized as part of a larger precursor molecule. The structure of the precursor has been deduced from the DNA sequence of the gene coding for the peptide, and consists of 92 amino acids (Fig. 2–1). This large molecule is broken down before release and both GnRH and the portion of the molecule distal to GnRH, a 56 amino acid peptide termed gonadotropin-releasing hormone associated peptide (GAP), are released. The precise biological role of GAP or fragments of it remains to be defined.

The human gene encoding GnRH has been isolated and is localized on the short arm of chromosome 8. In the mouse, a mutant has been discovered that lacks GnRH, the result of a deletion of the distal half of the GnRH gene. As a vivid illustration of the importance of GnRH as the primary instigator of gonadotropin secretion, this mutant remains hypogonadal. Of general interest is the experimental observation that the endocrine deficiency in this animal can be overcome following implantation in the brain of neural hypothalamic tissues from normal mice.

8

In the normal animal, inactivation of GnRH bioactivity following the administration of an antiserum to GnRH or of a GnRH antagonist results in a rapid decrease in gonadotropin secretion, again demonstrating that this neurohormone is essential for gonadotropin release.

GnRH: LOCALIZATION IN THE HYPOTHALAMUS

Peptidergic neurons synthesize peptidergic hormones such as GnRH within their cells. Surprisingly, it was found in lower mammals that GnRH cells do not originate in the brain, but rather migrate there from the embryonic olfactory placodes. This particular journey is one of the few examples of neurons developing outside the central nervous system and migrating into it. By the end of embryogenesis, the GnRH cells have reached the locations in the brain which they will occupy throughout reproductive life. This raises intriguing questions about *Kallmann's syndrome,* a syndrome in which idiopathic hypogonadotropic hypogonadism and delayed puberty are associated with anosmia. It is possible to speculate that defects in the paraolfactory area may account both for deficient olfaction and GnRH secretion, particularly if these prevent normal olfactory nerve and GnRH cell migration into their respective hypothalamic areas.

GnRH neurons in the hypothalamus usually appear as a dispersed population spread over several classic architectonic divisions of the brain. The degree of spread of the GnRH neurons varies with each species, and is most probably related to the extent of migration from the olfactory placodes to the hypothalamus. In the rodent, for example, migration is completed when the GnRH neurons reach the rostral hypothalamus, that is, the preoptic-anterior hypothalamic area. In the primate, migration proceeds further caudally, and GnRH neurons are seen in the medial basal hypothalamus and in the premammillary region. Particularly crucial in primates are GnRH neurons in the region of the *arcuate nucleus.* This nucleus is situated within the medial basal hypothalamus immediately above the median eminence (Fig. 2–2). The total number of GnRH neurons is small, approximately 1,500 (even fewer appear to be involved in the control of the gonadal axis).

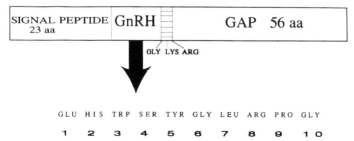

Fig. 2–1. The precursor to gonadotropin-releasing hormone *(GnRH)*. GnRH derives from a 92 amino acid precursor. It is released together with GnRH-associated peptide *(GAP)* of still uncertain function. *aa,* amino acid. GLU: glutamic acid, HIS: histidine, TRP: tryptophan, SER: serine, TYR: tyrosine, GLY: glycine, LEU: leucine, ARG: arginine, PRO: proline.

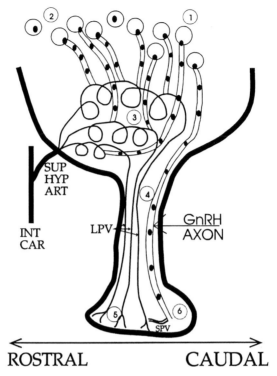

ROSTRAL   CAUDAL

Fig. 2–2. GnRH neurons and the hypothalamic-hypophyseal portal circulation. In the primate, many GnRH neurons are located within the *arcuate nucleus* (*1*), an important region for gonadotropin control. As in the rodent, however, GnRH neurons are also present rostrally within the *preoptic-anterior hypothalamic* area (*2*). (There is some discussion as to the functional role of this area in the primate; in the rodent, this rostral area is essential to reproductive function.) GnRH secreted by the peptidergic neurons is packaged in granules and transported by axonal flow to the *median eminence* (*3*) area. Within this area, GnRH is released into capillary loops derived from the superior hypophyseal artery *(SUP HYP ART)*, which itself is a branch of the internal carotid artery (int car). The capillaries collect into the *long portal veins (LPV)* which descend along the surface of the *pituitary stalk* (*4*) connecting the median eminence to the *adenohypophysis* (anterior pituitary) (*5*). In the primate, a few GnRH-containing axons also descend within the pituitary stalk to reach the *neurohypophysis* (posterior pituitary) (*6*), near the short portal veins *(SPV)*, which also irrigate the adenohypophysis. Abbreviations as in Figure 2–1.

In neurons, GnRH is packaged into granules within the Golgi apparatus. Granules are then transported by axonal flow to the axon terminal. The most prominent projections from arcuate neurons, as well as from other hypothalamic GnRH-producing neurons, are to the *median eminence,* the final common pathway for the regulation of anterior pituitary function, and the area from which the vessels irrigating the pituitary gland originate.

THE HYPOTHALAMIC-HYPOPHYSEAL PORTAL SYSTEM

GnRH axons within the median eminence terminate in the vicinity of capillaries into which the peptide is secreted. These capillaries, derived from the superior hypophyseal artery, form loops that cover the entire area of the median eminence, thus allowing for extensive axonal–vascular interactions. They then collect into the *long portal veins* which terminate into another set of capillaries within the anterior pituitary gland (Fig. 2–2).

In the primate, there are usually six to ten long portal veins descending along the surface of the *pituitary stalk* which connects the median eminence to the pituitary gland. Unlike the posterior pituitary (*neurohypophysis*), which is derived entirely from neural ectoderm, the anterior pituitary gland (*adenohypophysis*) derives from the buccal epithelium and has no direct neural connection with the hypothalamus. Thus, the hypothalamic-hypophyseal portal circulation is crucial to the endocrine function of the adenohypophysis. The anterior pituitary does not appear to receive direct arterial supply.

The major direction of blood flow is downward from the brain to the pituitary gland (although there is evidence of upward flow). This direct vascular connection between the brain and anterior pituitary is essential because it allows for the rapid transport of minute amounts of neurohormones (GnRH is secreted in picogram amounts) undiluted to the target organ (the gonadotrope, in the case of GnRH). Section of the pituitary stalk and, thus, interruption of the portal vessels disrupts the trophic function of the anterior pituitary: it causes a cessation of cyclicity and of the secretion of all anterior pituitary hormones, except for prolactin which is under an overall inhibitory influence of the brain.

It is important to note that by the time GnRH reaches the peripheral circulation, its concentrations are too low to be measured accurately because of dilution. This is unfortunate because GnRH secretory patterns and hypothalamic function cannot be assessed directly in the human. The investigator must then depend on indirect approaches, such as the pattern of pituitary gonadotropin secretion which under some circumstances may not accurately reflect hypothalamic activity, or interpolate from direct observations in animal models.

In higher mammals such as the primate but not the rodent, a few GnRH axons also descend within the pituitary stalk to reach the posterior pituitary. These GnRH-containing axons terminate in the vicinity of the *short portal vessels,* which connect the posterior to the anterior pituitary. What specific role can be attributed to GnRH derived from this route remains to be elucidated.

THE GnRH PULSE GENERATOR

In the 1970s, the advent of radioimmunoassays allowed for the first time the measurement of a large number of samples and thus provided the ability to observe hormonal secretion frequently over periods of several hours. When this technique was applied to the measurement of luteinizing hormone (LH), the first investigators were originally surprised and concerned by the variability of hormone concentrations within the same individual. However, it rapidly became apparent that these seemingly erratic LH concentrations were not related to the imprecision of the method but to the fact that LH is released intermittently, that is in a *pulsatile* rather than in a continuous fashion. These ultradian (less than 1 day) fluctuations are superimposed on the long-term rhythms (days, weeks) which are illustrated in Figure 1–1 for the same hormone measured on a daily basis during the menstrual cycle. LH ultradian fluctuations were first described in detail in the ovariectomized rhesus monkey, where plasma concentrations oscillate with a period of about 1 hour (circhoral). Each hourly pulse of LH consists of the abrupt release of the hormone from the gonadotrope into the peripheral circulation, followed by the exponential decline representative of the half-life of the pituitary hormone.

It is now well established that each LH pulse is the result of a GnRH pulse released by the hypothalamus into the hypothalamic-hypophyseal portal circulation; animal studies have shown a good synchronization between pulses of the neurohormone and of LH (Fig. 2–3). These observations have led to the concept of the *GnRH pulse generator,* a still not well-defined brain entity responsible for the pulsatile signal.

In the monkey, and presumably in the human, the GnRH pulse generator appears to be located in the medial basal hypothalamus within or in the vicinity of the arcuate nucleus. In the monkey, abrupt changes in multiunit electrical activity have been monitored within this area which are synchronous with pulses of LH in the periphery. Surgical isolation of the medial basal hypothalamus from the remainder of the brain that retains connections to the pituitary stalk allows for continued pulsatile LH release; however, lesion of the arcuate region of the monkey results in an abrupt cessation of pulsatile gonadotropin secretion.

THE CONTROL OF GnRH PULSATILITY

GnRH neurons are scattered throughout the medial basal hypothalamus rather than neatly arranged in a nucleus, a peculiar arrangement for neurons that need to be discharged synchronously. What accounts for the synchronous discharge of GnRH remains unknown and the subject of active research and speculation. Synchronized release from these neuroendocrine neurons could be, in theory, obtained in different ways. For example, GnRH neurons may have little interaction but individually receive a synchronized input; alternatively, the neurons may communicate with each other, so that when one or more generates a burst of activity, the others will follow. Recent examination at the cellular level has demonstrated several types of interactions between GnRH cells, such as axosomatic and axodendritic synapses which certainly would allow for communication to occur.

The question as to whether the GnRH cell is inherently pulsatile or whether other neurosecretory systems are implicated in the generation of GnRH pulses cannot be entirely resolved at present. There is, however, mounting evidence for interaction between neurotransmitters and GnRH release. Several neurotransmitters, among which the catecholamines norepinephrine and dopamine are included, have been shown to influence GnRH and gonadotropin secretion. The interpretation of the considerable literature related to the subject is complicated by observations that dual types of effects (e.g., stimulatory/inhibitory) are frequently reported for the same compound depending on the experimental and endocrine parameters. Thus, it is not possible yet to formulate a comprehensive concept of GnRH control.

At present, the best evidence in the primate suggests that a hierarchal network of norepinephrine-GnRH cells may form a core component of the pulse generator. This is supported by the observations that

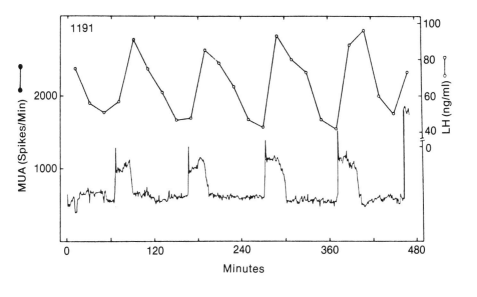

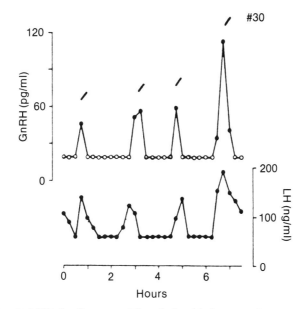

Fig. 2–3. The *GnRH* Pulse Generator. The relationship between GnRH pulse generator activity and luteinizing hormone *(LH)* release in the ovariectomized rhesus monkey: GnRH and LH pulses coincide, indicating a one-to-one causal relationship. *Upper panel:* The pulse generator is monitored by electrodes recording multiunit activity *(MUA)* in the arcuate region *(bottom)* (From Wilson RC, Kesner JS, Kaufman JM, Uemura T, Akema T, Knobil E 1984: *Neuroendocrinology* 39:256. Reprinted with permission from S Karger AG Basel. *Lower panel:* The pulse generator is monitored by radioimmunoassay measurements of GnRH *(top).* Abbreviations as in Figure 2–1. (From Van Vugt DA, Diefenbach WD, Alston E, Ferin M 1985: GnRH pulses in third ventricular cerebrospinal fluid of ovariectomized rhesus monkeys: correlation with LH pulses. *Endocrinology* 117:1550–1558. Copyright © by The Endocrine Society.)

13

1. administration of α-adrenergic (but not β-adrenergic) blockers to the monkey results in a suppression of GnRH and LH pulsatile activity. In the human, pharmacological studies using α-adrenergic blockade have yielded negative results, perhaps reflecting inadequate dosages of the pharmacological compound, as rather large dosages were needed in the animal model to demonstrate this effect. Alternatively, these studies may indicate a lesser dependence of the GnRH pulse generator on neurotransmitter control in the human.

2. release of norepinephrine in the vicinity of the pulse generator is pulsatile and appears to be synchronous with GnRH release from the median eminence. Complicating the interpretation of these observations, however, is the fact that, although noradrenergic innervation of the arcuate hypothalamic region arises from outside the hypothalamus, complete medial basal hypothalamic disconnection from the rest of the brain, which interrupts noradrenergic pathways into the region, does not interfere with pulsatile LH release in the monkey. While this observation does not necessarily negate a role for noradrenergic pathways, it certainly suggests that there may be more than one component to the pulse generator. Another candidate may well be dopamine, although, in the primate, this catecholamine is generally thought of as an inhibitor rather than a stimulator of LH release.

In the rodent, it appears that a population of preoptic/anterior hypothalamic neurons containing the neurotransmitter gamma-aminobutyric acid (GABA) may be associated with pulsatile release: each LH episode is preceded by an abrupt local hypothalamic drop in GABA release, suggesting the periodic removal of an inhibitory influence by GABA. The physiological importance of this relationship remains to be investigated in the primate, in which the preoptic/anterior hypothalamic area appears to play a lesser role in GnRH pulsatility and in the reproductive process.

THE ANTERIOR PITUITARY GLAND

THE GONADOTROPINS

There are two gonadotropins of pituitary origin: LH and FSH. Both are glycoproteins. A third gonadotropin, chorionic gonadotropin (CG) is of chorionic or placental origin and thus only secreted in pregnancy.

Each gonadotropin consists of two dissimilar peptide chains or subunits (α and β), which are synthesized as precursors that undergo posttranslational alterations. Glycosylation occurs on both subunits. The α subunit is common to LH, FSH, human CG (hCG), and thyroid-stimulating hormone (TSH). The β subunits of these hormones are different in sequence, and thus characterize each hormone. Individual subunits have little or no biological activity on their own: hormonal activity requires association of the α and β subunits. Each subunit is coded by a different single gene; α and β subunit genes are located on different chromosomes (α on chromosome 7, β on chromosome 19).

The *gonadotropes,* the cells within the adenohypophysis in which the gonadotropins are synthesized, are distributed throughout the glandular parenchyma. In general, the gonadotrope is thought of as multihormonal, in that it has the functional capacity of producing both LH and FSH. Although several studies report cells containing only one of the two hormones, these monohormonal cells are probably bipotential and may produce the other hormone under the appropriate conditions. GnRH, for instance, increases the percentage of gonadotropes containing both hormones, while causing a corresponding decrease in monohormonal cells.

Castration is followed by morphological changes within the gonadotrope, presumably reflecting the absence of the long loop negative feedback. So called *castration* cells appear, which are characterized by dilation of the endoplasmic reticulum. Overall, there is an increase in visible gonadotropes.

GnRH AND GONADOTROPIN RELEASE

Gonadotropin response to GnRH is rapid. Within minutes of a single injection of GnRH, both LH and FSH release occurs, to peak within 15–30 minutes. Because of the short half-life of the neuropeptide (3–5 min), gonadotropin concentrations decrease thereafter.

The interaction of GnRH with its plasma membrane receptor on the gonadotrope is the first step leading to gonadotropin release. The receptor is coupled to a calcium ion channel, and calcium is required for release: it is mobilized in response to GnRH and can activate LH release. Calmodulin (an ubiquitous intracellular Ca^{2+} receptor) appears to behave as an intracellular messenger for calcium mobilized in response to GnRH.

OVARIAN STEROID MODULATION OF THE GONADOTROPE'S RESPONSE TO GnRH

Early attempts to compare gonadotropin responses to single injections of GnRH at various times during the menstrual cycle revealed impressive fluctuations in the gonadotrope's sensitivity to GnRH under different endocrine conditions. When GnRH tests are performed during the follicular phase, there is a progressively greater and more sustained LH response from the early to the late follicular phase (Fig. 2–4). Maximal sensitivity to GnRH occurs at midcycle, with a tenfold increase in responsiveness on the day of the midcycle gonadotropin surge. These changes in pituitary sensitivity to GnRH during the follicular phase are the result of the progressively increasing levels of estradiol; the augmented response at the time of the high estradiol secretory phase can be completely eliminated following the administration of clomiphene citrate, a compound that competes with estradiol for its receptors. Estradiol, at its peak physiological concentration, requires about 12 hours to exert this midcycle enhancement of responsiveness. Pituitary sensitivity to GnRH during the midluteal phase is as great as that seen in the late follicular phase.

Precisely how steroids alter the sensitivity of the gonadotrope to GnRH is not entirely known. Results in the rodent and the primate suggest that estradiol-induced amplification of gonadotropin release requires the presence of normal or perhaps increased concentrations of GnRH in hypophyseal portal blood. This GnRH "priming" effect, that is, the capacity of GnRH to increase the respon-

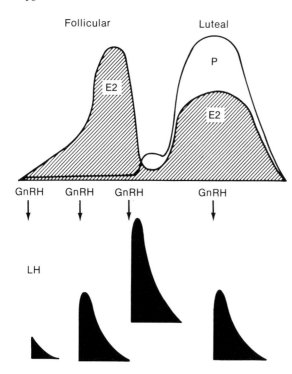

Fig. 2–4. Ovarian steroid modulation of LH reponse to GnRH. LH response to identical injections of GnRH at different times of the menstrual cycle. LH release is rapid at all times, but note the increased sensitivity to GnRH in the presence of estradiol *(E2)* alone or in association with progesterone *(P)*. Comparatively little gonadotropin is released in the early follicular phase when ovarian steroid secretion is minimal. Changes in sensitivity of the gonadotrope to GnRH play an important role in the sequence of events that leads to the midcycle gonadotropin surge. Abbreviations as in Figure 2–3. (Adapted from Wang CF, Yen SSC, 1975: *J Clin Invest* 55:201.)

siveness of the gonadotrope to the steroid, appears to be associated with a significant migration of secretory granules containing gonadotropins to a zone close to the plasmalemna, from which the granule can be easily released. This phenomenon could thus increase the *"readily releasible"* pool of LH and FSH available for rapid release. In turn, estradiol may increase the *"storage"* pool of LH and FSH, by increasing the synthesis of these hormones and therefore their availability for transfer to the readily releasible pool. Because of these complexities, the results of GnRH testing in patients with abnormalities of the cycle are difficult to interpret.

DESENSITIZATION OF THE GONADOTROPE

Several groups have observed that GnRH receptor occupancy by the natural neurohormone or by its agonists can produce "desensitization" of the gonadotrope. This specific effect can be observed both in vitro and in vivo and whether it occurs depends on the nature of the GnRH challenge. In superfusion systems, continuous exposure of dispersed pituitary cells to high doses of GnRH rapidly produces desensitization which leads to a lowering of LH release, whereas pulsatile GnRH administration prevents this phenomenon. In immature and adult animals or in women with reproductive deficiencies, attempts at maintaining gonadotropin secretion with continuous GnRH infusions or with long-acting GnRH analogs have been largely unsuccessful: following an initial release of

gonadotropins, secretion of LH wanes rapidly. With pulsatile GnRH administration, normal gonadotropin levels can be sustained indefinitely (Fig. 2–5). This
is not surprising since it has been shown that a pulsatile GnRH stimulus is
required to increase transcription of the gonadotropin subunit genes.

The cellular mechanism of desensitization remains to be elucidated. This process cannot be explained in terms of depletion of cellular LH and is probably
calcium independent. It has been suggested that constant GnRH stimulation
may induce internalization and degradation of GnRH receptors on the surface
of the gonadotrope, thus reducing the ability of the cell to control GnRH input.
However, the changes in GnRH receptor number and affinity do not appear to
be proportional to the induced changes in pituitary sensitivity, and, thus, desensitization cannot be explained solely by loss of GnRH receptors. At the moment,
it is best explained by postreceptor biochemical alterations, which are as yet not
well understood.

These observations clearly indicate that an intermittent or pulsatile pattern of
GnRH release is crucial for normal gonadotropin function; thus, the gonadotrope appears to be preprogrammed to respond only to intermittent stimulation.

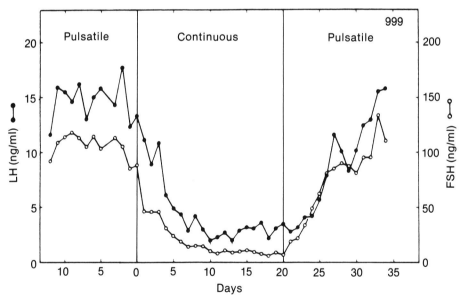

Fig. 2–5. Desensitization of the gonadotrope. A pulsatile pattern of GnRH stimulation
of the gonadotrope is essential for normal gonadotropin secretion. This concept is illustrated in this experiment in a monkey bearing a lesion of the arcuate region and therefore
lacking endogenous GnRH secretion, in which the effects of a *pulsatile* and *continuous*
GnRH infusion are contrasted. Note the "desensitization" of the gonadotrope during the
continuous infusion, resulting in a rapid decline in gonadotropin levels. *FSH,* follicle-
stimulating hormone; other abbreviations as in Figure 2–3. (From Belchetz PE, Plant TM,
Nakai Y, Keogh EJ, Knobil E, 1978: *Science* 202:631. Copyright 1978 by the AAS.)

In fact, in a normal individual, continuous chronic GnRH stimulation may lead to a significant deficiency in gonadal function. This, of course, bears significant therapeutical implications; thus, the desensitization phenomenon can be used clinically to suppress gonadotropin secretion when needed, such as, for example, in the treatment of premature puberty, hormone-dependent tumors or, experimentally, in contraceptive approaches. For this purpose, long-acting analogs of the decapeptide are usually used. The stimulatory regimen needed in patients lacking endogenous GnRH and gonadotropin secretion evidently requires a pulsatile infusion of the decapeptide itself to augment gonadotropin release (see Chapter 13).

GnRH AND FSH RELEASE

It is clear from most studies that GnRH controls the release of both LH *and* FSH. The rapid release of LH following GnRH administration is accompanied by an increase in FSH, although in smaller amounts. In the monkey, administration of GnRH antibodies results in a decrease in both LH and FSH.

Most observations suggest that FSH release is also pulsatile; however, clear evidence for FSH pulsatile release is only seen in some subjects at specific stages of the menstrual cycle. On many occasions, it is not possible to observe FSH pulses or to quantify FSH pulse frequency because of the low amplitude of FSH fluctuations presumably reflecting smaller amounts of FSH released in response to the GnRH pulse, and more importantly, the longer half-life of FSH resulting in individual pulses masking subsequent ones. There is an inverse relationship between estradiol concentrations and FSH, as estradiol also appears to selectively suppress FSH at the pituitary level. Thus, pulsatile FSH activity is more evident in the early follicular phase when estradiol concentrations are low than in the later parts of the follicular phase. Of course, in postmenopausal or ovariectomized individuals where amplitude and mean levels of gonadotropins are substantially greater, FSH pulses become more evident. When detectable, the vast majority of FSH fluctuations are superimposable on the larger and easily identifiable LH pulses, further suggesting that GnRH concomitantly stimulates the secretion of both gonadotropins.

In the rodent, there is emerging evidence for the existence of a separate FSH-releasing hormone (FSH-RH). This as yet uncharacterized compound, which appears to originate from the anterior hypothalamus, has been postulated to play a role in the control of pulsatile FSH release. Its function in the primate, in view of the decreased role of the anterior hypothalamus in the reproductive process, remains to be determined. There are, however, physiological instances of divergent LH and FSH secretion and of varying FSH:LH ratios in this species which are difficult to explain if a single neuropeptide stimulates both gonadotropins. Of significant interest in this regard are recent observations suggesting that the *frequency* of the GnRH pulse signal can selectively regulate gonadotropin subunit gene transcription, such that a fast GnRH pulse frequency favors LH β-messenger ribonucleic acid (mRNA), while a slow frequency favors FSH β-mRNA. The intracellular mechanisms remain uncertain, but several in vivo observations strongly support the concept that the hypothalamus can preferentially stimulate LH or FSH synthesis by varying GnRH frequency. This phenomenon was first demonstrated in experiments in the ovariectomized monkey bearing a hypothalamic lesion in which a slow GnRH pulse frequency replacement therapy favored FSH secretion, while a rapid pulse frequency decreased the FSH:LH ratio (Fig. 2–6). In later chapters, we will speculate that a similar mechanism may, in part, be responsible for the late luteal phase increase in FSH:LH ratio, an important feature of the menstrual cycle. In prepubertal children, in whom GnRH is presumed to be secreted at low frequency and amplitude, FSH secretion predominates. With the onset of puberty, GnRH pulse frequency increases and LH secretion is enhanced.

Thus, the control of FSH secretion is most probably multifaceted. Most important is the control of pulsatile FSH release by the GnRH pulse generator which, by modifying the frequency of the pulse signal, can influence the relative amounts of FSH secreted. In addition, FSH may be stimulated by a separate hypothalamic factor (FSH-RH), as well as controlled by newly characterized ovarian factors, such as inhibin or activin (see Chapter 4).

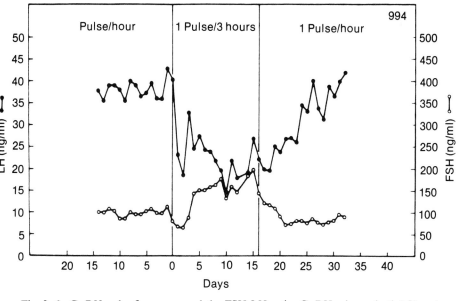

Fig. 2–6. GnRH pulse frequency and the FSH:LH ratio. GnRH releases both LH and FSH. This experiment in an ovariectomized monkey lacking endogenous GnRH illustrates the effect of changes in GnRH pulse frequency on the FSH:LH ratio; a slower frequency of the GnRH pulse signal favors FSH release, while a more rapid pulse frequency favors LH release. The effect is not instantaneous, but requires several days. Abbreviations as in Figures 2–3 and 2–5. (From Wildt L, Hausler A, Marshall G, Hutchinson JS, Plant TM, Belchetz PE, Knobil E, 1981: Frequency and amplitude of GnRH stimulation and gonadotropin secretion in the rhesus monkey. *Endocrinology* 109:376–385. Copyright © by The Endocrine Society.)

THE ENDOGENOUS OPIOID PEPTIDES AND OTHER NEUROPEPTIDES

Of all the neurotransmitter-like peptides implicated in the control of GnRH and gonadotropin secretion, only the endogenous opioid peptides have been proven at present to play a physiological role in the release of gonadotropins during the menstrual cycle. Thus, these compounds must be included in any review dealing with cyclicity.

THE ENDOGENOUS OPIOID PEPTIDES

Three distinct precursor molecules for the endogenous opioid peptides have been isolated: (1) *proopiomelanocortin* (POMC), the precursor for β-endorphin, adrenocorticotropin hormone (ACTH), α-melanocyte-stimulating hormone (α-MSH) and corticotropin-like intermediate lobe peptide (CLIP); (2) (*pre*)-*proenkephalin* A and B, precursors for methionine-enkephalin and leucine-enkephalin, and related products; and (3) prodynorphin, the precursor for dynorphin. Our present discussion will be restricted to POMC and its products.

The 31,000 molecular weight multifunctional prohormone, POMC, is processed into its metabolic products following cleavage by trypsinlike enzymes. Major central areas where POMC is synthesized include the corticotropic cell of the anterior pituitary, the melanotropic cell of the intermediary pituitary lobe in lower species and hypothalamic neurons within the arcuate nucleus (in close proximity to the site of the GnRH pulse generator). It is important to note that POMC processing and hormonal regulation of POMC gene expression vary with each site.

In the anterior pituitary, major end products are ACTH and β-lipotropin (β-LPH). Anterior pituitary POMC expression is controlled mainly by hormones of the adrenal axis: both ACTH and β-LPH are released simultaneously by corticotropin-releasing hormone (CRH) and their secretion is regulated by glucocorticoid feedback.

In the hypothalamus, processing yields mainly α-MSH and β-endorphin as main products. Similar end products occur in the intermediary lobe; however, the degree of acetylation of β-endorphin in the hypothalamus is much less than that in the intermediary lobe (nonacetylated β-endorphin has greater biological activity). In contrast to the anterior pituitary, hypothalamic POMC expression is controlled not only by the glucocorticoids but also by the gonadal steroids (Fig. 2–7).

β-ENDORPHIN AND GONADOTROPIN SECRETION

The predominant effect of the endogenous opiate, β-endorphin, on LH and FSH secretion is inhibitory. Acute inhibition of gonadotropin secretion following administration of β-endorphin results from a reduction in GnRH release into the hypophyseal portal circulation. There are, in fact, demonstrated connections between β-endorphin and GnRH neural networks.

Conversely, administration of naloxone, a general opiate antagonist, will increase gonadotropin release by decreasing the inhibitory endogenous opiate

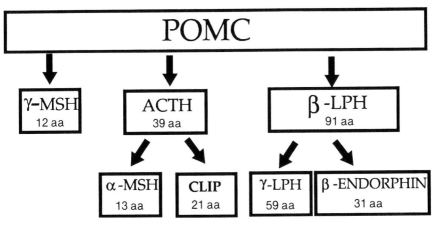

Fig. 2–7. Central processing of proopiomelanocortin *(POMC)*. POMC is a multifunctional precursor molecule, which, upon cleavage, yields several peptides. The precursor molecule is processed and modulated differently in the anterior pituitary and the hypothalamus. In the *anterior pituitary,* POMC yields mainly adrenocorticotropin *(ACTH)* and β-lipotropin *(LPH)* and POMC expression is controlled mainly by hormones of the adrenal axis. In the *hypothalamus,* α-melanocyte-stimulating hormone *(MSH)* and (nonacetylated) β-endorphin are the main end products, and POMC expression is influenced not only by glucocorticoids but also by gonadal steroids. *aa,* amino acids; *CLIP,* corticotropin-like intermediate lobe peptide.

tone. That naloxone is effective in this regard only under certain endocrine conditions in the primate reflects an important phenomenon that relates hypothalamic endogenous opiate activity to the ovarian endocrine status. For instance, there is a marked difference in β-endorphin release from the hypothalamus between intact and ovariectomized monkeys: in the ovariectomized group, β-endorphin is undetectable, suggesting that ovarian steroids are required for β-endorphin release. Low levels of β-endorphin are also observed at menstruation, at a time in the menstrual cycle when secretion of ovarian steroids is at a nadir. As the follicular phase progresses and with increasing estradiol concentrations, hypothalamic β-endorphin release increases. It is highest during the luteal phase in the presence of both estradiol and progesterone (Fig. 2–8).

Sequential estradiol and progesterone treatment of ovariectomized animals also results in very much enhanced β-endorphin release. These dramatic changes in β-endorphin reflecting the ovarian endocrine milieu are observed only centrally in the hypothalamus (as monitored in monkeys by measurements of β-endorphin in hypophyseal portal blood). Pituitary β-endorphin release (as monitored in the peripheral circulation) is not affected by changes in the ovarian status; β-endorphin concentrations in peripheral blood reflect principally adrenal axis dynamics, with release of the hormone paralleling that of ACTH.

These observations demonstrate a firm coupling between the hypothalamic endogenous opioid system and the ovarian steroids. Thus, if the effect of naloxone on LH is tested at different times of the menstrual cycle, the response is primarily influenced by the ovarian steroid milieu: at time of low endogenous

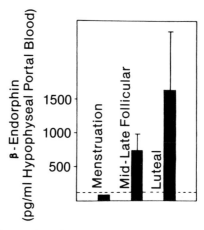

Fig. 2–8. Hypothalamic β-endorphin and the menstrual cycle. β-endorphin release by the hypothalamus (as measured in hypothalamic-pituitary portal blood of monkeys) is dramatically influenced by the ovarian steroids. β-endorphin levels are lowest in the early follicular phase when steroid secretion is at a nadir, increase at midcycle with the release of greater amounts of estradiol by the maturing follicle, and are maximal during the luteal phase in the presence of both estradiol and progesterone. Peripheral concentrations of β-endorphin, which reflect pituitary secretion, and the activity of the adrenal axis, remain largely unchanged. (From Ferin M, Van Vugt D, Wardlaw S 1984: *Recent Prog Horm Res* 40:441. Reprinted with the permission of Academic Press.)

opioid activity, such as after ovariectomy, at menopause, or in the early follicular phase, LH release by naloxone is minimal. In contrast, at times of significant endogenous opioid activity, especially during the luteal phase of the menstrual cycle or in the ovariectomized, menopausal, or hypoestrogenic individual on a steroid replacement schedule, naloxone causes a significant release of LH. This effect is especially marked in the presence of progesterone. Thus, the naloxone test is an indirect indicator of central opiate activity; it demonstrates the inhibitory influence endogenous opioid peptides exert on GnRH secretion. Maximal interaction between the neuropeptides and GnRH is seen in the presence of gonadal steroids; in their absence, the interaction is lost (Fig. 2–9).

OTHER NEUROPEPTIDES

Several neuropeptides other than the opiates have been implicated in the control of the GnRH pulse generator and of gonadotropin release, but a significant amount of experimental work remains to be done especially in the primate to determine their precise role. Two such neuropeptides are briefly reviewed here.

Substance P

Substance P is an undecapeptide initially described in the gastrointestinal tract and found to be widely distributed throughout the nervous system. Substance P has been shown to inhibit GnRH-stimulated LH and FSH release by the rat

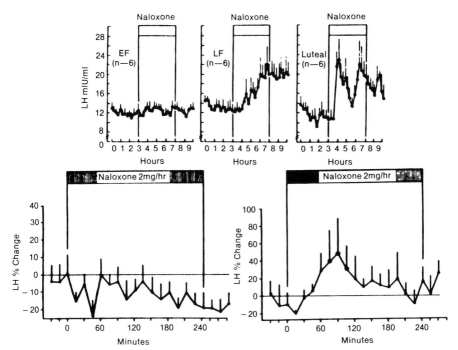

Fig. 2-9. LH Response to endogenous opioid antagonism under different endocrine conditions. There is coupling between the hypothalamic endogenous opioid system and ovarian steroids. Thus, the effects of naloxone (an opiate antagonist) vary with the endocrine environment. Naloxone releases LH only in the presence of ovarian steroids. *Upper figure:* Naloxone infusion into normal women during the early follicular *(EF)*, late follicular *(LF)*, and luteal phase of the menstrual cycle. LH response is absent in the early follicular phase when ovarian steroids are at a nadir; however, in the luteal phase, there is a rapid LH increase in response to endogenous opiate antagonism. (From Quigley ME, Yen SSC 1980: The role of endogenous opiates on LH secretion during the menstrual cycle. *J Clin Endocrinol Metab* 51:179-181. Copyright © by The Endocrine Society.) *Lower figure:* Naloxone infusion into ovariectomized patients, before hormonal replacement therapy *(left)*, and after 3 weeks of estrogen therapy. Note the absence of response prior to steroid therapy. Abbreviations as in Figure 2-3. (Adapted from Shoupe D, Montz FJ, Lobo RA 1985: The effects of estrogen and progestin on endogenous opioid activity in oophorectomized women. *J Clin Endocrinol Metab* 60:178-183. Copyright © by The Endocrine Society.)

anterior pituitary and administration of antiserum to the peptide increases LH and FSH secretion. In the rodent, this compound has been postulated to play a role in the ovulatory gonadotropin surge: hypothalamic release of substance P is inhibited by estradiol, thus facilitating the surge.

Neuropeptide Y (NPY)

Neuropeptide Y is a 36 amino acid peptide known to affect several functions of the organism. It has been shown to stimulate gonadotropin release from dispersed rodent pituitary cells, to enhance the gonadotrope's response to GnRH, to stimulate in vitro GnRH release from the hypothalamus, and to enhance the spontaneous gonadotropin surge. In the rabbit, NPY is released in parallel with GnRH during reflex ovulation. Yet, in the absence of gonadal steroids, NPY has also been shown to exert inhibitory influences on pulsatile LH release.

3

The Ovarian Component

There are two principal functional cyclic units within the ovary: the *follicle* and the *corpus luteum*. These two structures have different functions and are present and active at different stages of the menstrual cycle. Overall, the function of each follicle is to provide the necessary support to the oocyte, the female germ cell, and that of the corpus luteum to prepare for implantation of the developing embryo. Both structures secrete steroid hormones, which perform a large number of critical functions during the menstrual cycle. This chapter is divided into five sections: (1) The ovarian steroids; (2) folliculogenesis; (3) oogenesis; (4) the ovulatory process; and (5) the corpus luteum.

THE OVARIAN STEROIDS

OVARIAN STEROID BIOSYNTHESIS

All steroid structures derive from cholestane, a C27 compound and the parent of cholesterol. Sex steroids (i.e., steroids involved in the reproductive process) belong to three major classes, all metabolized from cholesterol and characterized by decreasing numbers of carbons: (1) the pregnane C21 series, the progestins; (2) the androstane C19 series, the androgens; and (3) the estrane C18 series, the estrogens.

The first step in the conversion of cholesterol to steroids is the cleavage of the C20,22 bonds that results in a C21 compound, pregnenolone, and a 6-carbon fragment. The multienzyme complex responsible for this step resides in the inner mitochondrial membranes of the cell. Pregnenolone is important because it occupies the key position as the precursor of *all* steroid hormones. It is converted to the following steroids within the agranular endoplasmic reticulum (microsome) (Fig. 3–1).

The Progestins

Progesterone is the most abundant member of this series. It is secreted mainly during the periovulatory period and the luteal phase of the menstrual cycle. Pregnenolone is converted to progesterone by the enzyme complex, delta^5-3β-hydroxysteroid dehydrogenase: delta$^{5-4}$-isomerase. Other progestins include 17-α-hydroxyprogesterone (a precursor of aromatizable androgens) and 20-α-dihydroprogesterone, secretory products of both the follicle and corpus luteum.

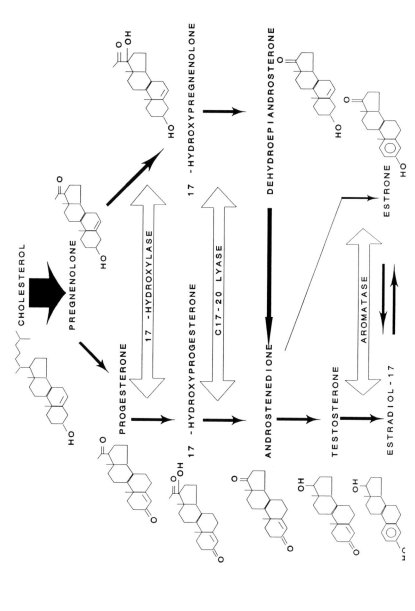

Fig. 3–1. Ovarian steroid biosynthesis. Three major classes of steroids are produced in the ovary: (1) the pregnane C21 series yielding the progestins (progesterone, 17-α-hydroxyprogesterone); (2) the androstane C19 series yielding the androgens (androstenedione, dehydroepiandrosterone, testosterone); (3) the estrane C18 series yielding the estrogens (estradiol-17β, estrone).

The Androgens

The two main androgens identified as secretory products of the ovary are andro-stenedione and testosterone. The rate limiting step in their biosynthesis is the microsomal enzyme complex: 17-α-hydroxylase: C17,20-lyase, which utilizes progesterone or pregnenolone as its substrate. This biosynthetic pathway results in the formation of androstenedione or dehydroepiandrosterone (DHEA), respectively, the first of which can be transformed into testosterone. The andro-gens are the immediate precursors of estrogens following aromatization (see later). However, the biosynthetic pathways in the ovary also yield a number of nonaromatizable (i.e., that cannot yield estrogens) C19 steroids, such as 5-α-dihydrotestosterone.

The Estrogens

The two main estrogens are estrone and estradiol-17β; the enzyme aromatase is responsible for the formation of the typical aromatic A ring.

STEROID-PRODUCING OVARIAN CELL TYPES

There are several major cell types in the ovary that are capable of producing ste-roids. They do so in response to stimulation by the gonadotropins, luteinizing hormone (LH) and follicle-stimulating hormone (FSH). Gonadotropin action is mediated via cyclic adenosine monophosphate (cAMP) and cAMP-dependent phosphorylation of proteins, with calcium playing a permissive role in the pro-cess.

The Granulosa Cells

These cells, which form the inner envelope surrounding the oocyte, are mainly FSH-responsive. Granulosa cells are principally organized to metabolize andro-gens to estrogens by aromatization and to synthesize progesterone and its metab-olites. The principal site of aromatase activity resides in the large antral and pre-ovulatory follicles that are found in the mid–late stage of the follicular phase. It is there that androgens are *converted* into estrogens under the control of FSH, which stimulates aromatase enzyme activity.

Late in the follicular phase, granulosa cells are also capable of de novo pro-gesterone synthesis in response to both FSH and LH stimulation (the preovu-latory progesterone rise; see Chapter 1). The metabolism of progesterone to 20-α-dihydroprogesterone in the granulosa cell appears to be influenced by FSH, but not LH.

The Theca Cells

These cells, which have an embryological origin distinct from the granulosa cell, differentiate from mesenchymal cells in the ovarian stroma. The theca layer sur-rounds the granulosa cell layer; it is not present in the small primary follicle and appears only when the follicle grows (see later). Theca cells synthesize androgens in response to LH stimulation, the major product being DHEA which is metab-olized to androstenedione. Lesser amounts of testosterone are synthesized because of a relative deficiency in 17-β-hydroxysteroid dehydrogenase. Theca cells appear to have much less aromatase activity than granulosa cells, and, hence, although they can produce estrogens, the quantity is much smaller than that produced in the granulosa cell.

Theca cells also produce progesterone in response to LH. The transient increases in 17-α-hydroxyprogesterone seen in the later part of the follicular phase also arise from theca cells at the time when the follicle is transforming from an estrogen to a progesterone-secreting tissue.

It is important to note that in estrogen production, a key concept in the synthesis and secretion of estrogens by the follicle (a crucial function) is that the process requires the interaction of two cell types. First, androgens must be synthesized in the theca cell under the stimulation of LH. Second, these androgens must diffuse across the basement membrane separating the theca from the granulosa layer to be used there for estrogen biosynthesis through an FSH-stimulated aromatic reaction; there is *little de novo production* of C19-steroid substrate in the granulosa cell (Fig. 3–2).

The Interstitial Cells

Specimens of interstitial cells are difficult to obtain without contamination with theca cells and, thus, their independent biosynthetic activity is not easy to study. In the adult, interstitial cells derive from theca cells in atretric follicles in which

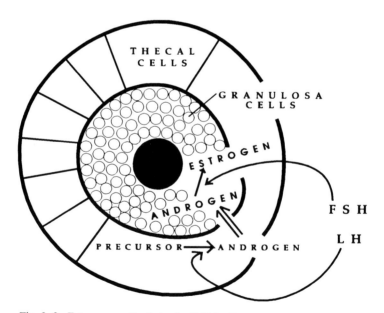

Fig. 3–2. Estrogen synthesis in the follicle. Estrogen synthesis depends on the interaction of two cells in the follicle: the theca cell which synthesizes androgens and the granulosa cell which aromatizes androgens into estrogens. Thus, androgens synthesized in theca cells diffuse to granulosa cells, where they are converted by the enzyme aromatase. *FSH*, follicle-stimulating hormone; *LH*, luteinizing hormone.

granulosa layer and oocyte have degenerated. Secretory products, stimulated by LH, are thought to be similar to those produced by theca cells.

The Luteal Cells

These cells are transient ones derived from the theca interna and granulosa of the graafian follicle in the process that ensues ovulation. Their main secretory product is progesterone, but they are also a source for estrogens. The most important endocrine factor controlling steroid secretion by these cells is LH.

FOLLICULOGENESIS

Folliculogenesis, the process of follicular growth, is continuous throughout life until menopause. Follicular growth is initiated when the oocyte of a small follicle in the resting pool begins to increase in size and the granulosa layer enlarges. Follicles grow sequentially through several stages until they ovulate or become atretic. It has been estimated that the time required from the primary follicle stage to ovulation is 40–90 days.

CLASSIFICATION OF FOLLICLES

The Primordial Follicle

Follicles recruited during the menstrual cycle derive from a stockpile of non-growing *primordial follicles* (Fig. 3–3). These follicles represent the pool from which all developing follicles will emerge. Primordial follicles consist of an association between the germ cell and a small layer of squamous epithelial or pregranulosa cells. Both are surrounded by a thin matrix, the basal lamina. At this stage, there is no zona pellucida to separate pregranulosa cells from oocyte, thus allowing for close contact within this microenvironment.

The Primary Follicle

When recruited, primordial follicles leave the nongrowing stockpile to be converted into primary follicles. The oocyte now starts to grow and becomes surrounded by a single organized layer of cuboidal granulosa cells. Glycoprotein material is used to form the zona pellucida that surrounds the oocyte and separates it from the granulosa layer.

The process of recruitment into folliculogenesis is already initiated during fetal life. Thus, at birth, the number of primordial follicles available for folliculogenesis will have been decreased from 2 million to about 500,000. Because the transition from quiescent primordial follicle to actively growing primary follicle is difficult to recognize, little is known about the mechanisms that control this important event. Yet, this would be a rich area of study, since the mechanisms that control this transition ultimately also determine the number of developing follicles in the ovary and the rate at which the finite pool of primordial follicles is exhausted. All in all, only a minority (400 or less) of these follicles will ever ovulate, and, of course, exhaustion of the stockpile signals the end of reproductive life or menopause.

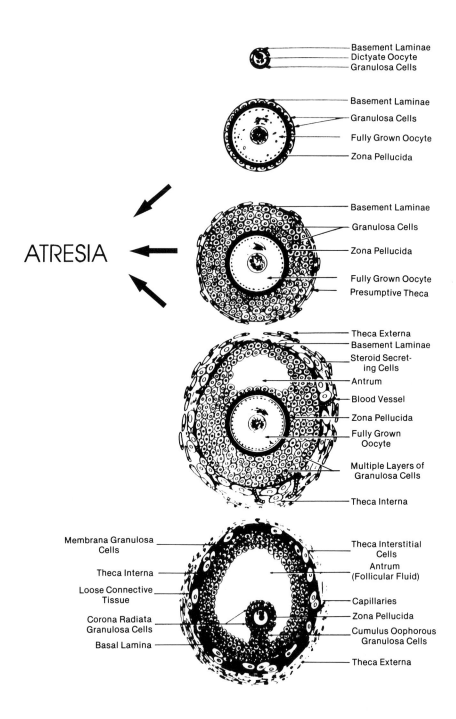

Fig. 3–3. The process of folliculogenesis. The primary follicle is recruited from a stockpile of primordial follicles. During its passage to a secondary follicle, it acquires a theca layer. The tertiary or antral follicle is characterized by the formation of an antrum. In its final stages of maturation at the end of the follicular phase, the graafian follicle undergoes a dramatic increase in growth. Folliculogenesis can probably proceed up to the antral stage in the absence of gonadotropins. Further differentiation requires FSH, while steroidogen-

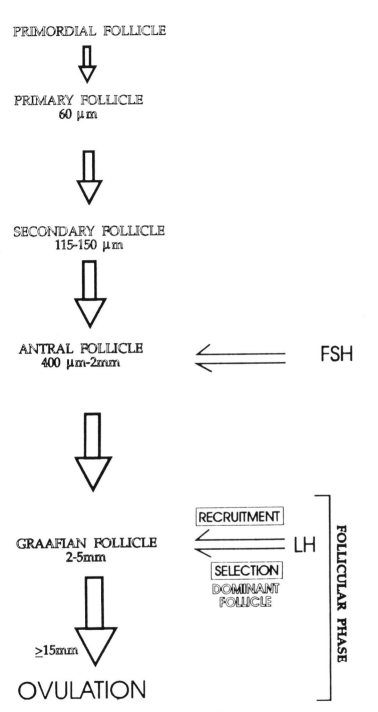

esis requires LH. In each menstrual cycle (for details, see Chapter 4), a cohort of tertiary follicles is recruited, one of which is to be selected to become the dominant follicle which will grow to full maturation and, at ovulation, yield a mature oocyte. Abbreviations as in Figure 3–2. (Drawings reproduced from Erickson GF, Magoffin DA, Dyer CA, Hofeditz C, 1985: The ovarian androgen producing cells: a review of structure/function relationships. *Endocr Rev* 6:371–371. Copyright © by The Endocrine Society.)

The Secondary Follicle

The primary follicle will grow into a secondary follicle: the granulosa cells proliferate into multilayers, and at the end of this stage, the oocyte becomes full grown. Events that characterize this transition include:

1. the organization of the theca layer. This begins with the migration of a group of stromal fibroblasts and epithelial cells to the basal lamina surrounding the follicle, and their arrangement all around the granulosa layer. This tissue will eventually be organized into a *theca interna* (next to the basal lamina), and a *theca externa* (the portion merging with the surrounding stroma).

2. the vascularization of the theca. Early on, the theca develops a vascular supply consisting of one or two arterioles terminating within the theca interna in a wreathlike network of capillaries. The theca interna vasculature is linked to another group of arterioles and venules in the theca externa. In contrast, the granulosa remains avascular. It is likely that transport of hormones and nutrients to the granulosa layer occurs through specialized structures, such as the well documented gap junctions.

The Antral Follicle

The follicle continuing its growth and reaching 400 μm in diameter becomes a tertiary or antral follicle. Characteristic features are:

1. the accumulation of fluid, resulting in the formation of a space (antrum) at one pole of the oocyte. Follicular fluid consists of plasma transsudate containing secretory products of the granulosa cells, including (at later stages of maturation) steroids at concentrations several orders of magnitude greater than in peripheral blood.

2. the development of a gap junction (i.e., specialized contact) between the granulosa and the oocyte, which mediates intercellular communication between the oocyte and the follicular cells.

3. the differentiation of the theca interna cells into a well-differentiated steroidogenic structure.

The Graafian Follicle

In its final stage of maturation, the tertiary follicle increases dramatically in size (from 400 μm to 15 mm or more in diameter). This large increase in growth results from the rapid mitotic proliferation of the granulosa cell layer and the rapid accumulation of follicular fluid in the antrum. The follicle is now referred to as the graafian follicle. It is a highly structured mass. The oocyte is enclosed at one pole of the antrum in a layer of specialized granulosa cells, the corona radiata which is connected to the remainder of the granulosa layer by the cumulus oophorus, the rest of the granulosa cells lining the remainder of the antrum. The vascularized theca interna is well differentiated into steroidogenic cells. The theca externa is also better differentiated; in it are some cells which show the ultrastructural characteristics of smooth muscle cells innervated by sympathetic and parasympathetic nerves and containing actin and myosin. Their precise role remains to be explored.

THE CONTROL OF FOLLICULAR GROWTH

The Primary and Secondary Follicle

The first step in folliculogenesis is the recruitment of the primordial follicle from the stockpile and its transformation into a primary follicle. The primary signal for this recruitment process most probably originates within the ovary, possibly a cue from the oocyte. If oocyte formation is abnormal, such as, for example, in the 45,XO chromosome Turner's syndrome, the organization of follicles is disrupted.

Gonadotropins do not play a major role in this process and, thus, early follicular growth can progress in the absence of the pituitary gland, although it is possible that *quantitatively* it may be hampered in this situation.

FSH receptors appear on the granulosa cell during the passage from primary to secondary follicle. The secondary follicle also acquires receptors for steroids.

The Antral Follicle

When the growing follicle reaches the early antral stage, there is no question that continued growth requires gonadotropins. Following differentiation, theca cells become endocrinologically active and secrete androgens in response to LH stimulation. Androgens, in turn, contribute to the secretion of estrogens through the aromatization process within the granulosa layer under FSH control. The vascularization of the theca interna plays an important role in this process, since it allows for a greater extraction of stimulatory hormones from the peripheral circulation.

Local Control of Follicular Growth

The early developing follicle generates its own estrogenic microenvironment. Estrogens, through their mitotic activity, are the main factor that promotes granulosa growth. All in all, the follicle undergoes a tremendous cell proliferation during its growth process: when it starts growing, at the primordial stage, it contains about fifty granulosa cells, but by the time it becomes a graafian follicle in the preovulatory state, there are more than 5×10^7 cells.

Current experimental studies suggest that not only estradiol but also several intraovarian peptides known for their tissue growth-promoting effects (*growth factors*) may be involved locally in the regulation and modulation of folliculogenesis. Judging from the current literature, their actions are complex, possibly intricately dependent on the maturation and endocrine status of the follicle, and there may be multiple components, some stimulatory, some inhibitory.

Most of these factors originate locally within the ovary. In contrast to the classical endocrine control, which requires that a hormone produced by a gland be secreted into the circulation so that it can affect distant target cells, action by these local growth factors may include other forms of control such as: (1) paracrine control in which a hormone produced by an organ influences another cell of the same organ by local diffusion; (2) autocrine control, in which a hormone synthesized by a cell exits the cell to bind to a membrane receptor on the same cell and reenters it to exert its action; and (3) intracrine control, in which a hormone synthesized within a cell acts without ever exiting the cell, a variation which remains to be experimentally demonstrated (Fig. 3–4).

At present, the most discussed ovarian growth factors include epidermal growth factor, fibroblast growth factor, and especially insulin-like growth factors (IGFs). *IGF-1* is synthesized by granulosa cells and has been detected in follicular fluid and in plasma. Recent research suggests that IGF-1 can act to regulate granulosa differentiation, perhaps by amplifying FSH action on aromatase activity or LH receptor induction. IGF-1 receptors are present on granulosa cells, suggesting a paracrine or autocrine mechanism of action. To complicate matters, however, it is now also known that IGFs in circulation are complexed to IGF-binding proteins. Several binding proteins have been characterized. It is thought that some IGF-binding proteins may act as inhibitors of IGF under certain circumstances, perhaps curtailing FSH action in some follicles and thus playing a role in the process of atresia (discussed later).

Compounds of the inhibin-activin family originally identified as ovarian-derived peptides that modulate pituitary FSH secretion (see Chapter 4) may also have a role in the local regulation of follicular development. Present evidence suggests that these compounds may act in a paracrine fashion to cause the growth of follicles into the recruited size class (inhibin) or to play a role in atresia (activin). No doubt that local control of folliculogenesis will be a rich area for future investigation; thus, the interested reader is referred to the literature for an updated view of this rapidly changing field.

An intriguing recent development is the suggestion that the resident ovarian blood cell population may function as a source for local hormones or growth factors. Macrophage populations vary with the phase of the menstrual cycle and are known to establish close contacts with ovarian cells. It has been proposed

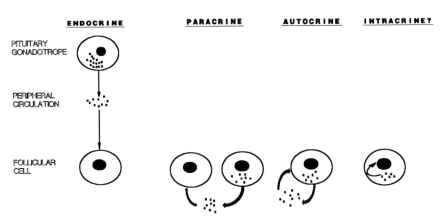

Fig. 3–4. General mechanisms of control of follicular growth and secretion. Classical examples of endocrine control of folliculogenesis are the gonadotropins, LH, and FSH. Examples of paracrine, and possibly autocrine, control within the follicle include not only estradiol, which through its mitotic activity is the primary promoter of granulosa growth, but also an expanding list of local growth factors. Intracrine control remains to be convincingly demonstrated in the follicle. Abbreviations as in Figure 3–2.

that cytokines, such as interleukin-1 or tumor necrosis factor, released by these components of the immune system, may influence local ovarian events. Again, we suggest that the interested reader refer to the current literature for an update on this very new area of investigation on the relationships between the immune and endocrine systems.

Surprisingly, several peptides, well known for their action in the brain, have also been isolated in the ovary. Proopiomelanocortin (POMC)-like messenger ribonucleic acid (mRNA) has been identified in the ovary and β-endorphin has been located in cells of the granulosa, luteal and interstitial layers in the rodent. POMC ovarian production appears to be controlled by gonadotropins. The physiological role of POMC in the ovary remains to be elucidated however. It should be pointed out that other steroidogenic organs, such as the testes and adrenals, also appear to produce these compounds (see Chapter 2 for a description of the role of POMC in the brain). Growth hormone-releasing factor (GRF) has also been detected in the ovary. FSH appears to promote the expression of GRF receptors in maturing granulosa cells through cAMP-dependent mechanisms. It has been suggested that locally produced GRF could accelerate follicular maturation by amplifying the granulosa cell response to FSH.

THE PROCESS OF ATRESIA

The process of folliculogenesis, whereby a primordial follicle grows to become a graafian follicle and goes on to ovulate, is of course crucial to normal reproduction. Yet, most growing follicles do not complete this sequence of events and degenerate, that is, undergo the process of atresia, at some stage of development. Of the estimated 2 million follicles formed in the human, only about 400 will reach the ovulatory stage. Thus, overall atresia rate is greater than 99%. The reasons behind this apparent "waste" and the fundamental nature of this degenerative process remain to be elucidated. Studies of this phenomenon are complicated by the high number of follicles at every stage of maturation within the ovary (a histological preparation of an ovary will usually reveal various cell complexes, from resting to growing follicles, from active to degenerating or atretic follicles), and by the difficulty in discerning the beginning stages of the atretic process.

Follicles can undergo atresia whether they belong to the nongrowing or growing pool. Thus, a follicle may degenerate before even being recruited into the process of folliculogenesis. Once a follicle enters the growing pool, either it goes on to ovulate or it becomes atretic. The chance is that the majority of follicles under observation will become atretic, since more follicles are recruited during a cycle than usually ovulate, even in animal species in which more than one follicle ovulates at each cycle. Follicular atresia occurs during all times of life (the disappearance of small follicles and oocytes is particularly high around the neonatal period) and during all stages of the ovarian cycle. It is most unlikely that, once the process of atresia has begun, the follicle can reenter the ovulatory pathway. Thus, once follicular growth has started, it is continuous until atresia or ovulation occurs.

The most dramatic sign of atresia occurs in the granulosa cell, in which the nucleus becomes pycnotic. An early increase of hydrolytic enzymes is also characteristic. In the antral follicle, LH and androgens may promote atresia. Premature induction of the LH surge in women may cause the rapid regression of the ovulatory follicle. Under LH influence, steroid production by the theca/interstitial cells is switched from an androgen- to a progesterone-producing tissue. In these follicles, it is thought that the decrease in local estrogen production, due to the loss of aromatizable androgens, is a primary event in atresia. The deficit in estradiol, of course, curtails mitotic activity of the granulosa cells, stunting the growth of the follicle.

OOGENESIS

DEVELOPMENT OF THE FEMALE GERM CELL

Oocytes originate from stem cells, the primordial germ cells, which arise extragonadally in the yolk sac entoderm. They are recognized at 4 weeks of gestational age. Primordial germ cells migrate by amoeboid movements along the wall of the hindgut to reach the genital ridges. Upon reaching the gonadal tissue, the cells are transformed into oogonia, which, characteristically, have a high mitotic activity, thereby leading to a rapid increase in their numbers.

In the interphase following its last mitotic division which occurs from the 3d–7th month of gestation, the oogonium is transformed into an oocyte (about 25 μm in diameter). Oocytes become surrounded by granulosa cells, and grow within follicles. The oocyte then begins the process of *meiosis.* It progresses through leptotene and zygotene in a few hours, at which time homologous chromosomes are paired allowing for crossing over of groups of genes. The oocyte then reaches a quiescent phase, the *diplotene stage,* in which meiosis is suspended until adulthood (*the first meiotic arrest*). Oocytes at this stage contain a nucleus, referred to as the germinal vesicle. In the human, all of these stages are completed by the time of birth.

It is important to remind the reader that, in contrast to the male germ cell, which is continuously produced throughout reproductive life, production of oocytes ceases by the 7th month of gestation, *never to be resumed.* This stockpile then represents the entire population of germ cells that will be capable of participating in the process of folliculogenesis.

Substantial growth of the oocyte is reflected by characteristic ultrastructural changes, for example, a marked increase in mitochondria, changes in the Golgi apparatus, and the appearance of cortical granules. The Golgi apparatus is associated with the processing of secretory products, among which are the glycoproteins that will form the coat surrounding the oocyte, the *zona pellucida,* whose appearance signals initiation of rapid oocyte growth. This impressive process of oocyte growth (to one of the largest cells in the organism) occurs while meiosis is arrested at the diplotene stage and the oocyte completes growth (to about 120 μm in diameter) by the time the follicular structure around it becomes a secondary follicle. Thus, the latter stages of folliculogenesis (to the antral follicle stage) occur after the oocyte has completed most of its growth; the diameter of the oocyte increases only slightly thereafter (see Fig. 3–5).

Oocytes, like the follicles in which they are contained, can proceed either to ovulation or to atresia. Only full-grown oocytes are ovulated. The fully grown oocyte in the graafian follicle responds to the preovulatory surge of LH by resuming meiosis (*meiotic maturation*). Separation of homologue sets of chromosomes without a centromeric division takes place: one set of homologues remains in the cell, the other set moves into a bleb of cytoplasm, the first polar body, which is extruded (reduction division). The oocyte, progressing from diplotene stage to metaphase II of the second meiotic division, is transformed into an *unfertilized egg*. The initial morphological feature of the meiotic maturation stage is the breakdown of the germinal vesicle. Passage through this stage is a necessary step prior to fertilization.

An interesting observation is that oocytes removed from antral follicles undergo spontaneous meiotic maturation in vitro. (This is not true for oocytes removed from preantral follicles.) This observation has led to the hypothesis of a local inhibitory control of oocyte maturation, which, in turn, is supported by the isolation of a factor, *the oocyte maturation inhibitor.* Oocytes cocultured with follicular wall are inhibited and do not resume meiosis. Significantly, the activity of the inhibiting factor is lower in graafian follicles than in some immature or atretic follicles. Further characterization of this or other factors is needed, however, before our understanding of this process can be completed.

At ovulation, meiosis is arrested again (*second meiotic arrest*). At this time, oogenesis has (1) provided for a mature egg, (2) produced a haploid cell (half of the normal number of chromosomes found in somatic cells), and (3) accumulated a store of macromolecules and organelles that will be involved in the fertilization process and support the fertilized egg during the preimplantation stages.

The *second meiotic division* (centromere division) will be completed at the time of fertilization. The division results in a mature egg (ovum) and a second polar body. Chromosome number, however, is not further reduced by this division: the nucleus of the egg is haploid. (DNA content, however, is again reduced, and is now at 25% of that in the oocyte.) After sperm penetration, the chromosomes in the egg become enclosed in a nuclear membrane to form the female pronucleus, which will fuse with the male pronucleus, to produce a diploid zygote.

THE OVULATORY PROCESS

Ovulation is the end process of a series of events initiated by the gonadotropin surge and resulting in the release of a mature fertilizable egg from a graafian follicle. Unfortunately, although there is a wealth of literature on the subject, the precise sequence of local events within the follicle that lead to rupture of the follicular wall and expulsion of the egg is not known. These mechanisms most probably relate to the interaction of a number of factors, each of which by itself may not be the primary mover, but which may complement each other's action.

There is no question that the process of ovulation is initiated by the gonadotropin surge, which occurs in response to the long loop estradiol positive feed-

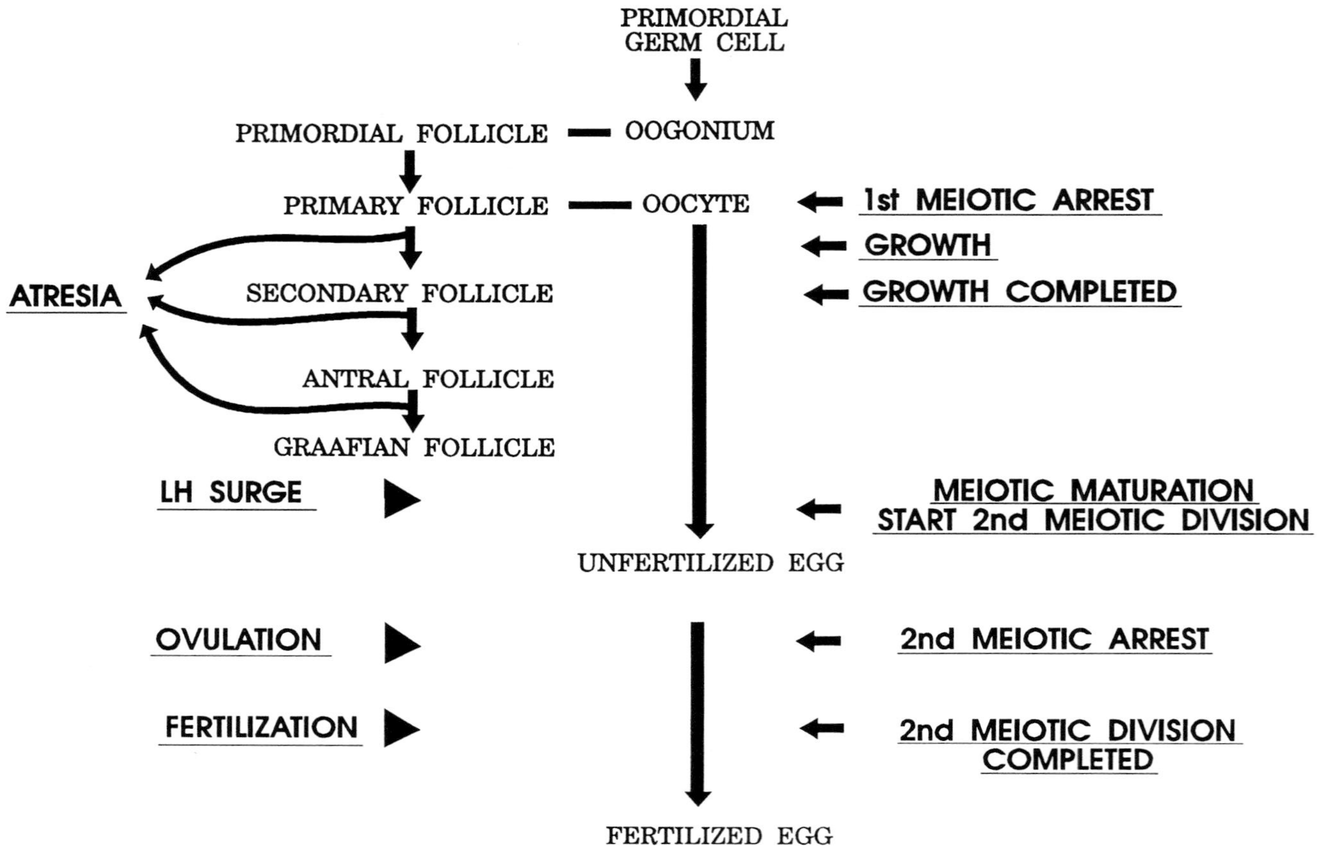

PRIMORDIAL
GERM CELL

PRIMORDIAL FOLLICLE — OOGONIUM

PRIMARY FOLLICLE — OOCYTE

1st MEIOTIC ARREST

GROWTH

GROWTH COMPLETED

SECONDARY FOLLICLE

ANTRAL FOLLICLE

GRAAFIAN FOLLICLE

ATRESIA

LH SURGE

MEIOTIC MATURATION
START 2nd MEIOTIC DIVISION

UNFERTILIZED EGG

OVULATION

2nd MEIOTIC ARREST

FERTILIZATION

2nd MEIOTIC DIVISION
COMPLETED

FERTILIZED EGG

38

back, the signal to the brain and pituitary that the dominant follicle has attained maturity (see Chapter 4). It should be emphasized that the occurrence of a gonadotropin surge does not guarantee ovulation. For instance, if the surge occurs before the follicle is mature and ready to release the egg, luteinization of the granulosa cells may occur without ovum release (luteinized unruptured follicle).

The gonadotropin surge terminates estradiol synthesis (see earlier discussion); the theca cell now changes from an androgen to a progesterone-secreting tissue (the preovulatory progesterone rise). What the role of this steroid is in the process of ovulation is unknown; however, it has been shown in the rodent that antiserum to progesterone can reduce the ovulatory rate. Whether this indicates a direct action of progesterone on the ovulatory process or whether progesterone acts through the regulation of other products, such as the prostaglandins (see later) is unknown.

Vascular changes in the preovulatory follicle occur within minutes of the LH surge. The multilayered capillary plexus within the theca dilates causing hyperemia, a prelude to the ovulatory process. This phenomenon is perhaps related to the rapid release of histamine and/or other kinins by local mast cells. About 6 hours into the LH surge, there is increasing ovarian blood flow due to decreased vascular resistance, increase in capillary and venule permeability leading to an increase in interstitial fluid volume.

Protein synthesis is largely initiated by the gonadotropin surge and remains an ongoing process throughout the ovulatory period. Ovulation can be blocked in experimental animals by agents that arrest protein synthesis. This increased synthesis may, in part, reflect the production of enzymes involved in follicle wall degradation. The release of proteolytic enzymes has been described and enzymatic degradation of the wall of the preovulatory follicle is a primary hypothesis to explain rupture. The enzyme plasmin may be a suitable candidate in this process. This protease is generated following secretion by the cell of plasminogen activator in response to FSH. This occurs within 2 hours of exposure to the gonadotropin surge. Plasmin in turn activates collagenase, which stimulates proteolysis and disintegration of collagen, the primary component responsible for the follicular wall tensile strength. This then probably results in a reduced tensile strength of the follicular wall to the point at which it ruptures. Whether this mechanism is true in the human as well has been questioned, however.

Whether ovarian innervation plays a role in ovulation is not really known. Main innervation of the ovary consists of adrenergic fibers, with nerves distrib-

←———————————————————————————————

Fig. 3–5. The process of oogenesis. Oogonia arise from extragonadal germ cells that have migrated into the gonadal tissue. Production of female germ cells ceases before birth. The oocyte undergoes meiotic divisions to reduce its genetic material before joining with the spermatozoon at fertilization. The first meiotic division starts during fetal life and is arrested at birth. It is completed only at the time of the preovulatory LH surge. At ovulation, a mature egg, with half the normal number of chromosomes, is released to be fertilized. The second meiotic division is completed at fertilization. Abbreviations as in Figure 3–2.

uted to the theca externa and theca interna. Adrenergic neurons within follicular walls are activated by LH and secrete norepinephrine in response. The contractility of whole ovaries is influenced by adrenergic compounds and adrenergic agonists can enhance the ovulatory response to the gonadotropin stimulus; yet, ovulation can occur even after denervation, thus casting doubt on a primary adrenergic role in the ovulatory process. The role of smooth muscles within the theca externa in follicular rupture is also questionable; it is possible, however, that these muscles may facilitate evacuation of follicular contents, once rupture of the wall has occurred.

Prostaglandins are another group of substances released by LH which have been implicated in the phenomenon of ovulation. The two main prostaglandins within the ovary are prostaglandin E2 (PGE2) and prostaglandin F2-α (PGF2-α). Local ovarian prostaglandin levels rise as the time of ovulation approaches. Blockage of prostaglandin synthesis by indomethacin prevents follicular rupture, without interfering with previous stages of folliculogenesis. Prostaglandins probably contribute to the process of ovulation through various pathways, such as affecting smooth muscle contractility. Contraction of smooth muscle in post-capillary venules may increase intracapillary pressure and increase transsudation, thus contributing to an increase in free fluid pressure within the follicle (however, PGF2-α increases contractility, while PGE2 decreases it), and by activating proteolytic enzymes especially those associated with collagen degradation.

THE CORPUS LUTEUM

After ovulation and expulsion of the unfertilized egg, a corpus luteum is formed. This new structure results from important LH-induced morphological changes in both the granulosa and theca layers of the graafian follicle after ovulation. The process of luteinization may be initiated once the granulosa cells have acquired receptors for LH and does not necessarily signify that ovulation has occurred.

Morphological changes that characterize the formation of the corpus luteum include:

1. the invasion of the previously avascular granulosa cell layer by a vascular supply. This vascularization process occurs immediately following the collapse of the follicular wall after expulsion of the egg.

2. the acquisition by the granulosa cell of the capacity of de novo synthesis of steroids. Previously during the follicular phase, granulosa cells had only the capability to aromatize delivered products, the androgens. The luteinization process involves the enlargement of the granulosa cell into the "large luteal cell," the largest endocrine cell in the organism, and its transformation into a structure containing all the elements of a typical steroid producing cell (principally progesterone and estradiol). This includes the presence of numerous mitochondria, extensive smooth endoplasmic reticulum and Golgi apparatus, and secretory granules. The theca cell becomes the "small luteal cell," which is much less active in steroidogenesis: it has no secretory granules.

THE PROCESS OF LUTEOLYSIS

The corpus luteum is a transient endocrine organ. Most observations are consistent with the notion that the corpus luteum has an inherent 12–15 day life span, and thus its regression (the process of luteolysis) is inevitable in the non-fertile cycle.

The corpus luteum attains maturation about 5 days after ovulation. At that point it is a quite large structure of about 15 mm in diameter, easily recognizable on the surface of the ovary. On about days 7–9 of the luteal phase, however, regression of the corpus luteum begins. This involves fibrosis of the luteinized cells, a dramatic decrease in the number of secretory granules with a parallel increase in lipid droplets and cytoplasmic vacuoles, and a decrease in vascularization. All these phenomena result in decreased secretion of steroids. (Factors controlling luteolysis will be reviewed in Chapter 4.) The defunct corpus luteum, referred to as the *corpus albicans,* becomes hyalinized within 6 months.

4

Hypothalamic-Pituitary-Ovarian Communication

It is clear from the preceding chapters that for normal reproduction, events must occur concurrently in various organs of the reproductive axis and that these events must somehow be synchronized. We must now understand how the hypothalamus, the pituitary gland, and the ovaries communicate with each other, so that an ovulatory menstrual cycle can occur. We will study the control of ovarian events by the hypothalamic-pituitary unit and examine how the ovaries modulate the activity of the hypothalamic-pituitary unit through the feedback loops.

HYPOTHALAMIC-PITUITARY CONTROL OF THE OVARIES

The hypothalamus, through gonadotropin-releasing hormone (GnRH), stimulates gonadotropin secretion. Luteinizing hormone (LH) and follicle-stimulating hormone (FSH), in turn, induce morphological and secretory changes in the ovaries: folliculogenesis is accompanied by increased estradiol secretion and corpus luteum activity by increased progesterone and estradiol release.

FOLLICULOGENESIS DURING THE CYCLE

Recruitment of the Cohort

During the luteal phase, the largest antral follicles are 2–4 mm in diameter. As suggested by the mitotic index of their granulosa cells, some of these follicles are active. These follicles, which number perhaps 3–5, contain high levels of aromatizable androgen, but low concentrations of estradiol and low aromatase activity. When tested in vitro, however, the granulosa of these follicles contains a very responsive FSH-stimulable aromatase system. Presumably, these follicles represent the *cohort* of follicles that will be recruited as the follicular phase starts and from which the *dominant follicle* (the antral follicle that will mature to ovulation) will be selected.

It is clear that FSH provides the fundamental signal for recruitment of the cohort. In fact, in the first stage of the follicular phase, the gonadotropin ratio clearly favors FSH (see Chapter 1). Experimental administration of inhibin, which diminishes circulating FSH levels, results in the deferral of new follicular growth and retardation or failure of final maturation. In contrast, multiple ovulation often follows administration of FSH at supraphysiological levels.

Selection of the Dominant Follicle

On day 1 of the follicular phase, the size of the largest follicle is still 3–4 mm in diameter; however, a couple of days later, one follicle, the dominant one, can be segregated, if not by size, at least by its higher granulosa cell mitotic index.

The nature of the selection process by which a follicle becomes the dominant one remains unknown. Does, for instance, the oocyte play a role? It is clear that FSH, and especially the early follicular phase FSH rise, facilitates the process: FSH stimulates granulosa cell mitosis and especially aromatase production, thereby facilitating the conversion of androgens derived from the theca into estradiol (see Chapter 3). Thus, the early developing follicle generates its own estrogenic microenvironment. This steroid, through its mitotic activity, promotes granulosa growth and thus further enhances estrogenic production in that particular follicle, setting it apart.

How can this process result in the development of only *one* follicle in the primate? The best developed follicle, in terms of granulosa cell number for its diameter, is the one logically most likely to be stimulated by FSH and to acquire aromatase activity and thus estradiol biosynthetic activity most rapidly. Granulosa cells increase in number by mitotic division; as they increase, so does the number of FSH receptors. Since FSH controls androgen to estrogen conversion, the number of granulosa cells within the follicle will influence the local amount of estradiol produced, and locally produced estrogens in turn induce FSH receptors in the granulosa cells in a self-propagating mechanism. This, then, may allow for the rapid growth of the dominant follicle and its preeminence (*dominance*) over the other follicles of the recruited cohort.

By developing sufficient aromatase activity to elevate *peripheral* estradiol concentrations, the dominant follicle, through the long loop negative feedback (see later), then suppresses peripheral FSH secretion to concentrations below those necessary for the growth of the other follicles. Studies in the monkey in which the gonadotropin-suppressing action of circulating estradiol during the follicular phase is interfered with by the administration of estradiol antibodies indicate that this normal selection process can be overridden. As a result, in this experimental condition, multiple follicles are brought to maturation.

Growth of the Dominant Follicle

By day 6, the dominant follicle is very much distinguishable from the other follicles in terms of cellular development and of vascularization. The density of capillaries surrounding the maturing follicle is at least twice that of less mature follicles; it has been shown that this change in vascularization results in a preferential delivery of gonadotropins to the maturing follicle. This may, in part, explain why the developing follicle continues to mature despite the overall reduction in peripheral FSH levels: such FSH concentrations are insufficient to initiate or maintain growth of the other less mature follicles.

Experimental removal of the dominant follicle in the midfollicular phase results in a delay in spontaneous ovulation of about 2 weeks (the length of a normal follicular phase), suggesting that *no surrogate follicle* present at that time is capable of substituting for the loss of the dominant follicle. A new cohort must be recruited (Fig. 4–1).

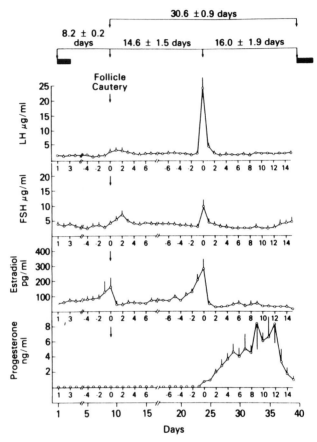

Fig. 4–1. The phenomenon of dominance. Soon after the follicular phase is initiated, one growing follicle has achieved complete dominance over the other follicles of the cohort (the dominant follicle): there is no surrogate follicle capable of taking over. This concept is illustrated in this experiment in normal cycling monkeys. The largest follicle is cauterized and destroyed during the midfollicular phase; as a result, the follicular phase is interrupted, and the spontaneous gonadotropin surge is delayed by 14 days in that cycle. This delay reflects the need for recruitment of a new cohort of follicles. *FSH,* follicle-stimulating hormone; *LH,* luteinizing hormone. (From Goodman AL, Hodgen GD 1979: Between-ovary interaction in the regulation of follicle growth, corpus luteum function, and gonadotropin secretion in the primate ovarian cycle. *Endocrinology* 104:1304. Copyright © by The Endocrine Society.)

The initial appearance and subsequent increase of *LH receptors* in granulosa cells of the growing follicle is a result of the synergistic action of estradiol and FSH. LH stimulates the production of aromatizable androgens in the theca, resulting in an exponential increase in estradiol concentrations (the midcycle estradiol peak). Very high levels of estrogens in follicular fluid, up to 2 μg/ml, parallel the high degree of aromatase activity in the preovulatory follicle. More than 90% of the circulating estradiol secreted during the late follicular phase originates from the one dominant follicle.

THE GONADOTROPIN SURGE

The ovulatory gonadotropin surge affects the structure of the graafian follicle and hence its secretory patterns (Fig. 4–2). The following phenomena occur in succession:

1. The LH surge suppresses granulosa cell proliferative activity and the cell begins to luteinize.

2. Within several hours of the initiation of the LH surge, there is a marked decline in estradiol secretion. This decrease in estradiol is the direct consequence of decreased androgen production in the theca, itself due to a selective inhibition of the enzyme 17-α-hydroxylase: C-17,20 lyase. It has been suggested that this is related to the relatively high levels and prolonged exposure to the LH surge which may induce a transient desensitization at the gonadotropin receptor level. During the gonadotropin surge, follicular fluid contains progressively decreasing concentrations of estradiol and androgens. The follicle now begins to secrete 17-α-hydroxyprogesterone.

3. A preovulatory rise in progesterone occurs, while estradiol synthesis remains low. This steroid, whose concentration in follicular fluid can be increased severalfold within 1 hour of the LH surge, is secreted by granulosa cells that acquired LH receptors during the late follicular phase and that become "luteinized" in response to LH binding to these receptors. With luteinization, new receptors form and the cells regain sensitivity.

THE CORPUS LUTEUM

Function

The main function of the corpus luteum is to secrete progesterone and estradiol, which, in combination, act on several reproductive tract target tissues to affect a variety of biological processes (see Chapter 5). Progesterone and estradiol, in turn, alter gonadotropin secretory patterns. This new gonadotropin environment is presumably inadequate to sustain growth of antral follicles, which then undergo atresia. Under certain experimental circumstances, it has been shown that follicular growth can also be inhibited directly by progesterone in the absence of a change in gonadotropins. This effect of progesterone may be exerted via a reduction of aromatization in the granulosa cell of the growing follicle. Progesterone also blocks the long loop estradiol positive feedback; thus, although estradiol concentrations are elevated during the luteal phase, LH surges do not generally occur.

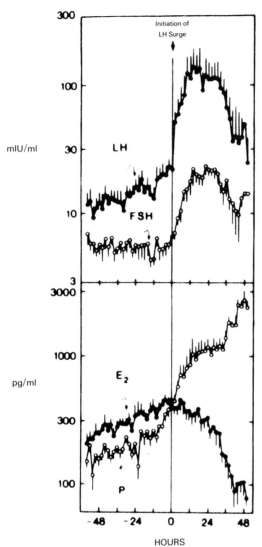

Fig. 4–2. Hormonal changes during the midcycle gonadotropin surge. Mean LH, FSH, estradiol *(E2)*, and progesterone *(P)*, measured every 2 hours during the midcycle period. Note the rapid changes in steroid secretion, which result in a decrease in estradiol and an increase in progesterone secretion. Abbreviations as in Figure 4–1. (From Hoff JD, Quigley ME, Yen SSC 1983: Hormonal dynamics at midcycle: a reevaluation. *J Clin Endocrinol Metab* 57:792–927. Copyright © by The Endocrine Society.)

Control of Luteal Function

It is important to point out first that adequate follicular maturation during the preceding follicular phase is an important determinant of the normal function of the corpus luteum, since this affects the number of granulosa cells that will be capable of luteinization. Women with abnormal luteal function (such as in the "inadequate luteal phase" syndrome) usually show lower concentrations of estradiol during the preovulatory estrogen peak, denoting insufficient follicular maturation. This defect, in turn, can usually be traced to a deficient FSH rise in the early follicular phase (see Chapter 10).

Although the luteal cell shows some capacity of secreting steroids on its own for a short period of time, a role for *LH as a luteotropic agent* has been well demonstrated; in fact, LH is necessary for the maintenance of the corpus luteum. In hypophysectomized patients subjected to a gonadotropin therapeutical regimen to promote folliculogenesis, the life span of the induced corpus luteum is abbreviated, unless several injections of LH are administered throughout the luteal phase. Interruption of LH secretion following administration of antiserum to LH or of a GnRH antagonist to monkeys during the luteal phase results in menstruation 2–3 days later, the result of an arrest in luteal activity. Most experimental evidence points to a dependence of the corpus luteum on pituitary gonadotropins *throughout* the duration of the luteal phase.

The Control of Luteolysis

In the primate, the process of luteolysis is unrelated to the presence or absence of the uterus. In contrast, a role for the uterus in the luteolytic process has been well documented in rodents and large domestic animals, in which hysterectomy results in a lengthening of the life span of the corpus luteum. This mechanism has been particularly well studied in the ewe, in which a uterine luteolytic factor, apparently prostaglandin F2-α, passes directly from the uterine vein to the ovarian artery to affect the life span of the corpus luteum.

Although a major progesterone-modulated decrease in LH pulse frequency occurs during the luteal phase (see below), this phenomenon does not appear to play a role in luteolysis in the primate. Increasing pulse frequency experimentally during the luteal phase does not succeed in prolonging corpus luteum survival long past its normal life span, nor does imposition of a decreased pulse frequency early on in the luteal phase accelerate luteolysis.

A frequently proposed candidate for an endogenous luteolytic agent in the primate is estradiol: the phenomenon of estrogen-induced luteolysis has often been reported experimentally. Initial studies have suggested that this effect may be exerted directly on the corpus luteum, perhaps by increasing prostaglandin secretion. Yet, although prostaglandins can exert a luteolytic effect when infused locally, the administration of indomethacin (a prostaglandin inhibitor) does not appear to prolong the luteal phase. Another explanation for the luteolytic effect of estradiol is that it may act, through its long loop negative feedback, to decrease GnRH and LH secretion and thereby the hormonal support to the corpus luteum. Recent experimentation regarding this hypothesis suggests that progesterone synergizes with estradiol to promote luteal regression, in the sense that estrogen appears to be luteolytic only in the presence of the slow LH pulse frequency instigated by progesterone. Yet, estrogen blockers do not prevent luteolysis, and thus the fate of this hypothesis remains uncertain.

Most recent evidence relates luteal regression most probably to an alteration in luteal cell responsiveness to LH. This is supported by data in experimental animals (Fig. 4–3) showing that reduction by more than half of the LH concentrations results in normal patterns of progesterone during the first 5–6 days of the luteal phase; however, thereafter, progesterone diverges drastically from the control, suggesting that an age-dependent alteration of the primate corpus luteum sensitivity to LH occurs midway through the luteal phase.

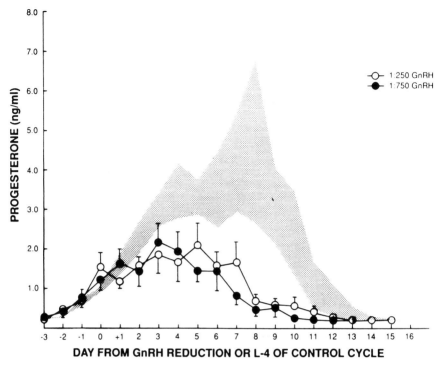

Fig. 4–3. The mechanisms of luteolysis. Recent evidence suggests that luteolysis during the nonfertile primate luteal phase may result from a change in the sensitivity of the luteal cell to LH midway through the luteal phase. In this experiment, monkeys bearing arcuate lesions and replaced with a pulsatile gonadotropin-releasing hormone *(GnRH)* infusion received a reduced GnRH dosage (1:250 or 1:750 th of control) during the luteal phase. Note the similar progesterone concentrations in these animals and in control receiving the full GnRH dose *(shaded area)* during the first days of the luteal phase. Note also the fall midway through the luteal phase in the animals receiving less than adequate amounts of GnRH. L-4: luteal phase day-4. (From Zeleznik AJ, Little-Ihrig LL 1990: Effect of reduced LH concentrations on corpus luteum function during the menstrual cycle of rhesus monkeys. *Endocrinology* 126:2237–2244. Copyright © by The Endocrine Society.)

PULSATILITY OF OVARIAN STEROID HORMONES

While pulsatility of GnRH and pituitary hormones is well documented (see Chapter 3), there are relatively few well-designed studies characterizing gonadal steroid release in relation to gonadotropin pulsatile activity. Best characterized is the midluteal phase of the menstrual cycle, at which time physiologic profiles of progesterone, estradiol, and LH exhibit discrete episodic pulses. Pulse analysis indicates that the occurrence of estradiol and progesterone pulses is simultaneous, which suggests that these two steroids are cosecreted by the corpus luteum. Furthermore, there is also a significant temporal relationship between LH and the steroid pulses, not necessarily proving, but certainly suggesting, a causal relationship between gonadotropin release and the ovarian response (Fig. 4–4).

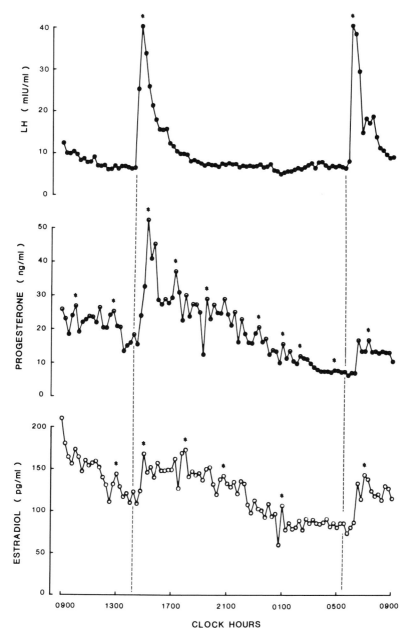

Fig. 4–4. Pulsatility of ovarian steroid hormones. Twenty-four-hour pulsatile profiles of
LH, estradiol, and progesterone in three women during the midluteal phase. *Asterisks*
indicate significant pulses and vertical lines identify the up-strokes of LH pulses and of
concomitant steroid pulses. Abbreviations as in Figure 4–1. (From Rossmanith WG,
Laughlin GA, Mortola JF, Johnson ML, Veldhuis JD, Yen SSC 1990: Pulsatile cosecretion of estradiol and progesterone by the midluteal corpus luteum: temporal link to LH
pulses. *J Clin Endocrinol Metab* 70:990–995. Copyright © by The Endocrine Society.)

THE FEEDBACK LOOPS

In order to avoid gonadotropin hyperstimulation of the target organ, that is, the ovaries, the output of the stimulatory hormone must be controlled. This is accomplished through the long loop feedback, an important concept in endocrinology. Usually, it is a negative or inhibitory feedback loop, whereby hormones secreted by the target organ "feedback" to the hypothalamic-pituitary unit to "readjust" neurohormonal and/or pituitary secretion (Fig. 4–5). Thus,

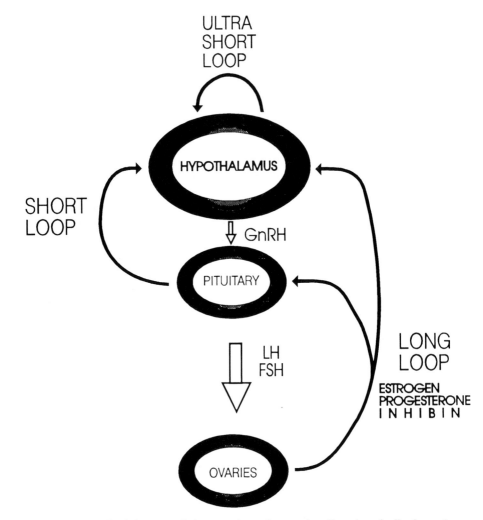

Fig. 4–5. Feedback loops regulating gonadotropin secretion. *Long loop feedback,* ovaries to hypothalamic-pituitary unit. Two types, negative and positive feedback, have been well demonstrated; *Short loop feedback,* pituitary to hypothalamus; *Ultrashort loop feedback,* hypothalamus to hypothalamus. The existence of the latter two loops has been demonstrated in lower species, but remains to be determined in the primate. Abbreviations as in Figures 4–1 and 4–3.

pituitary hormone levels are maintained within the normal range. An additional feature characteristic of the reproductive system is the long loop positive or stimulatory feedback; it is essential because it synchronizes follicle maturity and the signal to ovulation. The existence of additional feedback loops has been postulated, notably the short loop feedback (pituitary to hypothalamus) and the ultrashort loop feedback (hypothalamus to hypothalamus).

THE LONG LOOP STEROID FEEDBACKS

Long loop feedback, whether stimulatory or inhibitory, involves mostly the action of the ovarian steroid hormones estradiol and progesterone, although recent studies have supported the involvement of peptidergic hormones of ovarian origin as well.

The Long Loop Negative Feedback

One of the best demonstrations of the existence of the long loop negative (inhibitory) ovarian steroid feedback is the dramatic increase in gonadotropin concentrations that occurs after ovariectomy. In this case, the lack of ovarian steroid response to the gonadotropin stimulus induces the hypothalamic-pituitary unit to secrete more gonadotropins. Similar increases in gonadotropins are seen at menopause. In both situations, restoration of the negative feedback loop, for example by estradiol administration, results in a rapid decline in gonadotropins (Fig. 4–6). Estradiol is the principal component of the negative feedback loop and is the hormone responsible for maintaining gonadotropin levels within a concentration range representative of the menstrual cycle.

There are relatively few good studies on how the ovarian steroids affect GnRH secretion, since direct measurements of GnRH in the peripheral circulation are not possible. In the human, the study of gonadotropin pulsatility is the best and only tool available. Even such studies are difficult, since they require long experimental observation periods and frequent blood sampling. Nevertheless, there are sufficient data to conclude that estradiol and progesterone both affect pulse characteristics, and that they do so differently.

Estradiol and pulsatile LH release. LH pulse frequency during the follicular phase (close to 1 pulse/h) approximates the basic pulse frequency observed in the ovariectomized condition, suggesting that estradiol does not particularly affect pulse frequency. Rather, this ovarian hormone controls the *amplitude* of the LH pulse. Thus, although LH pulses are frequent during the follicular phase, they are of a small amplitude (Fig. 4–7).

Progesterone and pulsatile LH release. In contrast to estradiol, progesterone affects LH pulse *frequency*. A causative relationship between pulse frequency and this hormone has been clearly established in experiments in which progesterone administration to women in the late follicular phase is followed by a marked decrease in LH pulse frequency. Thus, during the luteal phase, when concentrations of progesterone are elevated, LH pulse frequency decreases. This effect is most dramatic toward the end of the luteal phase when, in some subjects,

OVX/MENOPAUSAL

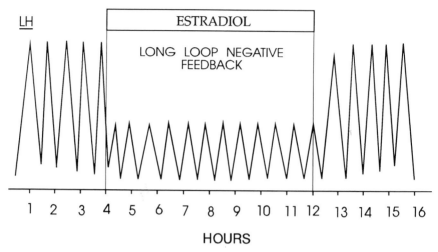

Fig. 4–6. The long loop estradiol negative feedback. In the absence of estradiol, such as after ovariectomy *(OVX)* or at menopause, LH and FSH concentrations are elevated due to the elimination of the long loop estradiol negative (inhibitory) feedback. The figure schematizes the effects of an 8-hour infusion of estradiol, at doses that mimic estradiol concentrations during the early–mid follicular phase of the cycle, in ovariectomized or menopausal subjects. Restoration of the long loop negative feedback results in a rapid (within minutes) decrease in gonadotropin pulse amplitude, and, hence, LH concentrations become comparable to those seen during the follicular phase. Gonadotropins will again rise immediately when estradiol replacement therapy is terminated. Abbreviations as in Figure 4–1.

there may be as few as 5 LH pulses/24 h. In concert with the decreased frequency, there is an augmented pulse amplitude over that seen during the follicular phase.

The interpretation of LH pulse characteristics during the menstrual cycle may be complicated by the following observations:

1. In some subjects, the large amplitude infrequent LH pulses observed during the luteal phase may be interspersed with small pulses, leading to some disagreements on "mean" amplitude LH pulse changes during that phase of the cycle.

2. Twenty-four hour pulsatility studies have reported subtle but definite circadian changes in LH pulse interval. For example, in some, but not all, women during the early follicular phase of the cycle, there is a nocturnal slowing of LH pulse activity with a concomitant increase in LH pulse amplitude. In rare individuals, this pattern extends to the midfollicular phase. Whether this event is triggered by sleep remains a matter of speculation; such a relationship is suggested, however, by anecdotal observations of clear episodes of LH release when subjects awake. The inconsistency of this circadian phenomenon across women of course complicates speculations on its significance. It is perhaps of interest to underline that this circadian pattern is opposite to that observed in the first maturational stage of puberty, at which time nocturnal pulse secretory activity is

FOLLICULAR PHASE   LUTEAL PHASE

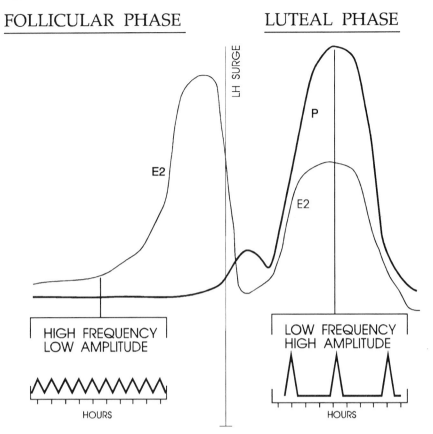

Fig. 4–7. Pulsatile LH patterns during the menstrual cycle. Estradiol and progesterone influence pulsatile patterns differently. Estradiol reduces pulse amplitude while progesterone reduces pulse frequency. Thus, pulses are frequent but of low amplitude during the follicular phase, while during the luteal phase, pulse intervals increase dramatically *(insert illustrates a 10-h period)*. Abbreviations as in Figures 4–1 and 4–2.

increased (see Chapter 7). Also unknown are the mechanisms for this circadian activity, although a role for the endogenous opiates has been suggested.

The Long Loop Positive Feedback

Estradiol also exerts a positive (stimulatory) feedback effect on LH and FSH release. Under proper conditions, this effect of estradiol results in the midcycle ovulatory gonadotropin surge. The long loop estradiol positive feedback is important because it allows for the precise coordination between follicular maturation and the stimulus to ovulation; what better signal than estradiol, since secretion of this hormone parallels, and, in fact, signifies maturation of the graafian follicle. Thus, timing of the major event of the cycle, the gonadotropin surge and subsequent ovulation, is determined not by the brain or the pituitary gland but by the ovary itself. Precise coordination is essential, since a premature LH surge may irreversibly damage the still maturing follicle while a delayed surge may fail to induce ovulation as the follicle now has lost its ability to ovulate.

Activation of the estradiol positive feedback requires (1) a rise of estradiol above a threshold (about 300–500 pg/ml) and (2) persistently elevated concentrations above that threshold for about 48 hours. Provided these two conditions are fulfilled, LH and FSH surges can be experimentally induced following estradiol injection. Administration of estradiol will be immediately followed by a decrease in LH pulse amplitude through activation of the long loop estradiol negative feedback, while the surge will occur only after proper conditions have been met (Fig. 4–8). Brief exposure to estradiol, even at supraphysiological concentrations, will only result in a suppression of LH and FSH (negative feedback) and fail to provoke the surge, unless condition (2) has been met.

While an active estradiol positive feedback is all that is experimentally required for the induction of a gonadotropin surge, it has also been suggested that *low* progesterone levels, such as those observed during the preovulatory period (the "preovulatory progesterone rise"), serve to augment the dimension of the estradiol-induced LH and FSH surges. (Although progesterone can, on its own, induce short-lived increases in gonadotropins, these do not resemble in any manner the large, sustained estradiol-induced preovulatory gonadotropin surge

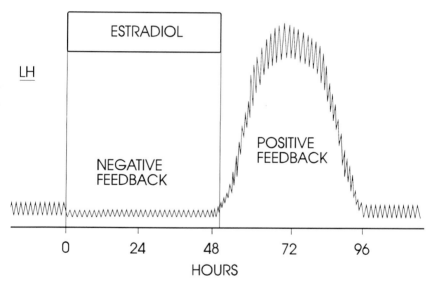

Fig. 4–8. The long loop estradiol positive feedback. A positive (stimulatory) feedback effect can be induced experimentally following estradiol infusion. In this figure, a gonadotropin surge was provoked in a subject during the early follicular phase, at a time when gonadotropin surges do not spontaneously occur. A surge occurs here because estradiol concentrations reach a threshold and remain elevated above the threshold for about 48 h (two conditions for the activation of the estradiol positive feedback loop). LH concentrations first decline because administration of *any* amounts of estradiol will rapidly activate the negative feedback loop. In the normal cycle, the long loop estradiol positive feedback coordinates follicular maturation and the stimulus to ovulation. Abbreviations as in Figure 4–1.

normally observed at midcycle.) In contrast, progesterone in *larger* but physiological amounts blocks the estradiol positive feedback. Thus, during the luteal phase, gonadotropin surges do not occur spontaneously even though estradiol concentrations may meet the conditions required for the activation of the long loop positive feedback, and it is not possible to induce a gonadotropin surge experimentally with estradiol.

Site of Action of the Long Loop Steroid Feedback

The question of the feedback action site of estradiol and progesterone on gonadotropin secretion is an important one, as it relates to the ultimate mechanisms that control the menstrual cycle. Steroid feedback action can be postulated to occur either at a hypothalamic or a pituitary site. At the level of the hypothalamus, feedback may modify the amount of GnRH released, by altering either frequency or amplitude of the GnRH pulse. At the pituitary, feedback may alter directly LH and FSH output or modify the responsiveness of the gonadotrope to endogenous GnRH stimulation. Unfortunately, experimental evidence to date in the primate does not allow unequivocal conclusions as to the precise site of feedback action. Most likely, feedback affects both sites and thus multiple mechanisms acting simultaneously or sequentially may have to be evoked.

Estradiol negative feedback. Because of the technical difficulty in measuring GnRH release over prolonged periods of time in nonstressed animals, data on the modulation of GnRH release by hormonal feedbacks are scant. At present, it appears that estradiol may act both at hypothalamic and pituitary sites, the combined actions of which result in a decrease in the amplitude of the LH pulse and diminished gonadotropin secretion. Cellular mechanisms remain to be identified.

Estradiol positive feedback. There is little doubt that the rising titers of estradiol at the end of the follicular phase act on the gonadotrope cell to enhance its responsiveness to GnRH (see Chapter 2). A further increment in pituitary sensitivity to GnRH follows the initiation of the preovulatory progesterone rise. It is evident that without this significant enhancement, the ovulatory gonadotropin surge may indeed not occur. That similar increases in the gonadotrope's ability to respond to GnRH are seen following addition of the two ovarian steroids to pituitary cells in vitro supports the concept of an important site of action of the positive feedback loop at the pituitary.

Does estradiol also act at a neural site to increase GnRH output? It is now apparent that the *degree* of concomitant hypothalamic involvement varies significantly among animal species.

In the rodent, there is overwhelming evidence of a central hypothalamic action of estradiol at the time of proestrus (the preovulatory period). Specifically, estradiol acts on GnRH neurons within the rostral hypothalamus (the preoptic/anterior hypothalamic area) to stimulate GnRH release into hypophyseal portal blood. In this animal species, the concentrations of GnRH increase significantly just prior to the LH surge. Functional connections between the preoptic/anterior hypothalamic area and the medial basal hypothalamus are required to elicit the positive feedback response to estradiol.

In the primate, it is known from experiments in the rhesus monkey model that intact connections between the anterior and mediobasal hypothalamus are not required, and that a substantial gonadotropin surge can be induced by estradiol in their absence. Recent results indicate that increases in GnRH follow estradiol administration when conditions for positive feedback are met, and precede the LH surge (Fig. 4–9). Similar increase in GnRH have been observed in the sheep.

It is important to emphasize that relatively small pulses of GnRH in the presence of estradiol can produce an ovulatory surge of LH, and, thus, the ovulatory surge is *not* dependent on a *massive* surge of GnRH. The physiological significance of the larger GnRH surge at proestrus in the rodent may be that it serves to ensure that the LH surge occurs at the proper time in relationship to the light–dark cycle. Such a mechanism is, of course, not required in the monkey, in which the timing of the ovulatory surge need not be tightly coupled to outside influences as it is in lower species.

In conclusion, the primary locus of estradiol in its positive feedback mode is at the pituitary level where it dramatically augments gonadotropin responsiveness to GnRH in all species. Increased pituitary responsiveness, however, requires the presence of GnRH. Thus, increased GnRH release by estradiol, the amount of which varies from species to species, could only facilitate this process.

Progesterone feedback. There is little doubt that alteration of pulse frequency during the luteal phase is the result of a central action of progesterone on the GnRH pulse generator. Decreased electrophysiological activity related to the pulse generator has been observed at that time of the cycle. It is also very well established that this effect of progesterone is not exerted directly but is mediated by the hypothalamic endogenous opioid peptides center. As related in Chapter 2, hypothalamic β-endorphin release is increased by progesterone. This enhanced β-endorphin activity is directly responsible for the decrease in LH pulse frequency; indeed, opiate antagonism by naloxone during the luteal phase increases LH pulse frequency to one that is more comparable to that seen in the follicular phase (Fig. 4–9). Thus, β-endorphin, released in the vicinity of the arcuate GnRH pulse generator, is a modulator of pulse frequency: periods of high pulse frequency are reflected by low endogenous opioid peptide activity in the hypothalamus (low progesterone) and periods of low pulse frequency by high endogenous opioid peptide activity (high progesterone).

Depending on its concentrations, progesterone can enhance or block the estradiol positive feedback. While the enhancing effect of small amounts of progesterone on the midcycle LH surge appears to be exerted at the level of the pituitary gland, the blocking effect of high amounts of progesterone on the LH surge is exerted centrally. This blockade cannot be observed in animals bearing hypothalamic lesions, and, importantly, cannot be overcome by pulsatile administration of GnRH. This latter observation suggests that progesterone action may well result in the release by the hypothalamus of a substance that prevents the LH response to GnRH. Recent efforts at characterizing such a putative substance have made some progress, but its structure remains to be elucidated.

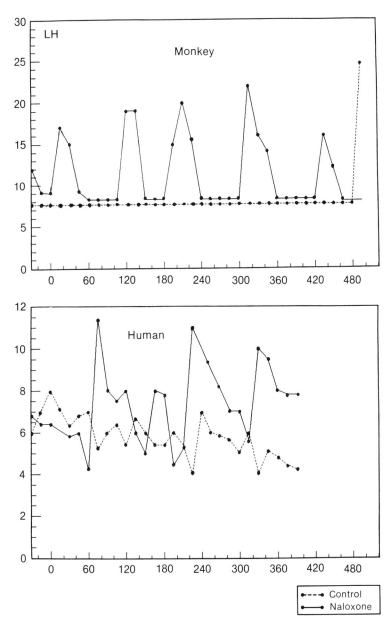

Fig. 4–9. Endogenous opiates and pulse frequency during the luteal phase. The low LH pulse frequency during the luteal phase, the result of increased progesterone concentrations, can be reverted following administration of naloxone, a general opioid antagonist. This suggests that progesterone, through its long loop negative feedback, stimulates the release of endogenous opioid peptides, which in turn are responsible for the decrease in pulse frequency. This figure illustrates the effect of naloxone infusion during the luteal phase in the monkey (From Van Vugt D, Lam NY, Ferin M, 1984: Reduced frequency of pulsatile luteinizing hormone secretion in the luteal phase of the rhesus monkey. Involvement of endogenous opiates. *Endocrinology* 115:1095) and in the human (From Cetel NS, Quigley MS, Yen SSC, 1985: Naloxone-induced prolactin secretion in women: evidence against a direct prolactin stimulatory effect of endogenous opioids. *J Clin Endocrin Metab* 60:191). Control LH values in the same individual are indicated by *interrupted lines.* Abbreviations as in figure 4–1. Copyright © by The Endocrine Society.

The various sites of action of estradiol and progesterone feedback are schematized on Figure 4–10.

THE LONG LOOP INHIBIN FEEDBACK

Inhibin is a long postulated gonadal factor thought to be particularly involved in the feedback regulation of FSH secretion. Several laboratories have now purified inhibin from ovarian follicular fluid of a number of species and its sequence has been derived by cloning techniques.

Structure and Site of Origin of Inhibin

Inhibin is a glycoprotein consisting of a dimer, in which two dissimilar subunits (α and β) are bound to each other by cysteine disulfide bonds. The two subunits are coded for by different genes. The genes code for larger precursor proteins, which are then processed proteolytically. The products are the subunits, which will combine at the time of release from the cell. Two forms of the β subunit have been isolated from follicular fluid, and their gene sequences identified; these are labeled βA and βB. Thus, inhibin can exist as α-βA or α-βB (Fig. 4–11).

There is good evidence that inhibin is produced by the granulosa and luteal cell and that its production is gonadotropin-driven. FSH appears to be the pituitary hormone that stimulates inhibin production. Local estradiol can augment FSH-stimulated inhibin production by the granulosa cell, but it has apparently no effect on its own.

Secretion of Inhibin

Recent data have shown that changes in inhibin concentrations in peripheral circulation can be observed during the menstrual cycle. Although the reader should update this information, secretory patterns are as follows:

1. During the early *follicular phase,* inhibin concentrations are low. This is consistent with the low biosynthetic capacity for inhibin of the small follicle. Inhibin levels rise during the late follicular phase, in parallel to the rise in estradiol. Large follicles have a high capacity for inhibin production. In this respect, inhibin concentrations may be a good marker of the number and functional capacity of the large antral/graafian follicles that are going to ovulate; greater amounts of inhibin are present following hyperstimulation with gonadotropins, reflecting the increased number of maturing follicles.

2. *At midcycle,* inhibin continues to rise past the estradiol surge in parallel to the gonadotropin surge. At ovulation, however, most probably because of architectural disruption of the follicle, there is an initial decline in inhibin from the high concentrations obtained.

3. Serum inhibin concentrations peak again during the *midluteal phase,* but decline at the end of the luteal phase. Removal of the corpus luteum results in a rapid decline of inhibin concentrations, demonstrating that not only the graafian follicle but also the corpus luteum is capable of producing inhibin.

Role of Inhibin

Inhibin inhibits gonadotropin secretion, and FSH preferentially. Although there is overwhelming evidence that circulatory gonadal steroids feedback loops

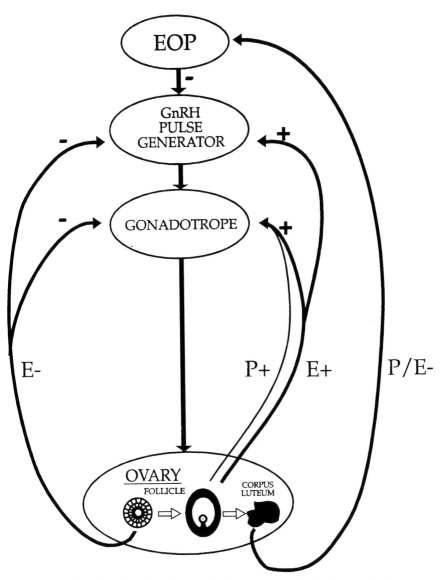

Fig. 4-10. Sites of action of ovarian steroid feedback. Estradiol in its negative feedback mode ($E-$), acts both at the hypothalamus to decrease GnRH pulse amplitude and at the pituitary to decrease the gonadotrope's response to GnRH. In its positive feedback mode ($E+$), it acts at the pituitary to increase the gonadotrope's responsiveness to GnRH, and at the hypothalamus to increase GnRH release, which in turn amplifies the gonadotrope's sensitivity. Progesterone, in its negative feedback mode—and in combination with estradiol *(P/E−)*—decreases pulse frequency by acting on the GnRH pulse generator through the endogenous opiate center *(EOP)*. In small amounts, progesterone enhances the estradiol positive feedback action at the level of the pituitary *(P+)*. In high amounts (not shown on schema), this steroid blocks the estradiol positive feedback (presumably by releasing a putative hypothalamic inhibiting factor that decreases the gonadotrope's response to GnRH). Abbreviations as in Figures 4-1, 4-2, 4-3.

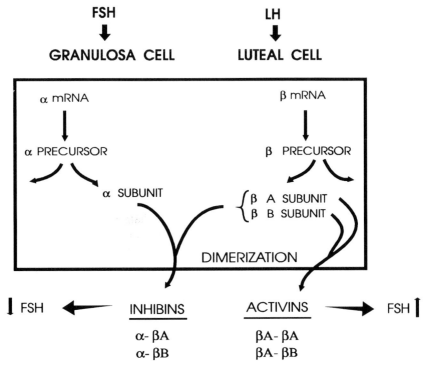

Fig. 4–11. Inhibins and related products. Inhibins are dimers of two subunits (α and β, the latter existing in two forms βA and βB). Inhibin is secreted by the follicle and corpus luteum into the peripheral circulation. Its main action is to decrease FSH secretion at a pituitary site (long loop inhibin feedback). Activins are dimers of the β subunits. These compounds have been shown to increase FSH secretion, but their physiological role remains to be determined. *mRNA,* messenger ribonucleic acid; other abbreviations as in Figure 4–1.

account for the greater portion of the inhibitory effects on gonadotropins, there is also increasing recognition that a portion of the negative feedback regulation of FSH may be mediated directly at the pituitary level by the inhibitory action of this nonsteroidal hormone (long loop inhibin feedback).

In considering inhibin secretory changes, it is plausible that, because of the inverse relationship between inhibin and FSH, this hormone may play a role in controlling FSH levels at the end of the luteal phase and during the passage from one cycle to the next: decreasing inhibin concentrations at that time may allow for the early FSH rise responsible for the recruitment and growth of the follicle cohort. This, however, remains to be conclusively demonstrated. In the rodent, immunization to inhibin increases both FSH levels and the number of follicles ovulating. On the other hand, the simultaneous peaks of inhibin and of FSH at midcycle would be contrary to a negative feedback role of inhibin, although other mechanisms may be at play at that time of the cycle.

It has also been speculated that inhibin may exert a local paracrine function within the ovaries, by mediating FSH-induced aromatase activity on LH-stimulated androgen biosynthesis. During the follicular phase, inhibin and estradiol are secreted in parallel, presumably under the influence of FSH. During the luteal phase, inhibin and progesterone are closely correlated, suggesting a dominant role for LH control at that phase of the cycle. Administration of a GnRH antagonist during the luteal phase results in a decrease of both progesterone and inhibin.

To complicate matters further, dimers of the β subunit have recently been found to *stimulate* FSH. These molecules have been labeled *activins:* the homodimer (βA,βA) is activin A; the heterodimer (βA,βB) is activin A-B (Fig. 4–11). The reader is referred to current literature for further update on this complex field and on the role of each compound of this extended family.

THE SHORT AND ULTRASHORT LOOP FEEDBACK

In addition to the long loop feedback mechanisms that involve hypothalamic-pituitary-ovarian relationships, the literature also describes a short loop feedback (pituitary to hypothalamus), and an ultrashort loop feedback (within the hypothalamus). In lower species, decreases in anterior pituitary hormone secretion (e.g., LH, adrenocorticotropin hormone [ACTH]) have been demonstrated following injection of large amounts of the respective hormone, suggesting that anterior pituitary hormones may directly influence their own release. Presumably, this may occur at a hypothalamic site by reducing the release of the respective releasing hormone (e.g., GnRH, corticotropin-releasing hormone [CRH]); however, evidence for the existence of a short loop feedback regulating LH secretion in the human is less than substantial. Although a few studies appear to indicate some degree of LH suppression following gonadotropin treatment, other well-controlled studies were unable to demonstrate any effect of high doses of exogenous human chorionic gonadotropin (hCG) (the gonadotropin used in many studies since it does not interfere with the immunoassay of LH) on LH secretion. Similarly in the monkey, prolonged elevations of LH do not affect the electrophysiological activity of the hypothalamic GnRH pulse generator.

Ultrashort loop feedbacks, that is, autoregulatory mechanisms whereby neuropeptides alter their own release, have been demonstrated in lower species for a number of hypothalamic hormones. Both in the sheep and rodent, centrally administered GnRH causes an inhibition of LH secretion. This most probably represents a central action of GnRH on its own secretion, since GnRH analog treatment influences directly GnRH release in vitro and in vivo. Thus central regulation of GnRH secretion by GnRH neurons, supported by the existence of numerous anatomical contacts between the neurons of the GnRH pulse generator, may represent a component of the complex mechanisms that regulate gonadotropin secretion. Perhaps, in unison with the endogenous opioid peptides, the ultrashort loop feedback may be part of an autoregulatory system that controls or synchronizes GnRH pulsatile release. At the moment, however, this concept requires experimental support in the primate.

5

The Genital Tract

The function of the genital tract is to transport the ovum, provide a place and milieu for fertilization, implantation, and embryonic development to a stage that permits the newborn to survive in the outside world. It also provides a receptacle where sperm can be deposited and survive until fertilization occurs. The steroid hormones produced by the ovary coordinate physiologically the various components of the genital tract. They affect the target organs through their action on specific receptor proteins; these receptors then function as signal transducers. Each ovarian steroid hormone exerts specific biological effects and, thus, the characteristics of the genital tract will fluctuate with the menstrual cycle. In this chapter, we will review the general characteristics of the steroid receptor and the cyclic changes that occur in the fallopian tube, uterus and vagina with the menstrual cycle.

THE STEROID RECEPTOR

In general, hormones affect their target organs by first binding or combining to specific protein structures or receptors. The receptor's hormone binding site possesses a very high affinity and specificity for the hormone, so that each receptor is very specific for its proper ligand. Thus, what characterizes a hormone responsive cell is the presence of a receptor. Estradiol and progesterone receptor concentrations are high in organs of the genital tract, such as the uterus, but also in the ovary, breast, and the hypothalamic-pituitary unit. It should be noted that, in some target tissues, receptors to two different but related hormones must be activated in a time sequence. In the follicle, for instance, the receptor to follicle-stimulating hormone (FSH) is present prior to the activation of the luteinizing hormone (LH) receptor. In many ovarian steroid-sensitive organs, estradiol must activate its own receptors in order to promote the synthesis of the progesterone receptor.

The amount of active hormone-receptor complex will depend on (1) the concentration of the specific hormone (2) the concentration of the receptor (which itself may also be the subject of intense regulation), and (3) the intrinsic affinity of the receptor protein for the hormone. The steroid receptor protein is found within the target cell; it is primarily located in the cell nucleus (Fig. 5-1), although in the absence of its ligand (its specific steroid), the steroid receptor may

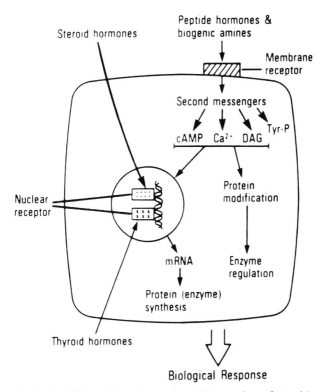

Biological Response

Fig. 5-1. Differential pathways for cellular action of steroid and peptide hormones. Peptide hormones bind to specific membrane receptors, while steroid hormones bind to nuclear receptors (thyroid hormones also bind to a nuclear receptor). Peptide receptor binding activates intracellular second messengers, which regulate the activity of protein kinase enzymes. Steroid hormone activates the receptor protein, which then binds tightly to nuclear chromatin, the site of action of the steroid. *CAMP,* cyclic adenosine monophosphate; *DAG,* diacylglycerol; *mRNA,* messenger ribonucleic acid; *Tyr-P,* phosphotyronine. (From Gill GN [ed] 1991: The endocrine system. In Physiological basis of medical practice [West JB ed], 8:782. Copyright © 1991 the Williams & Wilkins Co., Baltimore.)

also be present in the cytoplasm. Because they are lipid soluble, steroid hormones diffuse readily into cells to bind to the intracellular receptor. In contrast, receptors for peptide and protein hormones (e.g., gonadotropin-releasing hormone [GnRH], LH, FSH) are located on the cell membrane with the binding site on the exterior cell surface. Peptide binding elicits comformational changes in the surface receptor which induce the activation of intracellular second messengers, such as cyclic adenosine monophosphate (cAMP), cyclic guanosine monophosphate (cGMP), Ca^{2+}, or others. These messengers then activate specific protein kinase systems and synthetic pathways and the resultant physiological response occurs.

There is no second messenger activation following steroid binding to its intracellular receptor. Cloning of the steroid receptor genes and analysis of receptor sequences indicate the existence of a superfamily of receptors, which includes the steroids, vitamin D, thyroid hormone, and other related compounds. Within this superfamily, there is significant structural homology among three regions (identified as C1, C2, C3) (Fig. 5–2), which are highly conserved with a central DNA-binding domain containing Zn^{2+}-binding "fingers" characteristic of proteins that bind to DNA. In the absence of its specific ligand, the steroid receptor is inactive. This inactive state is thought to be due to its association with other proteins: dissociation of the complex results in activation. Steroid receptors function only after receiving an initial signal, induced by binding to the specific hormonal ligand. In the absence of its ligand, the receptor does not bind DNA or affect transcription, the two next essential steps in its action. One hypothesis is that the hormone-binding domain, usually the C-terminal portion of the receptor, functions as a repressor of receptor function.

The transformation process induced by the hormone results in a receptor molecule that binds tightly to chromatin in the nucleus. The resultant molecule is then capable of binding to specific DNA sequences (hormone responsive elements [HRE]), which allows for the regulation of transcription of specific genes. Region C has been identified as the DNA-binding domain. Transcription of messenger ribonucleic acid (mRNA) occurs which diverts protein synthesis and the manifestation of the biological responses characteristic of each hormone.

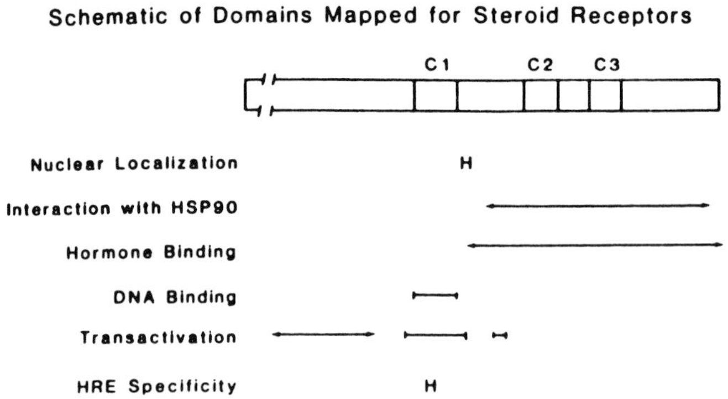

Schematic of Domains Mapped for Steroid Receptors

Fig. 5–2. Functional domains of steroid receptors. Steroid receptors are part of a superfamily of receptors, in which there is significant homology between three regions, labeled C1, C2, and C3. Indicated here are the domains required for the interaction with heat shock protein (HSP90), a protein thought to maintain the receptor in an inactive state. Hormone binding, DNA binding, and transcription of target genes occur through interaction with specific gene sequences *(HRE)*. (From Carson-Jurica MA, Schrader WT, O'Malley BW 1990: Steroid receptor family: structure and function. 1990: *Endocr Rev* 11:201–220. Copyright © by The Endocrine Society.)

CYCLIC CHANGES IN THE GENITAL TRACT

Estradiol and progesterone influence the genital tract differently, and, therefore, marked cyclic changes in its morphology and physiology occur during the menstrual cycle. Changes in the uterus, endocervical gland, and vaginal epithelium are generally well characterized, while those of the fallopian tube are less understood.

THE FALLOPIAN TUBE

The epithelial lining of the fallopian tube is comprised of several cell types. Among these are nonciliated secretory cells and ciliated cells. These two cell types respond to estrogen and progesterone. During the follicular phase, both ciliated and secretory cells are increasing in height; maximal epithelial thickness is seen at the time of ovulation. During the luteal phase, ciliated cells flatten somewhat, and, as a consequence, the secretory cells protrude over the ciliated cells giving the luminal epithelial border an irregular aspect. Cytoplasm of secretory cells can sometimes be observed to rupture into the lumen of the tube. At menstruation, both cell types are low and small.

Spermatozoa travel from the uterus and the ovum from the ovary to the site of fertilization within the fallopian tube. In the monkey, there is extensive ciliation at midcycle but sparse ciliation in the intercycle period, supporting a potential role of the tube in transport of gametes. However, changes in the degree of ciliation are much less extensive in the human, and apart from a role of ciliae in the ovum pickup through the tubal ostium, there is scant evidence for a role in transport. In fact, in the human, there is at present no definite proof that normal epithelial function is necessary to fertilization. Obviously, tubal physiology remains an area for future study.

THE ENDOMETRIUM

The endometrium is the mucosa lining the uterine cavity and served by a microvascular blood supply. It consists of a surface layer of columnar epithelial cells, some of them ciliated, and an underlying vascularized stroma made of connective tissue. Epithelial cells on the surface are interspersed with glands lined by similar epithelial cells and extending from the surface in a tubular shape into the stroma.

Follicular Phase

During the early follicular phase, with little ovarian steroid activity present, the surface epithelium is thin, the glands are short and narrow, and the stroma is compact. Later in the follicular phase, the endometrium comes under estradiol dominance: the main changes that occur relate to the stimulatory action of estradiol on DNA synthesis and on mitotic activity. As a result, the endometrium proliferates (*the proliferative phase*), the mucosa thickens, the glands acquire numerous mitoses and enlarge, and the stroma becomes well organized. By the end of the follicular phase, when estradiol secretion reaches its maximum, the

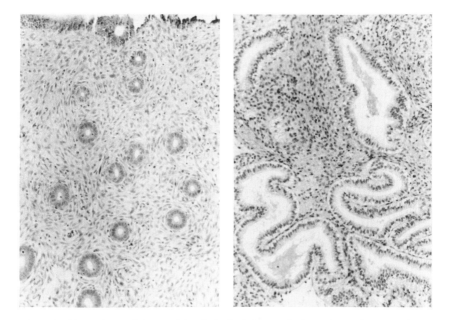

Fig. 5–3. The endometrial cycle. Morphological changes in the endometrium parallel the fluctuations in the secretion of estradiol and progesterone. *Left:* During the follicular phase, under the influence of estradiol, the endometrium *proliferates* and the endometrial glands acquire numerous mitoses and enlarge. *Right:* During the luteal phase, under the influence of progesterone, the endometrial glands undergo a *secretory* differentiation and secretory products are expelled into the lumen.

glands, because they are growing rapidly, become tortuous (Fig. 5–3). After menstruation, regeneration of the microvasculature is initiated from the remaining arteriolar stump in the basalis and is most likely controlled by several local tissue growth factors such as angiogenic growth factor, epidermal growth factor, fibroblast growth factor, or transforming growth factor.

Luteal Phase

Few changes in the morphology of the endometrium occur during the first 2 days following ovulation while the corpus luteum is forming. As the corpus luteum matures and with increased progesterone secretion, the endometrium undergoes a secretory differentiation, an important event in preparation for implantation (*the secretory phase*). Glycogen begins to be synthesized and to accumulate in the basal portion of the glands (it appears as vacuoles in fixed material). This intracellular product will gradually move to the apex of the glands and relegate the nucleus to the base of the cell. By day 6–7 of the luteal phase, these secretory products will be extruded into the glandular space by apocrine-type secretion (Fig. 5–3). Rising progesterone levels will also arrest glandular proliferation. The peak of intraglandular secretion occurs on day 7. If fertilization has taken place, it coincides with the time of implantation of the blastocyst. Increased vascularization occurs and transudation of plasma from circulating blood also contributes to secretory fluids. These fluids, for what they contain, are probably important in supporting the changes prior to implantation and in the early stages of development. It is of interest to note that the inhibitory effect that progesterone exerts on mitosis in glandular epithelial cells does not apply to the arteriolar component nor to the same epithelial cells in the basal regions of the gland. This provides for continued growth of the arteriolar system.

Progesterone has recently been shown to act on the estrogen-primed endometrium to induce the expression of an array of steroid regulated genes. The products of these genes are presumably important for the success of implantation. This remains an important area for future investigation.

The superficial stroma cells surrounding the spiral arterioles enlarge by day 9 of the luteal phase and come to resemble decidual cells characteristic of early pregnancy (see Chapter 6), even if fertilization has not occurred. Decidual differentiation is accompanied by a progressively increasing number of extravasated polymorphonuclear leukocytes and granulocytes.

Menstruation

During the final days of the luteal phase and in the absence of implantation, estradiol and progesterone secretion decreases dramatically. As a consequence of this hormonal withdrawal, the endometrium undergoes gradual necrotic ischemic changes leading to multifocal and progressive exfoliation of all cells except those lining the depths of the tubular glands and necrosis and shedding of the vessels, resulting in menstrual bleeding. Vessel necrosis is preceded by an intense vasospasm, possibly stimulated by prostaglandin F2-α. Concentrations of this prostaglandin increase significantly in the secretory endometrium by day 12 of the luteal phase and reach maximal concentrations at the time of menstruation. With the decrease in estradiol and progesterone concentrations, there is also a release of lysosomal lytic enzymes, the amount of which had been stimulated during the follicular phase by estradiol. These enzymes help in the digestion of the tissues. Each menstruation consists of approximately 35–45 ml of nonclotting blood (due to the presence of a fibrinolysin) and lasts an average of 4 days.

THE ENDOCERVICAL GLANDS

The epithelium of the cervical glands shows cyclic changes similar to those in the vagina (discussed later).

Characteristic changes in the production and properties of *cervical mucus,* the secretory product of the endocervical glands, also parallel the menstrual cycle.

1. In the absence of ovarian steroids, or when levels are very low such as in the early follicular phase, only small amounts of viscous mucus are produced.

2. With increasing *estradiol* concentrations during the late follicular phase, important changes occur.

a. Mucus becomes more abundant (up to a thirty-fold increase), its water content increases (the "wet days"), and its pH becomes alkaline.

b. The mucus shows increasing elasticity. Evaluation is provided by the spinnbarkeit test: the ability to stretch a small drop of mucus into a long, fine thread of about 10–12 cm indicates high estradiol secretion.

c. The ferning capacity of the mucus increases and a characteristic fern pattern (+ fern test) appears at the time of high estradiol secretion on microscopic observation of a dried-up smear of cervical mucus. Ferning or crystallization is caused by the interaction of high concentrations of salt and water with the glycoproteins in the mucus.

d. The cervical canal is broadened and the glycoproteins in the mucus appear to align in parallel filaments within the endocervical canal. This is thought to facilitate sperm passage through the canal.

3. With increasing *progesterone* concentrations during the luteal phase, different characteristics appear.

a. The amount of secreted mucus decreases (the "dry days"), and its pH becomes acidic.

b. The mucus becomes more viscous, elasticity decreases. In the spinnbarkeit test, the column of mucus breaks rapidly and cannot be stretched over more than 3 cm.

c. The fern test becomes negative.

d. The cervical canal narrows and glycoprotein filaments form a mesh that presumably impedes passage of spermatozoa into the uterus.

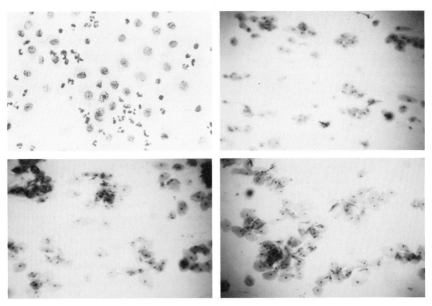

Fig. 5–4. The vaginal smear and the cycle. *Upper left:* In the absence of estrogens, mostly parabasal cells are seen (atrophic smear from a postmenopausal woman). *Upper right:* In the presence of low concentrations of estradiol (early follicular phase), basophilic cells with vesicular nuclei dominate. *Lower left:* With increasing concentrations of estradiol during the late follicular phase, keratinized cells with pycnotic nuclei appear. *Lower right:* With highest estradiol concentrations during the late follicular phase, keratinized cells predominate.

THE VAGINAL EPITHELIUM

The adult human vagina is lined with stratified squamous epithelium that consists of several layers. During the early follicular phase, basophilic cells with vesicular nuclei dominate. During the mid–late follicular phase, increasing estradiol secretion stimulates proliferation of superficial layers. As the vaginal epithelium thickens, the superficial layer is removed further away from blood vessels and keratinizes; these cells with a pycnotic nucleus are then sloughed off. Thus, at midcycle, the vaginal smear offers a predominant picture of cells with pycnotic nuclei that are acidophilic. During the luteal phase, both pycnotic and basophilic cells regress, the epithelium becomes thin allowing for the escape of polymorphonuclear leukocytes which now appear in the vaginal smear (Fig. 5–4).

6

The Fertile
Menstrual Cycle

If fertilization of the ovulated egg occurs, the sequence of events that characterizes the second part of the menstrual cycle is modified. The principal objective
now is to maintain the activity of the corpus luteum, so that hormones condu-
cive to implantation of the fertilized egg are secreted. This chapter briefly
describes the events surrounding fertilization and the first weeks of pregnancy.

EVENTS AT FERTILIZATION

SPERM TRANSPORT

Following ejaculation, spermatozoa must ascend into the female genital tract to
escape the lethal acidity of the vagina and to survive. The buffering capacity of
the seminal plasma (the bulk of which is derived from the seminal vesicles [60%]
and the prostate [30%] and which has an alkaline pH) is lost within minutes of
ejaculation. Several factors influence passage of spermatozoa through the cervix:

1. The physical properties of the cervical mucus: at midcycle, the mucus is
very fluid, plentiful, and at a neutral pH, thus providing a receptive environment
for spermatozoa; the parallel orientation of the glycoprotein micelles channels
sperm passage into the uterine cavity (see Chapter 5).

2. The mechanical interactions of the cervix and uterus during orgasm: contractions may propel spermatozoa to the uterotubal junction within minutes of
intercourse.

3. The colonization of the cervical crypts: spermatozoa may invade cervical
crypts from which they are slowly released over the next 2–3 days.

4. The motility of spermatozoa: deficient spermatozoa do not complete
migration.

Sperm transport through the uterus is aided by contractions of the myome-
trium, possibly influenced in part by the large amounts of prostaglandins present
in the ejaculate. After migration through the uterus, spermatozoa accumulate at
the uterotubal junction. The latter forms an important barrier to sperm transport: less than 200 of the 200–300 million spermatozoa will enter the fallopian
tube (Table 6–1). The filtering mechanism that controls entry into the tube
remains to be investigated.

Table 6–1. A Barrier to Sperm Transport: the Uterotubal Junction

Animal	Average Number of Sperm Sperm/Ejaculate (millions)	Site of Sperm Deposition	Number of Sperm in Ampulla of Oviduct
Mouse	50	Uterus	<100
Rat	58	Uterus	500
Rabbit	280	Vagina	250–500
Ferret	—	Uterus	18–1,600
Guinea pig	80	Vagina and uterus	25–50
Cattle	3,000	Vagina	A few
Sheep	1,000	Vagina	600–700
Pig	8,000	Uterus	1,000
Man	280	Vagina	200

Note: Although the cervix acts as a major barrier to sperm migration, considerable numbers of spermatozoa reach the uterus. The number of sperm entering the fallopian tube, however, is relatively constant.

Source: [Harper MJK 1982: *Sperm and Egg Transport, in Reproduction in Mammals, Germ Cells and Fertilization,* 2d ed. (Austin CR, Short RV, eds) Cambridge U Press, Cambridge, UK, 102.]

During transit through the female genital tract, spermatozoa will undergo capacitation, which is a process of gradual removal of some of the surface proteins that are acquired during transport through the male genital tract. In some species, this process is a prerequisite for fertilization. The necessity or extent of capacitation in the human has been debated, since fertilization of human ova can be obtained in vitro with sperm that has not come in contact with the female genital tract.

OVUM TRANSPORT

At ovulation, the ovum is released from the ovary surrounded by follicular cells: the corona radiata, a clump of cells closely attached to the zona pellucida, and the cumulus oophorus, cells surrounding the corona. The existence of this rather gelatinous cellular mass may play a role in ovum pickup by the fimbriae of the fallopian tube. Ovum pickup is also facilitated by the contractions of the oviduct, fimbriae, and ovarian ligaments, which may bring these structures in close apposition. Beating of cilia within the fimbriae may also allow for more efficient pickup.

FERTILIZATION

The egg possesses, in its outer coat, specific molecules that serve as receptors to sperm and to which the spermatozoon attaches itself firmly. In general, the binding of the spermatozoon to its receptor in the egg is species-specific. The binding of the sperm to the zona pellucida is followed by the acrosome reaction, which involves the fusion of the outer acrosomal membrane and the plasma membrane, a process that allows the release of stored enzymes, such as hyaluronidase. This reaction aids the penetration of the spermatozoon through the outer coat of the egg. Although the intimate mechanisms of penetration remain to be studied in detail, it probably results from the combined action of the propelling movements of the flagellum and of the dispersing enzymes released from the acrosome. Penetration is completed within 3 hours, at which time the entire spermatozoon, including the tail, has entered the egg, and fusion or mixing of the genetic materials of both parents has occurred. At that moment, a rapid and dramatic change in the properties of the egg occurs, the zona reaction; modification of zona materials is such that, in most species, attachment to and penetration of the zona pellucida by other spermatozoa are now precluded (Fig. 6–1).

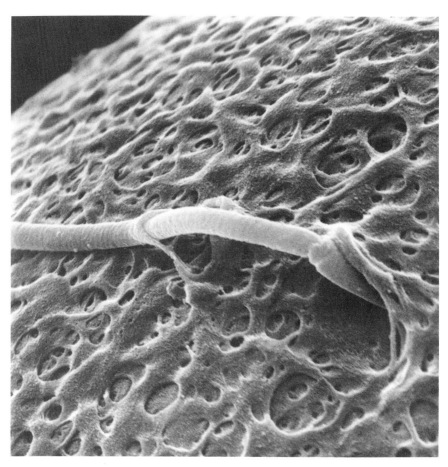

Fig. 6–1. Binding of spermatozoa to the egg. Several spermatozoa can bind to the zona pellucida, which contains sperm-binding receptors. Upon binding, the acrosome reaction will occur, allowing for penetration. Only one spermatozoon will fuse with the plasma membrane surrounding the egg. Upon fusion (fertilization), the zona reaction will prevent penetration by other spermatozoa. This is a scanning electron micrograph (courtesy of DM Phillips) of a hamster spermatozoon that has penetrated the zona pellucida. (From Yanagimachi R, Phillips DM, 1984, *Gamete Res* 9:1–19.)

Upon sperm–egg fusion, the second meiotic division, which before fertilization of the egg was arrested at metaphase (see Chapter 3), is resumed. The resulting female haploid nucleus becomes the female pronucleus. Chromosome duplication occurs in both female and male pronuclei. These pronuclei then fuse, and their chromosomes mingle for the first mitotic division. Cleavage to a two-cell stage occurs about 12 hours after penetration of the zona pellucida. The fertilized egg remains within the fallopian tube for 3 days. By day 4 after ovulation, the conceptus, now referred to as blastocyst, enters the uterus.

THE FIRST WEEKS OF PREGNANCY

MATERNAL RECOGNITION OF PREGNANCY

If fertilization has occurred, it is essential that the fertilized egg signal its presence in order to interrupt luteolysis or the demise of the corpus luteum that is about to occur at that time of the cycle. This must be done to allow continuing secretion of estradiol and progesterone to ensure uterine receptivity to the nidating egg. The embryo signals its presence through the secretion of several proteins, steroids, and other hormones, which are the subject of numerous ongoing studies.

In regard to the maintenance of the corpus luteum, the main hormone is chorionic gonadotropin (CG). Human chorionic gonadotropin (hCG) is a glycoprotein that consists of two nonidentical subunits: α (92 amino acids) and β (145 amino acids). The subunits are associated covalently. As is the case for luteinizing hormone (LH), α and β genes are located on different chromosomes; however, there appear to be several β subunit genes, all on the same chromosome. Subunit association is required for biological activity, because neither subunit alone binds to the CG receptor. It is of interest to note that there is considerable amino acid sequence homology between β-CG and β-LH, and, thus, in regard to its biological activity, hCG is very similar to hLH, although it has a substantially longer half-life.

The fertilized egg starts secreting CG from the time it becomes attached to the uterus, although some investigators have reported that the hormone may be secreted even before attachment, after the zona pellucida is shed. Actual secretion of CG precedes at least by 2 days the time at which it can be detected in the peripheral circulation. Appearance of CG coincides with the time at which estradiol and progesterone normally start to decline during the luteal phase. Presumably, the more intense CG stimulus can overcome the relative reduction in luteal cell sensitivity that occurs at that time of the luteal phase. Thus, luteolysis is prevented and the secretory capacity of the corpus luteum is maintained. As a consequence, estradiol and progesterone secretion continues and menstruation does not occur (the "missed menses") (Fig. 6–2). If at this time antibodies to CG are administered in the experimental animal, steroid secretion declines and implantation is prevented.

hCG concentrations in peripheral plasma increase significantly from the time of implantation until about the 8th week of pregnancy. They then plateau and decline afterwards until about week 18 (Fig. 6–3). Beyond week 18, hCG con-

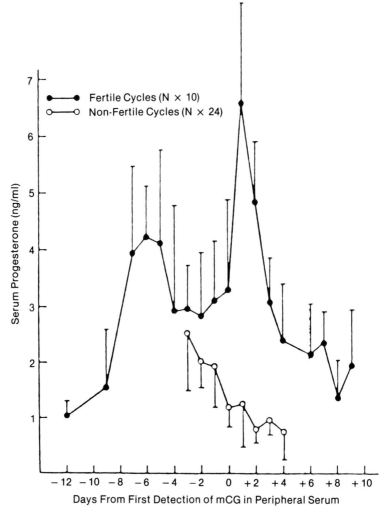

Fig. 6–2. The rescue of the corpus luteum in the fertile cycle. In the fertile cycle, chorionic gonadotropin "rescues" the corpus luteum and prevents luteolysis. As a consequence, ovarian steroid secretion persists. This figure compares progesterone concentrations in fertile and nonfertile cycles of rhesus monkeys. Time 0 denotes the detection of monkey chorionic gonadotropin *(mCG)* in peripheral serum. (Actual secretion of CG precedes detection by about 2 days.) (From Hodgen GD, Tullner WW, Vaitukaitis JL, Ward DN, Ross GT 1974: Specific radioimmunoassay of chorionic gonadotropin during implantation of rhesus monkeys. *J Clin Endocrinol Metab* 39:457–464. Copyright © by The Endocrine Society.)

centrations remain relatively constant, but low, for the remainder of pregnancy. (Since CG is of placental origin, it is secreted only in pregnancy. CG has also been measured in the nonpregnant state. This molecule, however, appears to be structurally different from placental CG, possibly in the amounts of carbohydrates it contains, and has a different half-life.)

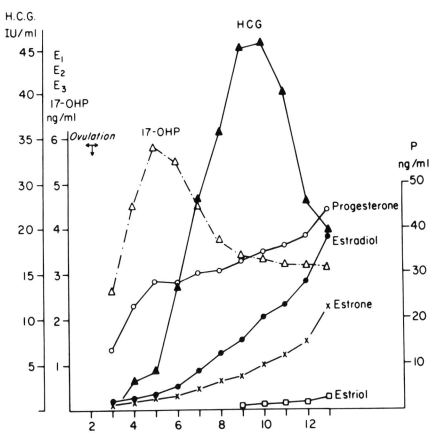

Fig. 6–3. Hormone secretion during early pregnancy. Plasma values of human chorionic gonadotropin *(hCG)*, progesterone (*P*), 17-α-hydroxyprogesterone *(17-α-OHP)*, estrone *(E1)*, estradiol *(E2)*, and estriol *(E3)* during the first 3 months of pregnancy. (From Tulchinsky D, Hobel C 1973: *Am J Obstet Gynecol* 117:884.)

IMPLANTATION

During the preimplantation period, various chemicals of blastocyst origin may interact with the endometrium to stimulate necessary changes in the uterus. These may include, apart from the aforementioned CG, steroid hormones, secretory proteins, and prostaglandins. As a whole, these compounds play several roles, for example, mediating endometrial vascular changes, increasing blood flow, facilitating the passage of nutrients into the lumen of the uterus, and protecting the fetal allograft from immunological rejection.

General hormonal requirements for the development of uterine receptivity to implantation necessitate, of course, a particular sequence of events that includes: (1) the priming of the uterus by estradiol (the proliferative estradiol effects during the follicular phase), and (2) the conditioning by progesterone (the stimulation of secretory activity during the first days of the luteal phase). Successful implantation of ova fertilized in vitro has been obtained in ovariectomized animals and in women with ovarian failure following a sequential pretreatment with estradiol and progesterone to simulate normal menstrual cycle hormonal changes. The crucial role that progesterone plays in early pregnancy is underscored in studies in which a progesterone antagonist, RU 486, was used. Such a compound, by antagonizing the action of endogenous progesterone on its target organs, terminates early pregnancy.

In the normal cycle, the endometrium appears to have a temporally restricted capacity to sustain implantation, such that receptivity to the fertilized ovum is most probably limited to a 3-day period. This is important to remember in in vitro fertilization procedures. It is not clear, however, at present, what uterine receptivity represents at the cellular level.

The implantation process requires first that the fertilized egg shed its zona pellucida. Attachment of the egg to the uterine epithelium involves a progressively increasing intimacy of contact, requiring first apposition, then investment of the embryo with maternal epithelium, thereby immobilizing the egg within the uterus. This is followed by a progressive interdigitation of microvilli and the attachment reaction. Once the uterine epithelium and its associated basal lamina are penetrated, a definitive vascular relationship with the mother is established. The earliest macroscopic sign of pregnancy is an area of increased endometrial vascularity in the vicinity of the blastocyst, resulting in local tissue edema due to changes in permeability, and the decidual transformation of the endometrium characterized by increasing proliferation and differentiation of the local stromal cells. The function of these cells, the decidua, is not entirely known, but it is generally thought that this specialized tissue is a critical component of the mother's response to the fertilized egg: it provides a solid mass of cells into which the conceptus becomes embedded.

THE LUTEOPLACENTAL SHIFT

Under the influence of hCG, the corpus luteum is maintained and there is a continuous rise in estradiol and progesterone during the first 4 weeks of pregnancy. The corpus luteum of pregnancy also secretes 17-α-hydroxyprogesterone. Four weeks after ovulation, a decline in luteal steroidogenesis starts to occur: this is

Table 6–2. Sequence of Events in Early Pregnancy

Day 0	Ovulation
Day 3	Fertilization
	Completion of the second meiotic division
Day 5–6	Shedding of the zona pellucida
Day 6–7	Attachment to the uterine epithelium
Day 7–12	Differentiation of the trophoblast
Day 8–10	hCG first detected in the peripheral blood
Day 12	Decidual reaction
Day 28	Luteoplacental shift begins
Day 49	Luteoplacental shift completed

hCG, human chorionic gonadotropin.

signaled by a marked decrease in the secretion of 17-α-hydroxyprogesterone. The other two steroids, however, continue to increase, but at a slower rate, reflecting increasing secretion and takeover by the placenta. This tissue, however, has little capacity for 17-hydroxylation, thus explaining the decline in 17-α-hydroxyprogesterone. The luteoplacental shift is completed by 7 weeks after ovulation (Table 6–2). Removal of the corpus luteum at that time does not affect the outcome of pregnancy. In contrast, luteectomy prior to 6 weeks of pregnancy results in a substantial decrease in progesterone concentrations and abortion.

The placenta is the source of several steroid, protein, and polypeptide hormones. In addition to hCG are human placental lactogen (hPL), a hormone that shows considerable homology to growth hormone and, to a lesser degree, to prolactin; gonadotropin-releasing hormone (GnRH), whose potential function may be to stimulate hCG secretion; adrenocorticotropin hormone (ACTH) and related proopiomelanocortin (POMC)-derived peptides, and corticotropin-releasing hormone (CRH) and thyrotropin-releasing hormone (TRH)-like peptides, whose precise role remains to be determined.

7

The First Menstrual Cycle: Adolescence and Puberty

Adolescence is the period of growth and maturation of the reproductive system that culminates in puberty. Secretory and morphological activities of the gonads reach the adult stage, and menarche, the first menstrual period, occurs. Average age of menarche in the United States is 12.8 years. A number of processes have been shown to advance or retard menarche in normal girls. For example, the progressive decline in the age of menarche noted in western Europe and the United States is thought to be due to improvement in socioeconomic circumstances, nutrition, and general health. Particular conditions reported to advance the age at which menarche occurs include blindness, obesity, urban residence, and hypothyroidism. Early menarche is also seen in bedridden retarded children. Conditions reported to retard the age of menarche include poor nutrition, altitude, number of children in family, thyrotoxicosis, excessive muscular development, and strenuous exercise such as ballet dancing.

We will review the mechanisms that control the onset of puberty, physiological aspects of sexual maturation at puberty, and the pathology of puberty.

MECHANISMS CONTROLLING THE TIMING OF PUBERTY

The precise mechanism that controls the timing of the sexual maturation process is still not well understood, although it is clear that an hypothalamic input is primary. Normal adult function of the reproductive system, as reviewed in the preceding chapters, requires interactions between the brain, the pituitary gland, and the gonads and their target organs.

THE NEURAL INPUT

There is no doubt that the initial step, and probably the key factor, in the series of events that culminate in puberty is an increase in the pulsatile release of the neurohormone gonadotropin-releasing hormone (GnRH), leading to enhanced secretion of gonadotropins. Surprisingly, recent studies have led to the notion that the neuroendocrine GnRH system is fully mature at birth and is capable of sustaining "quasi" adult levels of gonadotropins at that time. Yet, in the normal individual, sexual maturity fails to occur because pulsatile GnRH activity declines in late infancy and a prepubertal phase of relative hypothalamic quiescence occurs during which gonadotropin secretion is suppressed (the prepubertal hiatus). This period lasts until adolescence, at which time normal pulsatile GnRH activity is restored and the pubertal process initiated.

The nature of the inhibitory influence(s) that prevent adult GnRH pulsatile activity during infancy remains unknown. What is certain is that the inhibitory influence is not of gonadal origin, since agonadal subjects show a qualitatively similar course of gonadotropin secretion throughout infancy as the intact individual. Experimentally, these phenomena have been well illustrated in the rhesus monkey. Gonadectomy in the newborn monkey results in a postcastration rise in gonadotropins, similar to that seen in the adult following the interruption of the negative gonadal steroid feedback loop. In these animals, the GnRH pulse generator exhibits a pulse frequency typical of the adult castrate. Yet, gonadotropin secretion becomes suppressed during infancy; normal activity resumes at about the same time as in the normal animal (Fig. 7–1). Thus, both quiescence and recovery occur independently from the ovary.

Interestingly, hypothalamic GnRH and GnRH messenger ribonucleic acid (mRNA) are present in similar amounts in infant and adult monkeys. Premature GnRH pulsatile activity and, hence, gonadotropin release and sexual maturation can be activated by various hypothalamic lesions, primarily in the caudal region, thus suggesting that disinhibition from a neural inhibitory input responsible for the prepubertal hiatus may determine when the chain of events is initiated. It has also been suggested that the absence of GnRH release during the prepubertal hiatus may be related to a lack of an excitatory afferent input to the GnRH system. GnRH release can be obtained in a prepubertal monkey by intermittent stimulation of the hypothalamus with N-methyl-D-aspartate (NMDA), a central excitatory amino acid. In the male monkey, treatment with this compound results in the onset of precocious puberty and sexual maturation. This observation suggests that proper release of GnRH may require synchronous activity of specific neuronal systems, a process that would recur during the maturation process in the juvenile.

The Pubertal Nocturnal Luteinizing Hormone (LH) Increase

Reinitiation of pulsatile gonadotropin secretion in pubertal children follows a particular pattern: while gonadotropin secretion is relatively low during the daytime, it is increased during the night at which time large amplitude LH pulses, presumably the reflection of large GnRH pulses, are observed. This nocturnal increase in gonadotropins is usually the first sign that the process of sexual maturation is being initiated. In later stages of puberty, the nocturnal increase is replaced by gradually increased levels of gonadotropins which occur around the clock in an episodic manner (Fig. 7–2).

Because of the circadian rhythm of release in the first stage of puberty, several investigators have, over the years, studied the possibility of a relation between the pineal gland and its product of secretion, melatonin, and the onset of puberty; there is at present no evidence that would suggest a role of this gland in the initiation of puberty. On the other hand, there is good evidence for an asso-

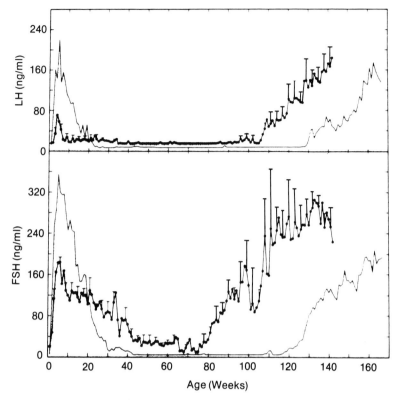

Fig. 7–1. The prepubertal hiatus in gonadotropin secretion in the gonadectomized animal. Time courses of LH *(upper panel)* and FSH *(lower panel)* secretion in ovariectomized
(solid circles) and orchidectomized *(stippled area)* rhesus monkeys. While gonadotropins
are actively released at birth, their secretion is suppressed during infancy, only to resume
in the first stage of puberty. The factors responsible for this hiatus in secretory activity
remain to be determined, but are not of gonadal origin since these agonadal monkeys
show a pattern similar to intact ones. *FSH,* follicle-stimulating hormone; *LH,* luteinizing
hormone. (From Plant TM 1988: Puberty in primates. In: *The Physiology of Reproduction* [Knobil E, Neill S eds], Raven Press, NY, 1763.)

ciation between the nighttime LH increase and sleep stages. In fact, the increase
can be delayed if the subject is kept awake. The significance of this association
with sleep is unknown.

THE METABOLIC INPUT

Metabolic factors are important in the timing of puberty. It is well known that
good nutrition advances the onset of puberty and that starvation delays it. In
undernourished girls, puberty can be delayed by a number of years. In rats, even
moderate food restriction can delay the onset of sexual maturation, while severe
food restriction completely prevents the pubertal process. In these animals, pulsatile LH secretion is abolished, demonstrating a link between nutrition and the
activity of the GnRH pulse generator. Thus, it has been suggested that normal

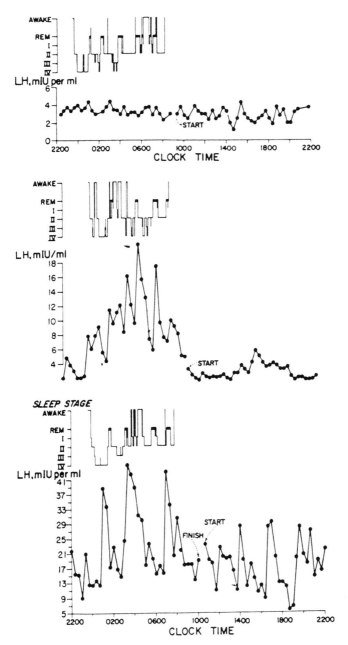

Fig. 7–2. Circadian gonadotropin concentrations at puberty. Plasma LH concentrations and sleep stage during three stages of puberty in girls: *prepubertal (upper panel), early pubertal (middle panel),* and *late pubertal (lower panel).* While pulsatile gonadotropin secretion is relatively low in infancy (the prepubertal hiatus), the first sign of initiation of the sexual maturation process is a nocturnal, sleep-related increase in pulsatile gonadotropin activity *(middle panel),* replaced in later stages of puberty by increased levels around the clock *(lower panel).* Abbreviations as in Figure 7–1. (From Boyar RM, Katz J, Finkelstein JW 1974: *N Engl J Med* 291:861.) Reprinted by permission of *The New England Journal of Medicine.*

81

changes in metabolic status or rate of growth in late childhood may participate in the stimulation of the central drive to maturation. Several investigators over the past three decades have advanced the hypothesis of a threshold of body weight, later refined to percent of body fat, critical for allowing initiation of the maturation process.

This concept, of course, is very attractive as it correlates early puberty in North American and European girls over the century with earlier age of the critical threshold weight in the later part of the century. It is, however, unlikely that body weight or body composition per se function as the causal factors triggering puberty, although it is probable that metabolic *cues* are relayed to the brain and provide signals that activate the GnRH pulse generator. Unfortunately, at present, few investigators have addressed the problem in a systematic fashion, and thus the nature of these putative metabolic changes remains to be elucidated.

THE PHYSIOLOGY OF PUBERTY

SEQUENCE OF EVENTS

Several physiological processes occur in sequence. These are summarized in Table 7–1.

Adrenarche

A change in the steroidogenic function of the adrenal gland usually precedes sexual maturation. This process results in an increase in the secretion of C-19 steroids of adrenal origin, such as dehydroepiandrosterone (DHEA) and its sulfate. An as yet unidentified adrenal androgen-stimulating factor of pituitary origin may be responsible for this phenomenon that normally occurs by 8 years of age. Thus, increases in these C-19 steroids are the earliest hormonal changes connected to puberty. It should be noted, however, that a role of adrenarche in the activation of the central drive for sexual maturation is unlikely, since puberty is not unduly delayed in children with primary adrenal insufficiency.

Table 7–1. Sequence of Events at Puberty

1. Adrenarche	→ C-19 steroids ↑
2. Sleep activation of GnRH pulse generator	→ FSH ↑ LH ↑ estradiol ↑
3. 24-h activation of GnRH pulse generator	→ FSH ↑ LH ↑ estradiol ↑
4. Decreased sensitivity to estradiol negative feedback	→ FSH ↑↑ LH ↑↑ → folliculogenesis → menarche
5. Maturation of estradiol positive feedback loop	→ FSH/LH surge → ovulation

FSH, follicle-stimulating hormone; *GnRH*, gonadotropin-releasing hormone; *LH*, luteinizing hormone.

Gonadarche

As mentioned earlier, the primary event in the initiation of puberty is the increased secretion of GnRH, initially at night, then throughout the 24-hour period. This increased activity of the pulse generator is, of course, followed by enhanced release of gonadotropins. Usually, in girls, baseline follicle-stimulating hormone (FSH) levels increase prior to LH, perhaps reflecting a low GnRH pulse frequency during the initial stage of puberty (slow GnRH pulse frequency favors FSH over LH secretion; see Chapter 2). Increased gonadotropin secretion in turn induces morphological and secretory changes in the ovaries (gonadarche). Morphological changes include the development of follicles. Secretory changes parallel the growth of the follicle and result in increased release of estrogens.

Changes in Sensivity of the "Gonadostat"

Although the hypothalamic-ovarian steroid feedback loops do not play a role in the initiation process of puberty, there appears to be, later as adolescence proceeds, a change in sensitivity of the hypothalamic-pituitary unit to the inhibitory feedback of gonadal steroids. This is expressed by a progressive decrease in sensitivity which would allow for increases in gonadotropin secretion in time as puberty progresses, even in the face of increasing steroid output (the "gonadostat" theory). It is thought that the timing of this decrease in estradiol inhibition of gonadotropin secretion sets the tempo of the final sexual maturation stages. There also appears to be a temporal association between increments in skeletal growth and the decrease in sensitivity to estradiol.

The best experimental demonstration of the gonadostat theory has been performed in animal models. Thus, in ovariectomized estradiol-replaced lambs or monkeys (Fig. 7–3), a spontaneous and progressive increase in gonadotropins occurs at about the time intact animals spontaneously begin to cycle, suggesting that initiation of cyclicity may be causally related to this change in estradiol negative feedback sensitivity. It is of interest to note that, in the sheep, similar changes in sensitivity to the estradiol negative feedback may underly the process of seasonal reproduction. (In the human adult, it is possible that alterations of sensitivity threshold may lead to pathological conditions in regard to menstrual cyclicity; see Chapter 10.) The precise mechanisms that underly this change in sensitivity remain to be understood.

PHYSICAL SIGNS OF PUBERTY: STAGING

Most of the clinical signs of puberty are related to the increased secretion of sex steroids from gonadal and adrenal origins. The sequence of physical events has been well categorized by Marshall and Tanner. On the average, progress from stage I to the adult stage (stage V) takes a minimum of 2 years. Staging is illustrated in Figure 7–4. The appearance of downy labial hair and budding of the breast are the first visible signs of puberty in girls, although the initial event is

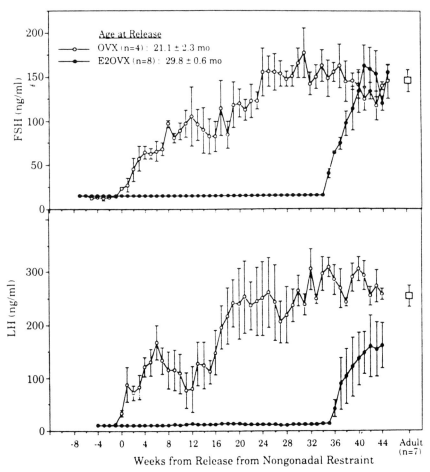

Fig. 7-3. The "gonadostat" theory. During the *later* stages of puberty, there appears to be a decrease in sensitivity to the estradiol negative feedback loop, thus allowing for increases in gonadotropin secretion in the face of persistent or even increasing steroid output. Changes in sensitivity of the "gonadostat" have been documented in ovariectomized (OVX), estradiol-replaced *(E2OVX)* pubertal monkeys *(solid circles)*. Despite administration of equivalent doses of estradiol over the entire experimental observation period which initially completely suppress LH and FSH secretion, a progressive increase in gonadotropin secretion is demonstrated, at about the time the later stages of puberty occur in the intact animal (week 30-36). This is presumably the result of a decrease in sensitivity to the estradiol negative feedback (the "gonadostat" theory). Abbreviations as in Figure 7-1. (From Wilson ME 1989: In: Control of the Onset of Puberty III [Delemarre-Vande Waal HA, Plant TM, Van Rees GP, Schoemaker J, eds], Elsevier Science Publishers Amsterdam, 137).

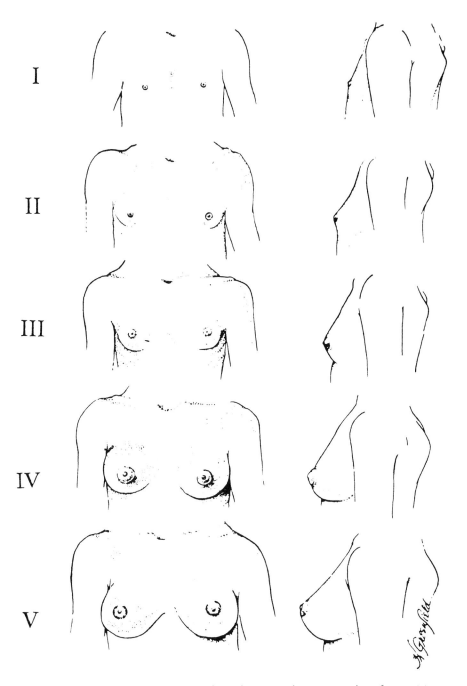

Fig. 7–4. Clinical signs of puberty: staging. Diagrammatic representation of stages 1 (pre-pubertal) to 5 (adult) of human breast maturation. *Stage I,* preadolescent, elevation of papilla only; *stage II,* breast bud stage, elevation of breast and papilla as a small mound, enlargement of areolar diameter; *stage III,* further enlargement of breast and areola; *stage IV,* projection of areola and papilla to form a secondary mound above the level of the breast; *stage V,* adult stage, projection of papilla alone. (From Ross GT, Vande Wiele RL 1981: The ovaries. In: *Textbook of Endocrinology* [Williams RH, ed] WB Saunders, Phil-adelphia, 355–399; as adapted from Marshall WA, Tanner JM 1969: *Arch Dis Child 44:291.)*

usually the appearance of the breast bud (thelarche). A large individual variation for these two pubertal events has been noted in normal girls, illustrating that these are two independently controlled phenomena. Appearance of pubic hair is related to C-19 steroid secretion, particularly from the adrenal gland (see earlier), while thelarche is influenced by the secretion of estrogen, in particular estradiol from ovarian follicles. Other factors, particularly growth factors, may also be involved.

Common indexes of estrogen secretion are summarized in Table 7–2. These indexes are the clinical measures used in evaluating girls to determine if estrogen secretion is present. Particularly valuable in the adolescent girl is the presence of a cornified vaginal smear and a bone age determining skeletal maturity.

The increase in body fat is the earliest change in body composition at puberty in females. The pubertal years in girls are marked by rapid gain in fat (an average of 11 kg). Lean body mass, skeletal mass, and body fat are equal in prepubertal boys and girls, but these proportions change postpubertally. Adult women have twice as much body fat as men; men have almost 1.5 times the lean body mass and the skeletal mass of women.

A growth spurt occurs during puberty. The time of most rapid growth in females is in the later stage of puberty, prior to the first menstrual period when females grow a mean of 25 cm. Growth slows rapidly after menarche (Fig. 7–5). (With a delay in this growth spurt, pubertal obesity may result.) Body proportions are also altered during this growth period. The upper to lower (U/L) body ratio in particular is changed. This ratio is defined as length from top of pubic ramus to top of head divided by the distance from the top of pubic ramus to floor. Early puberty is marked by elongation of the extremities. Later, the growth spurt equalizes growth of both the torso and lower extremities so that the U/L ratio decreases. The physiologic mechanisms governing these changes are still unknown although growth hormone secretion, gonadal and adrenal steroids all appear to be important.

The important bony changes that occur prior to menarche include epiphiseal fusion of different bone centers and osseous maturation, as evidenced by x-ray (usually of the wrist). Bone age is a very accurate index of physiologic maturation and correlates closely with menarche. It is a valuable tool in the evaluation of children with delayed puberty; bone age can also be used to predict final height.

Table 7–2. Indexes of Estrogen Secretion

1. Body fat distribution
2. Breast development
3. Bone maturation
4. Vaginal cell cornification
5. Cervical mucus
6. Proliferative endometrium
7. Withdrawal bleeding after progesterone administration
8. Plasma estradiol measurement

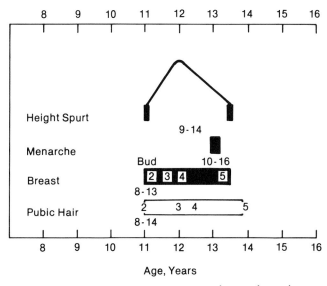

Fig. 7–5. Sequence of events at puberty. *Numbers under each representation* indicate age span during which the phenomenon takes place. *Numbers inside representation* indicate stage. (From Marshall WA, Tanner JM 1970: *Arch Dis Child* 45:13.)

Puberty and the Menstrual Cycle

Menarche occurs late in the process of puberty. This event relates to the presence of maturing follicles within the ovary and the resultant endometrial stimulation by estrogens secreted by these follicles. There is, however, much variability between the time menarche occurs and the onset of fully normal menstrual cyclicity. In general, anovulatory cycles predominate up to 2 years after menarche. The reason for this usually relates to the immaturity of the long estradiol positive feedback loop. Occasionally, small LH and FSH peaks may occur, but are asynchronous with follicular maturity. In adolescents who show ovulatory cycles, follicular growth may be slow and the preovulatory phase may be prolonged. Short luteal phases may also occur, due to the immaturity of the developing follicle. In general, 80% of the cycles have become ovulatory 6 years after menarche.

THE PATHOLOGY OF PUBERTY

PRECOCIOUS PUBERTY

Pubertal changes before age 8 years are considered precocious. A sudden growth spurt is usually followed by breast development and pubic hair appearance. Occasionally, these events occur together; sometimes, menarche may be the first sign. *True precocious* puberty is diagnosed when the gonads are the source of the hormones, the result of premature activation of the hypothalamic-pituitary unit. In contrast, *pseudoprecocious* puberty is the result of a primary ovarian abnormality independant of pituitary stimulation or of hormones secreted from an extragonadal source. Other terms are also commonly used to describe precocious puberty: If sexual development is consistant with genetic sex, it is referred to as isosexual. Signs of virilism in a girl indicate heterosexual precocious puberty.

Most commonly, the etiology of the problem is idiopathic or constitutional; however, serious conditions should be ruled out including intracranial pathology, ovarian tumors, or diseases of the adrenal gland. A family history may be associated with the constitutional sexual precocity due to premature maturation of the hypothalamic-pituitary-ovarian axis. The McCune-Albright syndrome (polyostotic fibrous dysplasia) consists of multiple disseminated cystic bone lesions including sclerotic changes at the base of the skull, café au lait spots, and precocious puberty usually occurring after 2 years of age. The cause of the syndrome is unknown.

It is helpful to classify precocious puberty according to the site of secretion of hormone excess. Primary gonadotropin excess will encompass more than 75% of girls with this syndrome who have premature activation of the hypothalamic pituitary axis. However, a specific central nervous system (C.N.S.) pathology must be ruled out in this group; this may relate to trauma, infection (such as encephalitis), space occupying lesions including pinealomas and craniopharyngiomas, hydrocephalus, and other congenital brain defects. Brain cysts as well as hypothalamic harmatomas can also occur. It is important to remember that C.N.S. lesions usually manifest neurologic symptoms prior to the advent of precocious pubertal development.

Ectopic secretion of human chorionic gonadotropin (hCG) that has LH-like activity should also be ruled out. They are very rare but can originate from hepatomas, teratomas, or chorioepitheliomas.

Estrogen excess as a primary cause of precocious puberty is usually related to ovarian tumors (granulosa or theca cell). These are almost always palpable. Ovarian cysts may also occur. Feminizing tumors of the adrenal glands can sometimes present this way. Oral or topical estrogens can also be a cause of the syndrome.

Androgen excess will usually cause premature development of body hair, acne, and in some cases, virilization. Congenital adrenal hyperplasia, adrenal tumors as well as Cushing's syndrome, and rarely androgen-secreting ovarian tumors should be ruled out. Premature pubarche may also occur as a result of organic brain disease for reasons that are unclear.

The diagnosis of the patient with precocious puberty is heavily dependent on the results of hormonal evaluation, including FSH, LH, estradiol, and when indicated, testosterone, DHEA, and androstenedione. Pelvic ultrasound and neurological evaluation is also important.

DELAYED PUBERTY

Lack of physical manifestations of puberty in a child who is 2.5 standard deviations beyond the norm (13 years old in girls and 14 in boys) is generally considered abnormal. Organic causes for this delay in puberty must be separated from environmental causes.

Organic Causes

Organic causes include C.N.S. disorders and isolated gonadotropin deficiency, and gonadal failure or dysgenesis. By far the most common problem, however, is a constitutional delay in puberty which represents a genetic predisposition to a delay in activation of the hypothalamic pulse generator. Constitutional delay in puberty occurs in 0.6% of North Americans and is associated with delayed growth and often a positive family history. Adrenarche, thelarche, and bone age, compatible with the immature physical development, are delayed as well. In these cases, however, development will ultimately be completed and full genetically determined height reached.

In contrast, hypogonadotropic hypogonadism may occur with or without growth retardation and ultimate short stature depending on the type of deficiency. Some hypogonadotropic subjects have an isolated GnRH deficiency while others may have associated growth hormone (GH) or FSH deficiency. Gonadotropin deficiency may occur as a result of genetic or developmental defects, a mass lesion, trauma, inflammation, a vascular lesion, or radiation. Isolated deficiency is typically associated with a normal height and eunuchoid proportions: an increased span (fingertip to fingertip) and an increased U/L ratio. This is due to the relative lack of sex steroids that prevents fusion of the epiphyses at a normal age. In Kallman's syndrome, a GnRH deficiency occurs with anosmia or hyposmia due to agenesis or poor development of the olfactory lobes and abnormal migration of the GnRH neuron into the hypothalamus. (see Chapter 2).

Idiopathic hypopituitary dwarfism is a syndrome manifesting multiple endocrine deficiencies and growth failure which may be familial. The growth failure is profound, in contrast to patients with tumors. Miscellaneous uncommon conditions include the Prader-Willi syndrome and the Laurence-Moon-Biedl syndrome. The first is characterized by massive obesity, carbohydrate intolerance, short stature, and mental retardation. These patients have hypothalamic dysfunction; weight reduction can be associated with sexual development and the onset of menarche. The second consists of polydactyly, obesity, mental retardation, and retinitis pigmentosa, also associated with delayed puberty.

Hypothyroidism is commonly associated with delayed puberty; this reverses with thyroid treatment only. Excess secretion of any of the trophic pituitary hormones causing Cushing's syndrome (adrenocorticotropic hormone [ACTH]) or acromegaly (GH) can cause delayed puberty. In general, functional suppression of GnRH occurs with these illnesses and there is a reversion with treatment.

Severe chronic illnesses of any kind may be associated with delayed puberty, particularly those associated with weight loss and debilitation. These include renal disease, malignancies, regional enteritis, chronic cardiac or pulmonary disease, cystic fibrosis, sickle cell anemia, and diabetes mellitus.

Environmental Factors

Environmental factors may negatively affect the maturational events which span several years and which prepare the body for reproduction. These include nutrition, weight, stress, and exercise. Weight loss, particularly of a pathologic degree

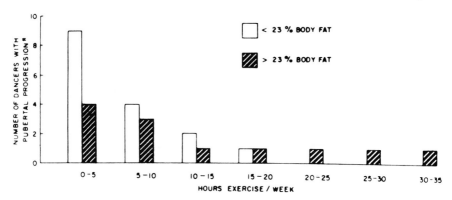

Fig. 7–6. Delay of puberty in ballet dancers. A typical example of the synergistic action of decreased body weight and exercise in delaying puberty in female ballet dancers. An increased number of exercise hours/week will result in a delay in pubertal progression, even in the dancers in whom weight is near normal. (From Warren M 1980: The effects of exercise on pubertal progression and reproductive function in girls. *J Clin Endocrinol Metab* 51:1150–1157. Copyright © by The Endocrine Society.)

as seen in anorexia nervosa, may delay puberty during growth. In general, weight loss will delay or arrest puberty if weight falls below 85% of ideal body weight. As in the adult (see Chapter 10), stress and exercise may have a negative impact on normal pubertal reproductive development. Typically, puberty may be arrested even with a less prominent weight loss if it occurs in the setting of endurance or vigorous exercise. This is commonly seen in ballet dancers (Fig. 7–6), figure skaters, gymnasts, and runners. This type of delayed puberty can be associated with skeletal complications due to the lack of folliculogenesis and estrogen secretion, and should be carefully monitored as hormonal replacement may be indicated (for additional details, see also Chapter 11).

THERAPY

Therapy depends on the etiology of the condition. Often treatment of the underlying disorder will resolve the problem. Recently, the treatment of constitutional precocious puberty has benefited greatly from the use of GnRH analogs (see Chapter 13 for mode of action) which suppress gonadotropin secretion and arrest skeletal maturation, and, at present, this is the treatment of choice. GnRH agonists are effective subcutaneously or nasally with few side effects, but must be administered chronically. (Monthly depot injections are also available.) Medroxyprogesterone acetate, cyproterone acetate (an androgen receptor blocker) and danazol (an isoxazole derivative of the synthetic steroid 17-α-ethinyltestosterone, with antigonadotropic activity) are alternative therapies; however, they all have undesirable side effects as they may cause bloating and weight gain. Danazol, in addition, may have androgenic effects such as acne, hirsutism, and voice changes.

Delayed puberty can also be treated generally by addressing the underlying condition. Treatment with pulsatile GnRH administration, whether intravenously or subcutaneously, has been used to induce puberty. This treatment stimulates the gonadotrope to secrete LH and FSH which then enhance ovarian steroid secretion. Of course, upon discontinuation of this treatment, gonadotropins regress to prepubertal levels, unless the normal process of puberty has finally started. Occasionally, steroid hormone replacement is indicated to prevent complications associated with hypogonadism and the social consequences of delayed maturation.

8

The Last Menstrual Cycles: The Climacteric and Menopause

The climacteric is a period of physiologic waning of ovarian function and of corresponding endocrine, somatic, and psychological changes. It covers the perimenopausal years in a woman's life in a broad sense. The term *menopause* more specifically denotes the cessation of menses, and is the traditional marker of reproductive senescence in women ("meno" + "pause"; *menses,* Latin for month; *pausis,* Greek for cessation). However, menopause is only one event in a sequence that extends from conception to advanced age. The changes leading to menopause precede by many years the actual cessation of menses and are part of the general process of senescence. We will review the physiology and etiology of menopause, the clinical symptomatology that accompanies menopause, and the management of the menopausal woman.

PHYSIOLOGY AND ETIOLOGY OF MENOPAUSE

AGE AND ONSET

The human female, contrary to females of other species, has a life span that extends considerably beyond reproductive age. In the industrialized world, the median age at menopause lies within a narrow range. For instance, in the Netherlands, the median age at menopause is 51.7 years while that in the United States is 49.8. In developing countries, however, the median age at menopause is less than 44 years. Menopause at an earlier age has been reportedly related to lower socioeconomic class, smoking, and late onset of menarche, while menopause at a later age may occur in women who experienced early onset of puberty or were at an older age at the time of the last pregnancy. Premature ovarian failure is a rare syndrome characterized by secondary amenorrhea before the age of 40 years and is probably genetically determined.

PATTERNS OF CYCLICITY

The cyclic changes associated with the climacteric are generally not sudden. Although some women stop menstruating abruptly, a prodromal period of decreasing ovarian function may last 5 to 10 years before complete cessation of menses occurs. During this time, fertility declines progressively despite continuing or intermittent ovulation. Prospective studies of menstrual cycles during the years before menopause have shown a marked increase in the variability of intermenstrual intervals. Usually cycles become shorter as a result of a decrease in the length of the follicular phase. Later, cycles may lengthen because of a failure of ovulation, and ovulatory cycles may become interspersed with anovulatory ones. Episodes of prolonged bleeding may occur due to progesterone deficiency (dysfunctional uterine bleeding). Eventually, menses stop altogether.

ETIOLOGY

The stockpile of primordial follicles and oocytes in the ovaries is maximal before birth; however, a steady depletion of primary ovarian follicles begins during fetal life and continues throughout reproductive life with a dramatic acceleration in the last decade of menstrual life. At menopause, this irreplacable supply of oocytes is exhausted (Fig. 8–1). In a recent study in a group of seventeen women between the ages of 45 and 55 years, follicular reserve ranged from a mean of 1,392 in those still cycling to a few hundred in the perimenopausal and to none in the menopausal state (Fig. 8–1). Thus, morphologically, the ovary will look very different in an adult cycling than in a menopausal woman (Fig. 8–2), and

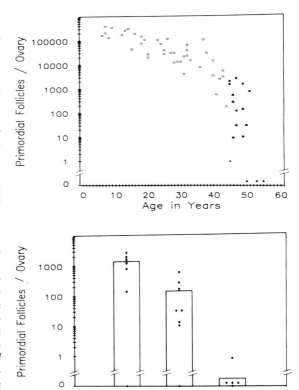

Fig. 8–1. Follicle number and the menopausal transition. Follicular depletion, which is initiated during fetal life, accelerates dramatically in the last decade of menstrual life. *Left,* comparison between age and the number of primordial follicles in the human ovary. *Right,* relationship between menstrual status and number of primordial follicles in age-matched women aged 45–55 years. *circles,* cycling; *squares,* perimenopausal; *triangles,* menopausal; *peri,* perimenopause; *post,* postmenopause. (From Richardson SJ, Senikas V, Nelson JF 1987: Follicular depletion during the menopausal transition: evidence for accelerated loss and ultimate exhaustion at menopause. *J Clin Endocrinol Metab* 65:1231–1237. Copyright © by The Endocrine Society.)

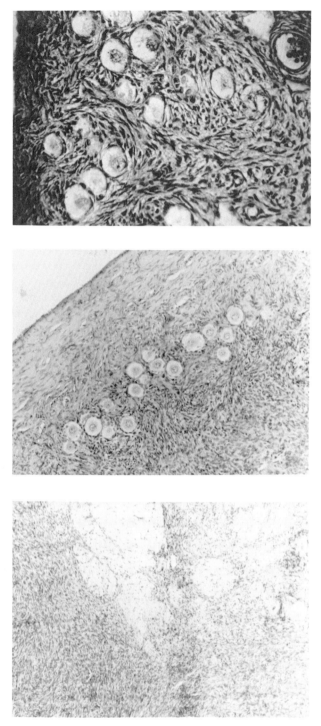

Fig. 8–2. Ovarian morphology before and after menopause. Note the presence of multiple primordial follicles in an ovary of a 1 year old *(top)*, and of several follicular structures during reproductive life *(center)*, and the absence of follicles after menopause *(bottom)*. (Photographs courtesy of Dr. Steve Lewis.)

there is no doubt that follicular exhaustion plays the key role in reproductive senescence.

In turn, changes in ovarian steroid secretory patterns that accompany ovarian senescence alter feedback relationships between the ovaries and the hypotha-lamic-pituitary unit and thereby affect brain-pituitary function. In the rodent, it has been shown that these changes may lead to altered neurosecretion, neuro-transmitter imbalance, variations in brain steroid receptor levels, and changes in behavior. In addition, it has become clear that aging of the reproductive sys-tem may involve a cumulative impact of ovarian steroids on the hypothalamus and pituitary and, therefore, although depletion of oocyte reserves is the domi-nant factor in the timing of acyclicity onset, primary hypothalamic changes also occur with senescence. In the human, however, the relative importance of changes in neuronal morphology and function in the process of menopause remains to be determined.

ENDOCRINOLOGY

In perimenopausal women who are menstruating regularly, estradiol concentra-tions are usually found to be lower and follicle-stimulating hormone (FSH) higher, while luteinizing hormone (LH) levels remain within the normal range. The reason for an increase in FSH before actual menopause is not completely understood. Since estradiol levels, although diminished, remain substantial, an explanation other than that of estrogen feedback inhibition is needed for the dis-cordant regulation of FSH and LH. Evidence that FSH is more sensitive than LH to the suppressive effect of exogenous estradiol argues against an increase in FSH caused by a decrease in estrogen concentration; moreover, at menopause, FSH and LH appear to decrease proportionally when estrogen is given. Although it is possible that an altered sensitivity of the aging hypothalamic-pituitary unit to sex steroids may manifest itself in the perimenopause by differential regula-tion of the gonadotropins, a more plausible possibility is that this phenomenon reflects decreased follicular inhibin levels, a consequence of the reduced number of follicles with aging. A decline in circulating inhibin concentrations would explain the elevated FSH in older women who have relatively normal estrogen and LH concentrations, as well as the considerable fluctuations in concentra-tions of FSH observed in the presence of very small changes in estradiol in peri-menopausal women. This hypothesis remains to be documented however.

Shorter duration menstrual cycles encountered in the premenopausal period most probably reflect the relative increase in FSH concentrations (Fig. 8–3). FSH will accelerate follicular recruitment and maturation and thereby shorten the follicular phase. Later on, however, as the follicular reserve pool shrinks and the number of follicles recruited in each cycle decreases, the period required to reach the minimum threshold for the triggering of the long loop estradiol posi-tive feedback increases, thereby lengthening the cycle. In time, synchronization between follicular potential for ovulation and the positive feedback loop may be lost and anovulatory cycles become interspersed in between ovulatory ones. It should be pointed out that, in contrast to the rodent, the ability to respond to an estradiol stimulus is not lost in the menopausal woman: exogenous estradiol administration can still trigger a proper gonadotropin surge.

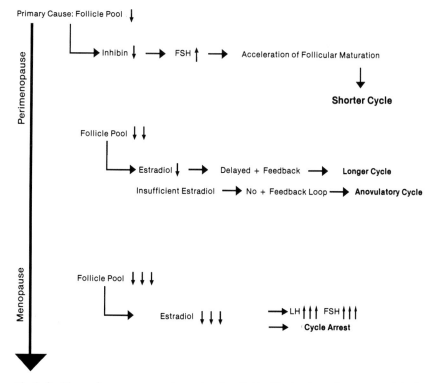

Fig. 8–3. The perimenopause and menstrual cyclicity. Mechanisms that may explain the sequence of events that characterizes changes in cyclic patterns before and after menopause are outlined. See text for details. *FSH*, follicle-stimulating hormone; *LH*, luteinizing hormone.

After menopause, ovarian production of estradiol and progesterone ceases. The remaining circulating estrogens (mostly the biologically less active estrone) are a result of peripheral conversion of androgens, which are still secreted in substantial amounts by the postmenopausal ovary. As in the castrate, both plasma LH and FSH are elevated severalfold over concentrations seen in the early follicular phase because of the inactivity of the long loop negative feedback. Pituitary response to gonadotropin-releasing hormone (GnRH) is not impaired by menopause.

THE LOSS OF FERTILITY

Demographic studies have shown that there is a progressive decline in fecundity after 30 to 35 years of age. Recent data suggest that the median age of sterility antedates the age of menopause by an average of 10 years. This is a complex issue, however, as most women complete childbearing before age 35 years, and, furthermore, the use of contraception, abortion, and sterilization may distort natural fecundity patterns. Social and economic factors are also important determinants. In "natural" societies where contraception is not practiced, fertility declines markedly during the fourth and fifth decades of life. Fertility in the 40–44 year age group is 40–50% lower than in the 35–39 year age group. Among the Hutterites of North America, who have one of the highest fertility rates ever recorded, the mean age of last confinement is 40.9 years. The oldest woman whose age at delivery was well documented was 57 years old.

One of the causes of infertility is, of course, the degree of irregularity of the menstrual cycle, and particularly the occurrence of cycles in which ovulation does not occur. Age-related changes in fertility may have, however, a multifactorial etiology, which may include age-related changes in the male partner, decreased frequency of intercourse, aging of the oocyte population resulting in increased frequency of chromosomal disorders, and improper secretion by the corpus luteum (the inadequate luteal phase) which may lead to innappropriate hormonal conditions for implantation. The premenopausal years are characterized by a marked increase in spontaneous abortion. Between 40–44 years of age, the spontaneous abortion rate is 34%, while over age 45 years, it rises to 53%.

CLINICAL SYMPTOMS OF MENOPAUSE

The major symptoms of menopause are the result of a decrease in estrogen levels. These include vasomotor instability (manifested as hot flushes and profuse sweating), vaginal dryness and irritation, osteoporosis, and decrease in the size of the breasts and uterus. However, not all women develop menopausal symptoms. The reason for this is not yet clearly understood, but it is possible that in some women increased peripheral conversion of androgens to estrone prevents their appearance. Other symptoms that may appear at menopause are nervousness, anxiety, irritability, depression, and insomnia. Insomnia is one of the most troublesome symptoms because it leads to sleep deprivation and chronic fatigue.

VASOMOTOR SYMPTOMS

Approximately 65–70% of women have hot flushes, and in the majority, the flushes last for more than 1 year. Studies of the mechanism of hot flushes have shown that they follow a typical pattern, starting with a sensation of pressure in the head associated with a headache, occasionally accompanied by palpitations. The actual flush proceeds from the head down through the neck, and may progress in a wavelike fashion over the entire body. The subject complains of a feeling of heat or burning that is immediately followed by an outbreak of sweating, particularly involving the head, neck, chest, and back. The length of a flush varies from a few seconds to 30 minutes.

Although the cause of hot flushes is still unknown, recent studies have elucidated profound physiological changes associated with them. Measurement of core temperature as well as levels of various hormones reveals that there is a hiatus between the prodromal symptoms and the actual flush of up to 3 minutes. Skin conductance, a reflection of perspiration, is the first quantifiable sign, followed by an increase in skin temperature reflecting cutaneous blood vessel dilatation. The subject starts to perspire and as a result, core temperature drops an average of 0.2°C. In addition, there is an increase in pulse rate (Fig. 8–4). Mea-

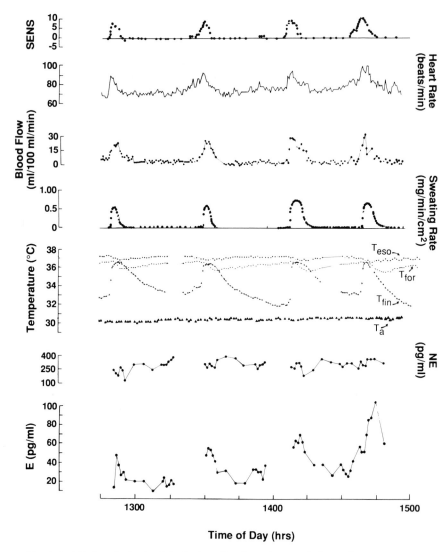

Time of Day (hrs)

Fig. 8–4. The hot flush physiological profile. Four characteristic hot flushes over a period of 2.5 hours in a menopausal woman. *From top to bottom,* patterns of changes in sensation *(SENS),* heart rate, finger blood flow, sweating, temperature (T) (esophageal [*eso*], forehead [*for*], finger [*fin*], arm [*a*]), and epinephrine (*E*) secretion. Many subjects experience a premonition (aura) of an impending hot flush, described as a feeling of unease or anxiety. Heart rate and skin blood flow increases occur rapidly and peak within 3 minutes of onset. The rise in finger temperature follows the vasodilation. The onset of sweating is rapid and occurs primarily on the chest and upper torso, but it may be profuse on the face and scalp. As vasodilation and sweating occur, esophageal (internal core) temperature falls. Each hot flush is usually associated with a sharp rise in epinephrine and, not shown here, with a LH pulse. (From Kronenberg F, Downey JA 1987: *Can J Physiol Pharmacol* 65:1312–1324 with modification.)

98

surement of hormone levels has demonstrated a correlation between pulsatile LH release and the occurrence of hot flushes, although the relationship is not causal. Cortisol, dehydroepiandrosterone (DHEA) and androstenedione are also found to increase with the hot flush, but there is no change in estrogen levels.

While the underlying dynamics of the hot flush are not clear, it appears that estrogen deprivation affects central thermoregulatory function possibly through changes in catecholamines in the central nervous system that control both temperature regulation and GnRH production. This can be reversed by estrogen treatment.

OSTEOPOROSIS

Osteoporosis is one of the most important changes associated with menopause because it has long-range consequences for general health. Maintenance of bone mass is a dynamic process in which bone is constantly being remolded by resorption and reformation. In women, peak bone mass occurs around 30–35 years of age, after which time bone replacement does not keep up with bone resorption, leading to a gradual decrease in skeletal mass with age. The rate of bone loss increases considerably after menopause. The loss is most rapid during the first 3–4 years after menopause, reaching an annual rate of loss of about 2.5%. Thereafter, the rate decreases to about 0.75% per year for the remainder of life. Accordingly, by age 70 years many women have lost 30–50% of their bone mass (Fig. 8–5).

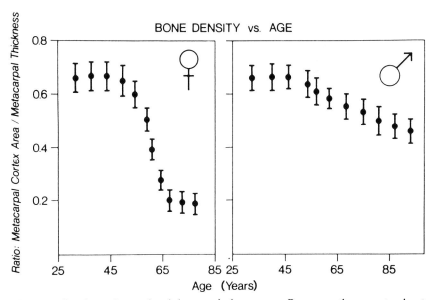

Fig. 8–5. Gender and age-related decrease in bone mass. Bone growth occurs to about 30–35 years of age. After that, loss of bone mass occurs with increasing age in both sexes. In women, there is a profound increase in the rate of decline of bone density after menopause. As a consequence, postmenopausal women have a much higher incidence of fractures than do men of comparable age. (From Soules MR, Bremner WJ 1982: *J Am Geriatr Soc* 30:547. Copyright © by American Geriatrics Society.)

The most striking changes are seen in trabecular bone in which there may be a loss of 50% with aging. Loss of cortical bone tends to develop later than that of trabecular bone and to a lesser extent (approximately 5% of cortical bone is lost). In the early stages of menopause, increased osteoclastic function is accompanied by increased osteoblastic activity (high turnover state), while later, there is a decrease in osteoclastic activity, but osteoblastic function can still not keep up (low turnover state).

It is of interest to note that osteoporosis is less frequent in black than white women and more common in fair-skinned and slim than obese women. Obese women have a higher conversion of androgens to estrogens, which is probably the reason why they are protected to a certain degree against osteoporosis. There is some evidence that smoking increases osteoporosis. Its incidence is lower in areas with high fluoride content in the water. Sodium fluoride concentrates in bone and decreases osteoclastic activity, resulting in calcium retention.

Estrogens are known to play an important role in maintaining normal bone. Most recent available data strongly suggest a decisive role of estrogen deficiency in the development of postmenopausal osteoporosis; however, estrogens are only one of the factors involved in bone metabolism. Further factors involved are parathyroid hormone (PTH), vitamin D, calcitonin, and others. A detailed discussion of all the factors involved in bone metabolism is beyond the scope of this text.

The major effect of estrogens is to inhibit osteoclastic activity and reduce bone resorption; thus, it is antagonistic to the action of parathyroid hormone. Estrogen exerts little effect on osteoblastic function. A decrease in estrogenic activity leads to a marked elevation in plasma calcium, resulting in hypercalciuria and a negative calcium balance. Increased plasma and urinary concentrations of calcium, phosphorus, and hydroxyproline have been reported in postmenopausal women. Several studies also found an increase in parathyroid hormone with age. These changes were reversed following estrogen treatment. Using morphometric techniques, it was found that in postmenopausal women, regardless of age, there is loss of bone mass related to the number of years after menopause. In general, these losses can be prevented by estrogen replacement therapy. Such a treatment results in decreased bone resorption and return of parathyroid hormone to normal levels. Long-term estrogen therapy reduces bone resorption to very low levels. These findings indicate that after menopause, disruption of the normal regulatory mechanisms of bone turnover by parathyroid hormone and lack of gonadal steroids plus an intrinsic abnormality of bone cell function are important in the pathogenesis of osteoporosis.

Osteoporosis is present when the demineralization process becomes severe and symptomatic. Osteoporosis is a major public health problem in the Western world and is becoming more so with increase in longevity. In the United States, osteoporosis may account for as many as 1–2 million fractures each year, including about 350,000 hip fractures, 85% of which are sustained by women. The vertebral body is the most common site of fracture in postmenopausal women. In northern Europe, 25% of women have vertebral fractures by 65 years of age and 50% by age 76 years. Our ability to treat established osteoporosis is very limited.

Prevention by prophylactic administration of estrogen is clearly the most promising approach and produces better results than therapy initiated after the onset of osteoporosis.

GENITOURINARY CHANGES

Some degree of urinary incontinence is common in elderly women. In most cases, this is not caused by gross anatomical changes, but is due to changes in the supporting structures of the bladder neck. Maximal urethral closure pressure decreases with aging, but is increased by estrogen, which probably has a stimulatory effect on the urethral mucosa and smooth muscles.

Lack of estrogens generally causes atrophy of the genital organs. The major problem is atrophy of the vaginal mucosa, which may constrict the vaginal introitus and cause dyspareunia and susceptibility to trauma and infection. Estrogen therapy reverses the atrophic changes.

ATHEROSCLEROSIS AND CARDIOVASCULAR DISEASE

The relationship between estrogens and the pathogenesis of atherosclerosis, myocardial infarction, hypertension, and stroke is still unclear. Several studies have found a possible relation between decreased estrogen production and increased incidence of atherosclerosis. Changes in blood lipids probably play an important role in the genesis of atherosclerosis and cardiovascular disease. An increase in very low-density lipoproteins (VLDL) and in low-density lipoproteins (LDL) appears to be associated with coronary artery disease, while high-density lipoproteins (HDL) appear to be protective. In premenopausal women, HDL levels are higher than in men of the same age and concentrations of VLDL and LDL are lower. After menopause, cholesterol, VLDL, and LDL increase and HDL decrease. Synthetic estrogens (found in oral contraceptives) exaggerate these changes while "natural" estrogens (conjugated estrogens) increase HDL and decrease the other fractions. Thus, conjugated estrogens are more beneficial. Oophorectomy before natural menopause is associated with an increase in coronary artery disease. In a British study, a marked increase in the incidence of coronary heart disease was found in women who stopped menstruating before age 40 years and who were followed for 10–20 years. Blood cholesterol and triglyceride levels in these women were significantly higher than in age-matched controls who continued to menstruate until normal menopause. Thus, there is a suggestion that estrogens have some protective effect; however, solid evidence is still lacking.

Blood pressure rises with age, although the increase in postmenopausal women is gradual and probably not related to estrogen deficiency.

SKIN CHANGES

With menopause, the skin becomes dry, the epidermis becomes thinner, and there is gradual increase in pigmentation, due to an increase in the rate of production of melanin. These changes are gradual and become more accentuated over the years. The skin contains estrogen receptors, and estrogen administration will induce edema of the dermis and increase proliferation of the epidermis.

Therefore, estrogen has a beneficial cosmetic effect. It is difficult, however, to distinguish between the effect of decreased levels of estrogen on the skin and the general effects of aging.

OTHER SYMPTOMS

Gallbladder disease generally increases with age. The risk in healthy women aged 45–69 years is 2.5 times that of younger controls.

Glucose tolerance decreases with age. Although basal insulin levels remain normal, the insulin response to hyperglycemia decreases. There may be a further decrease in the insulin response in women taking estrogen, although there have been no reports of estrogen-precipitated diabetes.

PSYCHOLOGICAL CHANGES

The climacteric is a period in a woman's life when physiological changes are often closely interwoven with psychological and social changes, and at times, it is difficult to separate their clinical effects. Though most of the physiologic symptoms can be explained by the lack of estrogens, understanding the psychological phenomena is more complicated. Many menopausal women report mood swings, depression, anxiety, a sense of frustration, feelings of inadequacy, loneliness, irritability, loss of a sense of well being, loss of libido, headaches, backaches, insomnia, palpitations, and diminished drive, interest, and energy.

While somatic symptoms are usually relieved by estrogen replacement therapy, psychological symptoms are not always alleviated. Many of the symptoms that appear around the climacteric have deep roots in the distant past and for various reasons surface after menopause. An issue commonly encountered at this time of life is that of loss: loss of the ability to reproduce, loss of children as they leave home, loss of the husband's interest, etc. These losses can be handled in a variety of ways, some positive and some negative. The husband's reaction to the wife's emotional strain associated with menopause may severely hinder or aid in her final adjustment.

Although depression may follow estrogen withdrawal, such as after pregnancy, at menopause, or after surgical castration, estrogen treatment does not always alter the psychological symptoms; many patients improve dramatically, but others will require additional therapy. When estrogen therapy does not produce positive results, the addition of minor tranquilizers and hypnotics and supportive therapy can be beneficial.

SEXUALITY IN POSTMENOPAUSAL WOMEN

Most women experience some changes in sexual function during the perimenopausal years and immediately after menopause. The most common sexual complaints include decreased sexual desire, diminished sexual activity and responsiveness, dyspareunia, and a dysfunctional male partner.

Sexual function is influenced by the changes in physiological, psychological, sociocultural, and interpersonal factors. Physiological changes occurring during menopause and related to sexual function include decrease in muscle tension, lack of increase in breast size during sexual stimulation, delay in reaction time of the clitoris, delay and decrease in vaginal lubrication, decrease in vaginal expansion, and many other parameters. Most of these changes are probably caused by alterations in sensory stimulation and blood flow secondary to a decrease in estrogen levels and can be reversed or improved by estrogen replacement. However, the issue is more complex because of the psychological and sociocultural factors involved. Nevertheless, these problems are as important as the other issues of menopause and have to be dealt with in the general management of menopause.

MANAGEMENT OF MENOPAUSE

Menopause is an integral part of the process of aging, and thus it should not be considered an abnormal state. Nevertheless, the menopausal syndrome is a state of hormonal dysfunction resulting from ovarian failure and as such it responds to substitution therapy. Estrogen administration alleviates most menopausal symptoms, including, as outlined earlier, the hot flush, atrophy of the genitourinary tract and, possibly, skin changes. More importantly, there is excellent evidence that estrogen treatment is effective in preventing osteoporosis, one of the main health hazards of older age in women. It is important to point out, however, that our ability to treat established osteoporosis is very limited. Thus, *prevention* is clearly the most promising approach. There is no doubt that prophylactic administration of estrogen produces better results than therapy initiated after the onset of osteoporosis.

The questions of who should be treated, how, and for how long are simple ones, but the answers are complicated. A rational approach to the management of the postmenopausal woman is difficult to adopt because there are no definitive data concerning the efficacy and safety of long-term treatment and the risk/benefit ratio. The major issue is whether long-term prophylactic treatment, mainly to prevent osteoporosis, is advantageous. At present, most physicians advocate prophylactic estrogen therapy to all women who are at risk with careful monitoring. Risk factors for osteoporosis include a small frame, a sedentary lifestyle, early menopause, nulliparity, poor nutrition, cigarette smoking, alcohol abuse, and Caucasian or Asian origins. For maximum benefit, estrogen replacement therapy should be initiated as soon as possible after menopause because once bone mass is lost, estrogen treatment will not replace it.

Most clinicians use oral conjugated estrogens, which are well tolerated. The standard dose for prevention of osteoporosis is 0.625 mg/day. Generally, this dose successfully controls the hot flushes as well as other symptoms. Although conjugated estrogens are most commonly used, other estrogen preparations are available. One to 2 mg of micronized estradiol can be given orally or intravaginally, and recently, topical transdermal administration has been utilized successfully. There are basically two regimens of treatment. In one, estrogen is given continuously and a progestin (medroxyprogesterone acetate, 5–10 mg/day for 10–12 days) is given at monthly intervals. This regimen simulates the ovulatory cycle, and women will have monthly withdrawal bleeding. In the other regimen, estrogen is given for 21–25 days (3 weeks on and 1 week off) and in the last 7 days of estrogen, a progestin is added (medroxyprogesterone acetate, 5–10 mg/day) after which the woman has withdrawal bleeding; a new cycle is started 5 days thereafter. The reason for this regimen is to decrease endometrial stimulation by estrogen. The disadvantage is that the patient is estrogen deficient one-fourth of the time and many women complain of menopausal symptoms during the week when estrogens are lacking.

One of the major issues in long-term estrogen replacement therapy is the relationship between estrogens and cancer. Because of its mitogenic properties on the endometrium, estrogen therapy may lead to an increased risk of endometrial carcinoma. A small focus of cancer, previously undetected, may grow rapidly under estrogen therapy. Overall, however, most studies have not shown estrogens to be carcinogenic. To prevent unopposed estrogenic stimulation and endometrial hyperplasia, a progestin can be added cyclically (as discussed earlier). The latest consensus is that estrogen treatment does not pose an increased risk of breast cancer. In a recent epidemiologic study from Sweden, there was no reported increase in breast cancer in women treated with conjugated estrogens. However, after at least 9 years of treatment with estradiol, the risk of breast cancer doubled. The most disturbing finding in this study was a fourfold increase in the risk of breast cancer in women treated for more than 4 years with estradiol and progestins (medroxyprogesterone). The authors speculated that the combination of estradiol and progestin may be more carcinogenic than estrogen alone. However, this is a study with a small number of patients and there are numerous other studies where no increased incidence of breast carcinoma was found. In the United States, the common practice is to add a progestin to the estrogen for long-term users in order to prevent endometrial hyperplasia and endometrial carcinoma. Nevertheless, a possible increase of breast cancer in postmenopausal women treated with estrogens and progestins must be considered in assessing the risk/benefit factor, particularly since endometrial cancer developing after estrogen treatment is always well differentiated and considerably less lethal than breast cancer; however, if women are followed closely with annual or semiannual physical examinations and mammograms, the risk is minimal.

Other factors are important in the management of postmenopausal changes. The average postmenopausal woman should attain a calcium balance on a daily intake of 1,500 mg calcium. In the United States, most women ingest about 600 mg of calcium daily, and thus may be viewed as calcium deficient. Theoretically, calcium supplementation should help preserve skeletal mass, but the issue of calcium supplementation is controversial and requires further evaluation. Other nutritional factors may enhance the risk of osteoporosis: bone loss is accelerated by excessive intake of alcohol, caffeine, and protein.

Life-style may affect the development of osteoporosis. Physical activity and exercise are extremely important. It is known that weightlessness and immobilization promote bone loss. Active exercise can retard bone loss.

Overall, the most commonly used prophylactic measures to prevent osteoporosis in the menopausal woman include primarily estrogen replacement therapy, supported by a program of regular weight-bearing exercise, adequate dietary measures, and most probably a supplementary calcium intake since calcium absorption declines with age.

9

The Abnormal Menstrual Cycle: Introduction

The first task in the evaluation of the patient consulting for infertility is to determine whether the menstrual cycle is "normal". Thus, the usual initial diagnostic steps include a review of the main physiological events that characterize the ovulatory cycle coupled with clinical observation and the use of simple clinical tests to pinpoint the event that may be deficient.

THE OVULATORY MENSTRUAL CYCLE: AN INTEGRATIVE DESCRIPTION

The normal menstrual cycle is the result of the precise coordination of various events or sequences of events taking place in different locations of the organism, most notably the hypothalamus, the pituitary gland, the ovaries, and the reproductive tract. Local cyclic events in each of these systems have been reviewed in separate preceding chapters. Here, we will provide an integrative schematic description of the normal ovulatory menstrual cycle. The events described here are represented in Figure 9–1.

1. The menstrual cycle is initiated when conditions allow for the preferential release of follicle-stimulating hormone (FSH), the hormone that promotes folliculogenesis. Consequently, a cohort of follicles is recruited from the follicle stockpile and the follicular phase starts.

2. FSH promotes granulosa cell growth and differentiation and stimulates the enzyme aromatase that converts androgens to estrogens. Estradiol concentrations increase slowly within the follicles and in the peripheral circulation.

3. Within a few days, one of the follicles in the cohort has become dominant. Increasing estradiol concentrations, through activation of the long loop negative feedback, decrease luteinizing hormone (LH) and FSH pulse amplitude. Diminished gonadotropin concentrations, in turn, will slow down the growth of all cohort follicles, but the dominant one: they become atretic. The dominant follicle continues to grow, presumably because critical stimulatory concentrations of gonadotropins are able to reach it, due to specific morphological characteristics acquired early on in the process of selection.

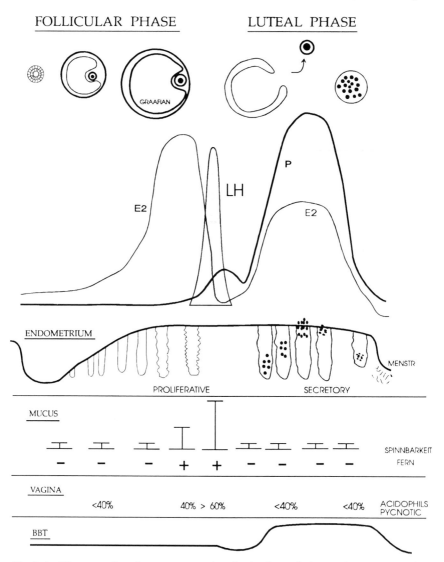

Fig. 9-1. The normal ovulatory menstrual cycle. A schematic integrative representation of the hormonal, morphological, and thermal (basal body temperature [BBT]) changes that characterize the normal ovulatory menstrual cycle. See text for details. *E2*, estradiol-17β; *LH*, luteinizing hormone; *MENSTR*, menstruation; *P*, progesterone.

4. The dominant follicle acquires LH receptors. LH stimulates the biosynthesis of androgens within the theca layer of the follicle; upon transport into the granulosa, these androgens are metabolized into estrogens. Estradiol is highly mitogenic and potentiates several local growth factors; thus, the selected follicle will grow rapidly and in a few days become a fully mature graafian follicle. Reflecting the dramatic maturational growth of the graafian follicle, estradiol

concentrations rise almost exponentially during the final stage of the follicular phase.

5. Maturity of the graafian follicle is marked by high circulating concentrations of estradiol, the signal to the hypothalamus and pituitary gland that the follicle is ready for the ovulatory signal. The long loop estradiol positive feedback is activated, and, as a result, the gonadotropin surge occurs.

6. The high gonadotropin concentrations during the surge arrest granulosa cell proliferation and secretory activity in the graafian follicle. Estradiol secretion declines rapidly. Granulosa cells begin to luteinize, and as a consequence, a small preovulatory rise of progesterone occurs. Ovulation, the release of the fully grown oocyte, occurs about 18 hours following the gonadotropin "peak", or at least 36 hours after the "initiation" of the surge. At ovulation, the oocyte resumes meiosis.

7. After release of the oocyte, the granulosa layer becomes vascularized, and the granulosa cell completes the process of luteinization, whereby it acquires de novo steroid synthesis capacity that it previously lacked. LH stimulates progesterone and estradiol secretion for this newly formed structure, the corpus luteum. Progesterone in combination with estradiol, in turn, activates the hypothalamic opiate center, the result of which is to decrease gonadotropin pulse frequency.

8. The corpus luteum is a transient organ that has an inherent 12–15 day life span. Thus, estradiol and progesterone secretion peaks about 7–9 days after its formation.

9. Luteolysis, the process of regression of the corpus luteum, results in a rapid decline in progesterone and estradiol concentrations. This leads to ischemia of the superficial layers of the uterine mucosa and necrosis of the uterine blood vessels with resulting menstruation.

10. Through a combination of several factors, which may include the long period of decreased pulse frequency during the luteal phase, a decrease in inhibin secretion and/or of estradiol and progesterone secretion, FSH concentrations increase relatively to those of LH, and a new cycle is initiated.

THE INITIAL CLINICAL EVALUATION OF THE ABNORMAL CYCLE

THE FIRST TWO ESSENTIAL QUESTIONS

In many cases, initial evaluation centers on the documentation of whether ovulatory or anovulatory cycles occur. Thus, the evaluation will require first the answer to two questions: (1) Does follicular maturation occur? and (2) Does the patient ovulate?

In the initial evaluation process, it is sufficient to remember that each of the two phenomena alluded to in these questions is characterized by a dominant steroid background: estrogen during follicular maturation, progesterone after ovulation. In turn, each steroid affects the organism, especially the reproductive tract, differently (see Chapter 5). Observation of these physiological effects provides the physician with a set of simple diagnostic tools, usually sufficient to answer these questions.

The Genital Tract

Under estradiol dominance, the mucus becomes fluid and abundant: greatest release of mucus and maximal spinnbarkeit (an elasticlike quality to the mucus) will occur simultaneously with the estradiol peak, and, hence, signify follicular maturation. Under progesterone dominance, the cervical mucus becomes acidic and viscous (the uterine cavity becomes effectively sealed in preparation for embryo arrival and implantation). The vaginal epithelium, as monitored by the vaginal smear, is similarly affected by the two ovarian steroids. In practice, the major usefulness of the vaginal smear as a diagnostic tool is to detect estradiol production.

Observations of significant quantities of watery endocervical mucus with ferning and high spinnbarkeit and vaginal smears with a high index of pycnotic and acidophilic cells provide good evidence of significant estradiol secretion; hence, these tests are excellent indices that follicular maturation is progressing successfully. This conclusion can be supported in the anovulatory patient by the progesterone withdrawal test which challenges the adequacy of estrogen production: in the presence of previous estrogenic stimulation of the endometrium, a treatment with progesterone (typically a 5-day treatment with medroxyprogesterone acetate, 10 mg/day) will, upon its termination, result in menstrual bleeding.

If these genital tract tests are negative, this may signify either low levels of estradiol secretion (as occurs normally during the early follicular phase, or as may be indicative of inadequate folliculogenesis), *or* an active luteal phase. Sequential observations can, of course, differentiate between a normal or interrupted follicular phase.

Basal Body Temperature

The presence of a luteal phase can be best established initially by monitoring the basal body temperature (BBT). Progesterone acts on the hypothalamic thermoregulatory center to increase BBT. Usually, a significant rise in temperature occurs about 2 days after the peak of the LH surge and remains for the duration of the luteal phase (14 $\pm$ 1.5 days). Thus, the BBT chart in an ovulatory cycle will always be *biphasic,* reflecting the higher baseline temperature during the 2-week life span of the corpus luteum (Fig. 9–2). A biphasic temperature curve signifies the presence of an active corpus luteum and, hence, indicates that ovulation has occurred. When the BBT curve is flat or erratic (e.g., temperature rises do not exceed a few days), the cycle can be described as anovulatory. A simple basal thermometer, a chart, and the willingness to take the temperature every morning is all that is required to assess this aspect of the cycle. The patient should be encouraged to record BBT for extended periods of time, even though this may become frustrating in the absence of results.

Ultrasonography

Recent developments in *ultrasonography,* particularly the transvaginal approach, are now allowing for accurate assessment of ovarian development and

BASAL BODY TEMPERATURE CHART

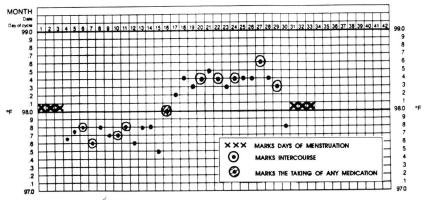

Fig. 9–2. A biphasic basal body temperature *(BBT)* curve, typical of a normal ovulatory cycle. Because the shift in temperature is modest, special care must be taken to monitor the BBT curve, which must be recorded daily in the morning before arising from bed. To be diagnostic of ovulation, the rise in temperature must last a minimum of 12 days, the lifetime of the corpus luteum.

this method is used extensively in the new reproductive technology. The transvaginal transducer enables detailed visualization of follicular development. In the natural cycle, usually only one follicle becomes dominant (see Chapter 4). Once the leading follicle reaches a diameter of 14 mm, the daily growth rate is approximately 1.5–2.0 mm until ovulation when follicular diameter is 20–24 mm (Fig. 9–3). With ovulation-inducing drugs, such as human menopausal gonadotropin (hMG), several follicles reach this stage (multiple ovulation) and this can also be accurately assessed sonographically. This technique may also be used to assist in egg retrieval in in vitro fertilization (IVF) programs (see Chapter 13).

The endometrium undergoes typical changes during the menstrual cycle (Chapter 5); these can also be assessed sonographically. From a thin echo during

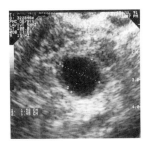 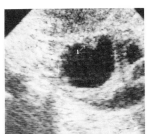 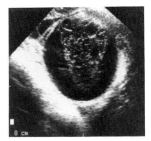

Fig. 9–3. Ultrasonography of the normal ovary. Ultrasonographical representation of the dominant follicle (day 12 of the cycle) *(left);* the preovulatory follicle *(arrow* indicates cumulus mass) *(center),* and of a corpus luteum *(right).* (From Timor-Tritsch IE, Rottem S 1987: *Transvaginal Sonography,* Elsevier, NY. Reprinted by permission of the publisher.)

menses, the endometrium gradually enlarges through the proliferative phase as indicated by changes in thickness and texture. Before ovulation, in the mid–late follicular phase, the endometrium is represented by three lines. An inner lumina interface is surrounded by the functional hypoechogenic endometrium and the echogenic myometrial-endometrial interface. Increasing thickness of the endometrium is associated with higher estrogen levels. An endometrial thickness of less than 5 mm usually indicates the early follicular phase. In the late follicular phase, endometrial thickness approaches 10 mm (Fig. 9–4). After ovulation has occurred, the rise in progesterone causes an increase in stromal edema that appears sonographically as an increase in echogenicity. The luteal phase begins with an increase in peripheral echogenicity that gradually progresses to the lumen and eventually causes its obliteration.

Other Clinical Tests

There are other clinical tests which, in practice, may be useful in the initial diagnostic procedures. Some are listed here.

Abnormal secretion of *androgens* clinically expressed as hirsutism, may interfere with the process of the normal menstrual cycle, and must be excluded (Chapter 12 deals specifically with this problem). Elevated concentrations of *prolactin* are usually accompanied by menstrual irregularity (see Chapter 10). This hormone should be measured during the initial evaluation process, if menses are irregular or absent.

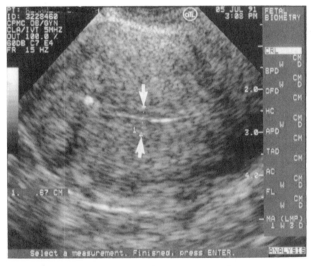

Fig. 9–4. Ultrasonography of the endometrium. Endometrium (arrows indicate thickness) in longitudinal section on day 12 of the menstrual cycle. (From Timor-Tritsch IE, Rottem S 1987: *Transvaginal Sonography,* Elsevier, NY. Reprinted by permission of the publisher.)

Postcoital test. The postcoital test is used to assess cervical mucus and semen, as well as the interaction between the two. The test should be carried out as close to the time of ovulation as possible, the period when the quality of cervical mucus is optimal for semen receptivity. Since spermatozoa can live in estrogen-ized midcycle mucus for at least 48 hours, this gives some leeway in coordinating the test with intercourse. (Too often, the patient is told to report for the test within 2–3 hours of intercourse, placing undue and unnecessary stress on the couple.) In a normal postcoital test, at least five to six actively motile sperma-tozoa per high power field are seen (magnification × 400). The test is considered abnormal if spermatozoa are absent, only dead spermatozoa are seen, sperma-tozoa are moving in place without progression, or the cervical mucus is too thick with poor spinnbarkeit at the time of ovulation.

The most common cause of abnormal or inadequate results is the improper timing of the postcoital test with regard to the menstrual cycle. If the test is ordered too early or too late in the cycle, the mucus will be inadequate for sperm survival: the test should be repeated at the appropriate time. Of course, this can-not be done if the patient fails to produce normal amounts of estrogen. Patho-logical causes for a poor postcoital test include cervicitis, abnormal semen, and, in rare instances, the presence of antisperm antibodies in the cervical mucus.

Hysterosalpingography. The hysterosalpingogram gives a radiographic evalua-tion of the anatomy of the genital tract, documenting the normal shape of the uterus and patency of the fallopian tubes. It should be performed in the early follicular phase of the cycle, as soon as menstrual bleeding has stopped. A small amount of radiopaque dye (3–5 ml) is injected transcervically and several x-rays are taken. The results will reveal the state of the uterine cavity, patency of the tubes and, sometimes, presence of peritubal adhesions. There has been some evi-dence that the procedure itself is therapeutic, in addition to being diagnostically accurate.

For best results, it is recommended that not only the radiologist but also the physician be present during hysterosalpingography. In this way, the actual pro-cedure can be adapted to specific needs as the path of the dye shows on the tele-vision monitor. The dye may be oil-based or water-based: there are as yet no definitive data to resolve this issue, although there are some indications that pregnancy rates are somewhat higher when an oil-based medium is used. Hys-terosalpingography can, in rare instances, result in allergic reactions or infec-tions. Women who are allergic to iodine or are suspected of having occult infec-tions should not undergo this procedure.

Endometrial biopsy. An endometrial biopsy provides another simple and useful index documenting endometrial development and, hence, the hormonal and ovulatory status. It should be done as close to menstruation as possible, but before the actual onset of blood flow. While other parameters have been used to assess ovulation (e.g., progesterone measurement or BBT records), the biopsy is more accurate and informative as it is a biological end point which reflects the various events of the ongoing cycle.

The biopsy is an easy office procedure, taking less than a minute to perform. The patient notes the day of onset of the next menstrual period and the dating of the tissue obtained is correlated with this information. During the cycle, the histological changes of the endometrium are typical and can be dated quite accurately. A discrepancy of more than 2 days between the actual day of the cycle and the day estimated on the histological slide occurring in consecutive cycles is diagnostic of an inadequate luteal phase.

Although small, there is a chance that the endometrial biopsy can abort an existing early pregnancy. A sensitive urinary pregnancy test (for β-human chorionic gonadotropin [hCG]) should be done prior to the biopsy, or the patient should be asked to use a barrier contraceptive in order to eliminate this concern.

Laparoscopy. The last test done in the regular infertility workup is a laparoscopy/hysteroscopy. It is performed when all other tests are normal, or when there is reason to suspect intra-abdominal pathology (such as endometriosis, or pelvic adhesions). Laparoscopy is scheduled in the early to midfollicular phase of the cycle in order to avoid disrupting a pregnancy. At this stage of the cycle, the endometrium is low, allowing for accurate tubal patency studies while minimizing false negative results. Hysteroscopy is also easier at this time of low endometrium. If focal endometriotic lesions are found, they are more prominent, easier to spot and to cauterize (using electric cautery or laser).

Since each of the tests mentioned must be carefully timed at different stages of the menstrual cycle, the infertility workup may take several months to complete. There is little reason to rush the procedures (especially laparoscopy) since about 25% of infertile patients conceive spontaneously with time. Additionally, many of these tests have some therapeutic value, and time should be allowed in order to take full advantage of it. In the case of older women (late 30s–early 40s), however, or when a particular problem is suspected, there may be a need to speed up the workup. In the rare instance where tumors are suspected, the diagnosis is more difficult: it may take time and require sophisticated and expensive tests. Recently, the use of ultrasound, magnetic resonance imagery (MRI), and selective catheterization techniques (in the case of adrenal tumors) have greatly improved diagnostic abilities.

Non-routine tests. Two other tests are available for the assessment of infertility. They are not part of the routine evaluation as they are aimed at specific, suspected problems. When a properly timed postcoital test reveals that, although the semen analysis is normal, spermatozoa are moving in place or are nonmotile within the mucus, or when long-standing unexplained infertility is present, the possibility of *antisperm antibodies* has to be contemplated. Specific tests for antisperm antibodies in cervical mucus, serum and seminal plasma are available. The significance of these tests in regard to infertility workup, however, is not always clear-cut: there can be poor correlation between antibody presence and infertility and some patients are known to conceive in the presence of these antibodies. Antisperm antibodies have also been found in idiopathic infertility with normal postcoital tests, but, again, it is not known if they are the cause of infertility. *The hamster egg penetration test* is aimed at assessing the ability of spermatozoa to undergo capacitation and achieve fertilization. Egg penetration that is equal to or greater than 10% is considered normal. In the absence of any other abnormal findings, low values on this test, which reflect poor penetration or a lack of sperm penetration into the egg, may suggest the existence of subtle factors that affect the ability of sperm to penetrate and fertilize the egg. Clinical relevance of such results remains to be established, however, especially since pregnancy can still occur under these circumstances.

10

Introduction to the Pathophysiology of the Menstrual Cycle

There are numerous conditions under which the menstrual cycle may become abnormal, that is, irregular, lengthened, shortened, anovulatory, or simply absent. In general, the diagnosis of the condition and the treatment of the resultant infertility are quite easy and successful. The search for the primary cause of the disorder, however, is frequently unsuccessful. In reviewing the normal physiology of the reproductive process, it is easy to understand the difficulty the clinician has in pinpointing the single factor originally responsible for the abnormal condition. For instance, a small deficiency in the estradiol signal could rapidly lead to inappropriate gonadotropin-releasing hormone (GnRH) and gonadotropin secretion, which in turn would result in further derangement of ovarian secretion, and further dysfunction of the hypothalamic-pituitary unit. By the time the patient seeks medical advice, anovulation may have set in, and the initial disturbance is impossible to trace. An additional problem is that neurohormones cannot be measured in the peripheral circulation, and thus categorizations such as hypothalamic amenorrhea are presumptive and sometimes do not reflect the primary disturbance responsible for anovulation.

In the last few years, however, attempts have been made to understand some of the pathophysiological mechanisms that may lead to cyclic disturbance, anovulation, and/or infertility. Although the experimental approach may not necessarily be relevant to successful therapeutical resolution of the infertility problem, it is of general interest to review some of the data at this point. We will review cyclic disturbances due to abnormalities in the function of the GnRH pulse generator, in hypothalamic-pituitary-ovarian communication, and in prolactin secretion.

ABNORMALITIES OF THE GnRH PULSE GENERATOR

Since the gonadotrope appears to be programmed to respond only to pulsatile (intermittent) GnRH stimulation (see Chapter 2), it is clear that an intact GnRH pulse generator is required for a normal menstrual cycle. Thus, in the absence

114

of a functional pulse generator, gonadotropin secretion is lacking and the ovaries remain unstimulated: this characterizes the hypogonadotropic hypogonadism syndrome. A particular variation of this dysfunction is Kallmann's syndrome, in which hypogonadotropism is accompanied by anosmia; possibly, the GnRH neuron's journey from the olfactory area (where it originates) (see Chapter 2) is halted with complete or partial failure to migrate into the brain. The neuron then may fail to establish its normal connections, with a resultant deficit in GnRH secretion. Similar defects may prevent olfactory nerve development, leading to the lack of smell.

In the presence of an active GnRH pulse generator, gonadotropin release is stimulated and the morphological and secretory processes in the ovary are initiated. Recently, it has become apparent that optimal follicular growth not only requires pulsatile gonadotropin release but also a proper pulse frequency. In GnRH-deficient monkeys, for instance, a normal follicular process can be restored with hourly GnRH pulses. Lower pulse frequencies will be less effective, and, at a frequency of 1 pulse/3 h, follicular maturation does not occur and of course the cycle is anovulatory (Fig. 10–1). This requirement for proper pulse frequency in regard to follicular maturation has been demonstrated in the human and other species as well, although the optimal frequency window varies with the species (1 GnRH pulse/90 min in the human, 1 GnRH pulse/45 min in the rat). This frequency is, of course, close to that which characterizes the follicular phase of the normal cycle.

"HYPOTHALAMIC" AMENORRHEA

Recent observations have clearly demonstrated that, while the hypothalamic-pituitary-ovarian axis is capable of maintaining ovulatory cyclicity on its own, multiple endogenous or environmental influences may impinge on the normal activity of the pulse generator usually to decrease GnRH pulse frequency and thereby induce cyclic dysfunction. These conditions are usually diagnosed as hypothalamic amenorrhea. Frequent causes of hypothalamic amenorhea are related to *exercise, diet,* or *stress.* Interference with normal cyclicity can be pronounced; however, normal cyclicity is readily restored in most patients following removal of the condition.

Exercise and Cyclicity

In women, exercise, particularly of a strenuous nature such as jogging, swimming, or ballet dancing, can have a profound effect on the reproductive cycle (and also on the sexual maturation process, see Chapter 7). The amount of exercise and its intensity, particularly of an endurance nature, appears to influence the reported frequency of the problem. In runners, for example, reproductive dysfunction occurs in 8–15% of women running less than 20 miles a week, but in 25–50% if running more than 70 miles a week.

Athletic training is associated with unambiguous reduced luteinizing hormone (LH) pulse frequency. Reduction in pulse frequency, of course, results in defects in the follicular maturation process, and, hence, cyclic abnormalities; the degree of pulse inhibition will determine whether the menstrual cycle will be

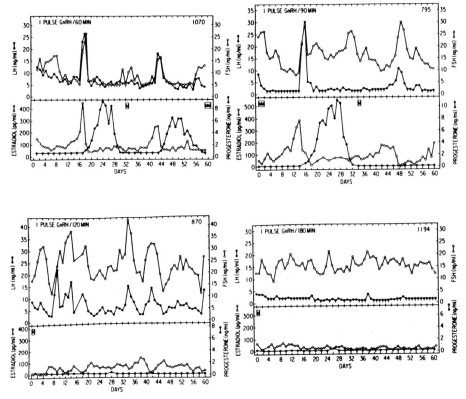

Fig. 10–1. Gonadotropin-releasing hormone (GnRH) pulse frequency and folliculogenesis. An optimal GnRH pulse frequency ensures proper follicular maturation. This is illustrated in an experiment performed in monkeys lacking endogenous GnRH following a lesion of the arcuate hypothalamic region. GnRH pulses were given for a period of 2 months at four different frequencies. With a 1 pulse/h frequency (the optimal pulse frequency in this species), normal folliculogenesis is obtained, and the two observed cycles are ovulatory, as indicated by the increase in progesterone. With slower frequencies, folliculogenesis deteriorates, and, at 1 pulse/2 h, the "cycle" becomes anovulatory. *FSH,* follicle-stimulating hormone; *LH,* luteinizing hormone; M or MM, menstruation. (From Pohl CR, Richardson DW, Hutchison JJ, Germak JA, Knobil E 1983: Hypophysiotropic signal frequency and the functioning of the pituitary ovarian system in the rhesus monkey. *Endocrinology* 112:2076–2080. Copyright © by The Endocrine Society.)

only slightly disturbed or whether the woman will be anovulatory, with several degrees of gradation in between (Fig. 10–2).

The amount of suppression of gonadotropin secretion will also determine the degree of inhibition of estradiol secretion, a potential worrisome feature for long-term well being, particularly in regard to premature osteoporosis.

Weight Loss and Cyclicity

There appears to be a correlation between weight loss and menstrual cycle abnormalities. In fact, amenorrhea appears to be more common in athletic groups, such as ballet dancers, where dieting may be part of the picture. In most species, inadequate nutrition is usually accompanied by a decrease in reproduc-

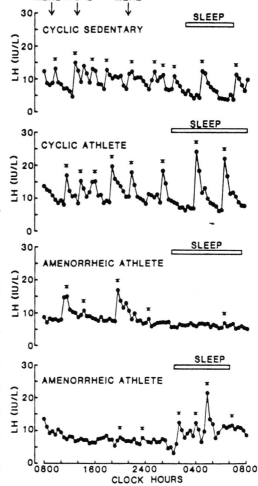

Fig.10–2. Athletic training and the menstrual cycle. Exercise influences pulsatile LH activity in women athletes, the severity of the inhibition depending on the strenuousness of the exercise and the particular sensitivity of each individual. With ongoing function of the GnRH pulse generator, the athlete continues to have normal ovulatory menstrual cycles. Menstrual cycle disturbances will parallel the severity of the decrease in pulse frequency Abbreviation as in Figure 10–1. (From Loucks AB, Mortola JF, Girton L, Yen SSC 1989: Alterations in the hypothalamic-pituitary-ovarian and the hypothalamic-pituitary-adrenal axes in athletic women. *J Clin Endocrinol Metab* 68:402–411. Copyright © by The Endocrine Society.)

tive function. In the adult, this is usually translated by a cessation of gonadotropin release, accompanied by decreased pituitary stores of the hormone, probably the result of a suppression of the activity of the GnRH pulse generator. In the *anorexia nervosa* syndrome, or starvation amenorrhea, behavioral changes and weight loss, both of which can be extreme, are always accompanied by amenorrhea. Endocrine studies in these patients reveal low gonadotropin concentrations and a decreased pulse frequency reminiscent of the prepubertal period. These are accompanied by extreme estrogen deficiency. With recovery, increased pulsatility occurs and menstrual cyclicity may return (Fig. 10–3).

Stress and Cyclicity

In various animal species, conditions such as high population density or environmental stress will interfere with the normal reproductive process. In the primate, physical or psychological stress may produce chronic amenorrhea. There

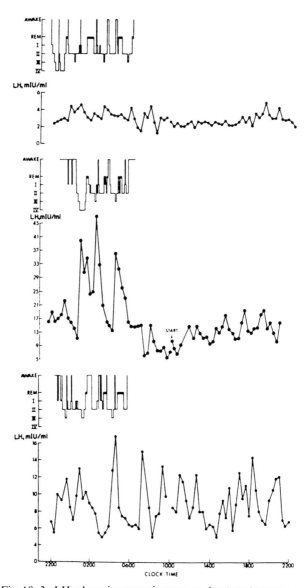

Fig. 10–3. LH release in anorexia nervosa. A return to prepubertal gonadotropin secretory patterns is usually seen during the active anorexia nervosa syndrome *(upper panel)*. Clinical remission and a return of body weight to normal will be accompanied by a return of gonadotropin secretion to a normal adult pattern *(lower panel)*. An intermediary stage, resembling stage 1 of puberty (nocturnal pulsatile increase, see Fig. 7–2), has also been documented and may represent an early stage of remission of the syndrome *(middle panel)*. This can also be observed in patients with excercise-induced amenorrhea (see Fig. 10–2). Abbreviation as in Figure 10–1. (From Boyar RM, Katz J, Finkelstein JW, Kapen S, Weiner H, Weitzman ED, Hellman L 1974: *N Engl J Med* 291:861. Reprinted by permission of *The New England Journal of Medicine.*)

118

have been several hypotheses as to the mechanism or chain of events whereby stressful stimuli decrease pulsatile LH secretion. In animals, a wide range of stimuli can modify catecholamines, not only peripherally but also locally within the hypothalamus. Psychological disorders which may produce amenorrhea may also mirror neurotransmitter pathology. Drugs, such as the phenothiazines, are known both to induce cyclic abnormalities and central nervous system (C.N.S.) catecholamines alterations. Stress, probably through the catecholamines, also activates the hypothalamic-pituitary-adrenal axis and hypercortisolism is associated with cyclic irregularities or anovulation.

A major progress in our understanding of how stress may influence gonadotropin secretion comes from the recent demonstration that corticotropin-releasing hormone (CRH), the major neurohormonal stimulus to the pituitary-adrenal axis, can inhibit the GnRH pulse generator (Fig. 10–4). Although CRH administration activates the adrenal axis and cortisol secretion, its acute inhibitory action on LH is exerted through a central effect on GnRH without the involvement of the adrenal gland. Interestingly, this inhibitory effect of CRH is the result of activation of central endogenous opioid peptide release; indeed, this CRH effect can be prevented by the simultaneous administration of an opiate

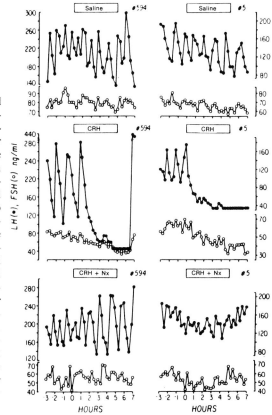

Fig. 10–4. The adrenal axis and gonadotropin secretion. Administration of corticotropin-releasing hormone *(CRH)*, the major neurohormonal stimulus to the pituitary-adrenal axis, results in an acute inhibition of LH secretion through a direct central effect. This is illustrated in two ovariectomized monkeys *(middle panel; upper panels* are saline control infusions). This inhibitory action of CRH is mediated by the endogenous opiates and can be reversed by the administration of naloxone *(Nx) (lower panel).* Abbreviations as in Figure 10–1. (From Gindoff PR, Ferin M 1987: Endogenous opioid peptides modulate the effect of CRH on gonadotropin release in the primate. *Endocrinology* 121:837–842. Copyright © by The Endocrine Society.)

antagonist. These experimental results suggest that cyclic irregularities during "stress" may in part reflect increased CRH activity within the C.N.S. and a resultant enhanced opiate tone. This conclusion finds support in observations that naloxone can restore normal pulsatile gonadotropin release in some patients with amenorrhea, and by measurements of increased levels of immunoreactive CRH in cerebrospinal fluid obtained from anovulatory patients with the anorexia nervosa syndrome, where, undoubtedly, stress plays a role.

Although interference with the reproductive cycle in hypothalamic amenorrhea induced by diet, exercise, or stress can be pronounced, normal ovulatory cyclicity is readily restored in most patients following removal of the condition. A particularly striking example is illustrated in Figure 10–3. There is no evidence that training leads to permanent menstrual dysfunction. It is of interest to note that return to normalcy in some of these patients is first expressed as a nocturnal sleep-related increase in pulsatile activity (see bottom panel of Fig. 10–2, or middle panel of Fig. 10–3). This type of circadian pulsatile release pattern is reminiscent of that which characterizes the first maturational stage at puberty (see Chapter 7), suggesting that the reactivation process that characterizes both pubertal development and improvement in the hypothalamic amenorrhea syndrome may represent facets of the same phenomenon. In this regard, experimental studies of the pubertal process and specifically the identification of the still unknown factor(s) that prevent(s) normal pulsatile activity throughout infancy will undoubtedly help in the diagnosis and possibly the therapy of the hypothalamic syndrome itself. These patterns have been well documented in patients with the anorexia nervosa syndrome, in whom weight gain reverses prepubertal LH secretion patterns (absence of pulsatile release), first to the pubertal (sleep-related night increases) then to the adult pattern (24 h pulsatility).

OTHER DISTURBANCES

Although abnormal pulsatile patterns usually translate into a decrease in pulse frequency, there have been sporadic observations of increased pulse frequency as well. For instance, a small percentage of patients with the polycystic ovarian syndrome have been described as having a higher than normal pulse frequency. Since it has been demonstrated that a high GnRH pulse frequency favors the secretion of LH over that of follicle-stimulating hormone (FSH) (see Chapter 2), it may be speculated that this may have played a role in the overproduction of LH. In turn, increased LH secretion may induce abnormally high androgen concentrations, a major characteristic of this syndrome (see Chapter 12).

ABNORMALITIES IN HYPOTHALAMIC-PITUITARY-OVARIAN
COMMUNICATION: ASYNCHRONY OF PITUITARY AND
OVARIAN EVENTS

A crucial step in the menstrual cycle is the precise synchronization between the process of follicular maturation and the signal to ovulation, that is, the gonadotropin surge. Synchrony is important, because the time frame within which a follicle can ovulate is limited. A premature gonadotropin surge occurring when the follicle has not attained full maturity may, in fact, destroy the follicle des-tined for ovulation, while a long delayed surge will find a mature follicle that has lost its ability to ovulate. Asynchrony may physiologically occur in the early phase of reproductive life because of immaturity of the long loop estradiol pos-itive feedback; hence, several of the first cycles that follow menarche are usually anovulatory. A similar phenomenon may occasionally be observed during the premenopausal period. Of course, one should also keep this synchronization process in mind in therapeutical approaches in which the ovulatory signal is administered in the form of human chorionic gonadotropin (hCG): injection of this hormone must be properly timed in regard to follicular maturation (see Chapter 13).

ABNORMALITIES IN THE LONG LOOP NEGATIVE
FEEDBACK

Studies of ovarian-pituitary feedback clearly suggest that slight disturbances in negative feedback regulation may result in abnormal menstrual cycles. For example, quantitative relationships between ovarian steroids and FSH release determine the amounts of FSH released at the end of a menstrual cycle: subnor-mal FSH release or abnormal FSH:LH ratios during the intermenstrual period may result in deficient follicular growth, a delay in ovulation, and/or deficiencies in the secretory activity of the corpus luteum (presumably because of decreased amount of tissue available for luteinization), decreased progesterone secretion (the inadequate luteal phase syndrome), and potential adverse effects on the implantation process.

Shifts in sensitivity of the neural structures responsive to the long loop estra-diol negative feedback are thought to participate in the later part of the pubertal process (the "gonadostat" theory, Chapter 8). They have also been shown to account for seasonal variations in fertility in some animal species. A good exam-ple of such a seasonal breeder is the sheep. In this animal, LH pulse frequency and amplitude vary with the time of year. These changes in pulse characteristics play a major role in switching the gonadal axis *on* or *off* depending on the season. During anestrus, photoperiodically controlled inhibitory neurons hold GnRH pulse frequency in check; thus, a slow pulse frequency prevents normal follicular recruitment and ovulation. This can be reverted experimentally by a proper GnRH pulsatile infusion, in which case a normal follicular phase ensues. A sim-ilar process, in fact, occurs spontaneously when the breeding season resumes, at which time the hypothalamic signal resumes a frequency compatible with follic-ular recruitment and maturation. Experimental results demonstrate that there is, in ovariectomized ewes, a major seasonal difference in serum LH concentra-tions in response to constant serum estradiol infusion levels (Fig. 10–5): LH lev-els in these animals are extremely low during the period when anestrus normally occurs, whereas they increase considerably during what should be the breeding season. These results illustrate how photoperiod-controlled changes in the sen-sitivity to the estradiol negative feedback loop govern seasonal reproductive function in this species. Of course, profound seasonality changes such as those observed in the sheep are not seen in the human; however, a shift in the sensi-

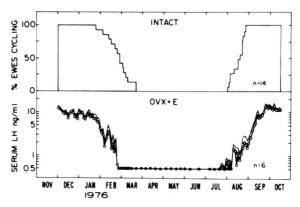

Fig. 10–5. Seasonal changes in sensitivity of the long loop estradiol negative feedback. The sheep is a seasonal breeder. *A*, incidence of estrous cycles in intact ewes with time of year; *B*, LH concentrations in ovariectomized ewes treated with the same amount of estradiol throughout the year. The inhibitory action of estradiol is much increased during the spring–summer anestrous months than in the breeding season, due to a change in negative feedback loop sensitivity. A low sensitivity allows for an increase in gonadotropins during the reproductive months (winter). *E* = estradiol, *OVX*, ovariectomized; other abbreviations as in Figure 10–1. (From Legan SJ, Karsch F 1979: *Biol Reprod* 20:74.)

tivity of the structures responsive to the estradiol negative feedback have been evoked in a few reports as a possible cause of anovulation in cases of amenorrhea. Reports of this type, however, are scant, and this phenomenon, although fascinating, remains to be confirmed in well-controlled studies in the human.

Abnormal feedback may also result from an inappropriate release of estrogens, either from ovarian origin, or from nonovarian origin. In pathological situations, such as Cushing's syndrome, congenital adrenal hyperplasia, the polycystic ovarian syndrome, or androgen-secreting tumors in the ovary or adrenals, estrogen precursor availability is increased and extraglandular production of estrogen may become excessive. Because the increase in estrogen is *acyclic* and not under the control of gonadotropins, the original estradiol feedback signals are distorted or masked, and menstrual irregularity may ensue.

THE INADEQUATE LUTEAL PHASE

The inadequate luteal phase syndrome occurs under various circumstances, most of which are not well understood. It is thought to reflect subtle changes in hormonal secretion during the follicular phase, an indication of a poor follicular maturation process. These changes may include a low FSH:LH ratio at the start of the follicular phase, altered follicular LH pulse frequency, and low estradiol or inhibin concentrations. These, in turn, lead to a deficient gonadotropin surge and inadequate luteinization. In general, this pattern results in blunted progesterone secretion (Fig. 10–6). The syndrome is observed with increased frequency in women at a later reproductive age, especially in the context of infertility (probably because of better analytic techniques). It is also a frequent occurrence in the

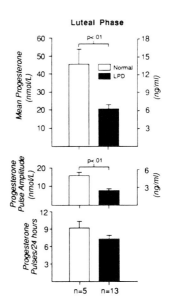

Fig. 10–6. The inadequate luteal phase. Luteal phase deficiency *(LPD)* is a reproductive disorder frequently associated with infertility and early abortion. The syndrome is characterized by deficient luteinization and formation of the corpus luteum, reflected in a significant decrease in the amounts of progesterone secreted. Insufficient progesterone, in turn, causes an abnormal secretory activity of the endometrium. (From Soules MR, Clifton DK, Cohen NL, Bremner WJ, Steiner RA 1989: Luteal phase deficiency: abnormal gonadotropin and progesterone secretion patterns. *J Clin Endocrinol Metab* 69:813–820. Copyright © by The Endocrine Society.)

initial stages of hypothalamic amenorrhea related to stress, exercise, or diet (discussed earlier). The relationship to infertility reflects interference with implantation or recurrent first trimester abortion, which results from deficient progesterone secretion by the corpus luteum and abnormal secretory activity of the endometrium. It has been estimated that the incidence of inadequate luteal phase in infertile women is about 3.5%, although it may be as high as 35% in habitual early aborters.

It is not possible to diagnose accurately an inadequate luteal phase by basal body temperature (BBT) measurements or assay of one plasma progesterone level. Increases in BBT may occur in the presence of subnormal progesterone concentrations. Serial daily progesterone measurements throughout the luteal phase would be diagnostic, but this is an expensive and impractical approach. Three low progesterone values have been used by some as a diagnostic tool. Endometrial morphology reflects overall progesterone activity and can actually serve as a more reliable bioassay end point for progesterone. Thus, an endometrial biopsy, taken 1–2 days before menstruation, will more adequately reflect steroidogenic function of the corpus luteum. Using fine, disposable small diameter cannulae, an endometrial biopsy is easily obtained with little discomfort to the patient. A single strip of endometrium is usually sufficient for diagnosis. As implantation occurs usually on the posterior surface of the uterus, the danger of interfering with an early pregnancy is minimized. (In case of concern, a sensitive pregnancy test should be performed beforehand.) BBT has to be recorded and the histologic dating is calculated from the onset of the next menstrual period as well as from the estimated date of ovulation. A biopsy out of phase by more than 2 days should be confirmed in a subsequent cycle. Occasionally, especially in younger women, an inadequate luteal phase will be interspersed with normal menstrual cycles. In the typical syndrome, however, the syndrome occurs repetitively.

HYPERPROLACTINEMIA

Increased prolactin (PRL) levels are frequently associated with disturbances of the menstrual cycle. Most commonly, these are seen in patients with a PRL-producing pituitary adenoma. Thus, in the initial evaluation process of the infertile patient with irregular menses or amenorrhea, it is always important to measure PRL concentrations. Because of its association with menstrual cycle pathology, PRL is reviewed here. Most probably, however, this hormone is not directly causally associated with the cyclic pathology; in most cases, hyperprolactinemia is the result of changes which are also responsible for acyclicity.

THE PHYSIOLOGY OF PRL

PRL consists of 198 amino acids in a single peptide chain. Close structural homologies between the growth hormone and the PRL molecules suggest that both may have evolved from an identical precursor. PRL appears to exert diverse actions on tissues, but these remain to be fully elucidated especially in the human. In some vertebrates, PRL plays a major role in osmoregulation. In other species, however, its main action appears to be on the reproductive process. In the rodent (but not in the human), PRL is luteotropic: it prolongs the secretory life of the corpus luteum in early pregnancy. In the human, the main function of PRL is to initiate and maintain lactation. Under the proper conditions, which require the hormone to act in concert with estradiol, progesterone, cortisol, and insulin, PRL stimulates the synthesis of the proteins, lipids, and carbohydrates characteristic of milk. Higher PRL secretion during the reproductive years in contrast to the prepubertal and menopausal periods may also suggest that minimum levels of PRL are required for the normal function of the hypothalamic-pituitary-gonadal axis, although this remains to be demonstrated convincingly.

THE CONTROL OF PRL SECRETION

Because experimental separation of the pituitary gland from direct hypothalamic influences (such as following pituitary stalk section or placement of the pituitary gland under the kidney capsule) results in a prolonged elevation of PRL secretion, it has been concluded that PRL release is under a tonic inhibitory control by the hypothalamus. Isolated pituitary cultures also secrete large amounts of PRL. Restraint on PRL release is exerted by a PRL-inhibiting factor (PIF). The main PIF is dopamine, a catecholamine which is secreted in sufficient amounts into the hypophyseal portal circulation to account for the inhibition of PRL release. There is also evidence that, under certain circumstances, PRL release is stimulated by a PRL-releasing factor (PRF). Several PRFs have been proposed, such as thyrotropin-releasing hormone (TRH), vasoactive intestinal peptide (VIP), oxytocin and β-endorphin, but their relative physiologic importance remains to be determined in the human (Fig. 10–7).

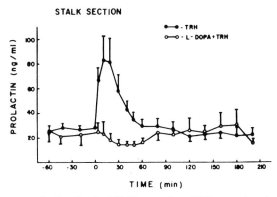

Fig. 10–7. The control of prolactin (PRL) secretion. PRL secretion is mainly under a tonic inhibition by the hypothalamus. This accounts for the elevated baseline PRL levels in these pituitary stalk sectioned monkeys, in which the pituitary has been physically isolated from hypothalamic influences (normal monkey basal PRL levels: 10 ng/ml). The main hypothalamic PRL-inhibiting factor is dopamine. Several factors are also known to release PRL, such as thyrotropin-releasing hormone *(TRH)* (shown here), vasoactive intestinal peptide, β-endorphin, and oxytocin. Coadministration of L-DOPA, a dopamine precursor, prevents the PRL-releasing activity of TRH. (From Diefenback WP, Carmel PW, Frantz AG, Ferin M 1976: Suppression of prolactin secretion by L-DOPA in the stalk-sectioned rhesus monkey. *J Clin Endocrinol Metab* 43:638. Copyright © by The Endocrine Society.)

PRL release is pulsatile. Since pulsatile release patterns are abolished by pituitary stalk section, the mechanism regulating pulsatile PRL secretion must be located within the C.N.S. rather than in the pituitary. Whether pulsatile PRL release reflects the intermittent inhibition of dopamine activity or the intermittent release of a PRF is not known.

PRL can also, to a certain degree, autoregulate its own secretion by stimulating neuronal activity of hypothalamic dopamine neurons. For example, following experimental administration of PRL, there follows increased synthesis and turnover of dopamine, and increased release of dopamine in hypophyseal portal blood.

The secretion of PRL is also influenced by several other factors.

Estradiol. The ovarian hormone estradiol augments PRL release. Estradiol action is probably responsible for the differences in PRL concentrations in the adult versus the prepubertal or menopausal woman. Some authors have reported increases in PRL at midcycle at the time of maximal estradiol secretion, but this is not uniformly observed. Estradiol also augments TRH-induced prolactin release. Progesterone does not appear to increase basal PRL levels.

Sleep. There is a moderate rise in PRL concentrations during sleep.

Stress. Several types of stress (e.g., cold, heat, physical aggression, intravenous catheterization, or surgery) are all known to increase PRL release. Similarly, certain types of exercise will also result in increased PRL levels.

Pharmacological agents. Several drugs increase PRL, mostly by decreasing dopamine activity through specific mechanisms. Tranquilizers may block dopaminergic receptors, such as the phenothiazine derivatives (chlorpromazine), the butyrophenones (haloperidol), or sulpiride, or inhibit dopamine reuptake from the interneuronal cleft, such as the tricyclic depressants. Opiates also increase PRL release, either by modulating dopamine or PRF release.

The suckling stimulus. The suckling stimulus is an important physiological releaser of PRL. The amount of PRL released is proportional to the frequency of the suckling stimulus; hence, levels of PRL characterizing the postpartum period are related to the amount of suckling. Initially, it was postulated that PRL release following suckling was the result of a reduction in tonic hypothalamic inhibition. In the rodent, however, changes in dopamine after suckling are rather sluggish and probably insufficient to explain the dramatic change in secretion of PRL. Thus, release of PRL during suckling may be provoked by a PRF (Fig. 10–8).

GnRH. Under certain circumstances, various investigators have reported coincidental LH and PRL pulses. In some superfused pituitary cell cultures, it was

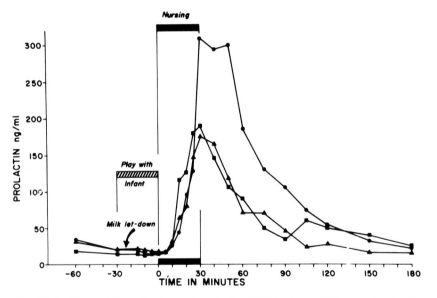

Fig. 10–8. The suckling stimulus and prolactin (PRL) release. PRL secretion in three nursing postpartum women (patient 1: triangles; patient 2: squares; patient 3: circles). PRL levels are moderately elevated between episodes of nursing, with a major rise after the onset of suckling. Milk letdown is a phenomenon that occurs in mothers who are anticipating nursing. It is an oxytocin-mediated phenomenon and is not associated with PRL release. PRL increase occurs only with the suckling stimulus (solid bar). (From Noel GL, Suh HK, Frantz AG 1974: Prolactin release during nursing and breast stimulation in postpartum and nonpostpartum subjects. *J Clin Endocrinol Metab* 38:413–423. Copyright © by The Endocrine Society.)

also found that GnRH can stimulate PRL release. This effect is not due to a direct action of the neurohormone on the lactotrope, but rather to the apparent production of a paracrine factor by the gonadotrope, which in turn stimulates the lactotrope to secrete PRL. The physiologic significance of this observation remains to be ascertained.

HYPERPROLACTINEMIC STATES AND AMENORRHEA

Hyperprolactinemic states are frequently associated with disturbances of the menstrual cycle and amenorrhea. Physiologically, amenorrhea is observed during the postpartum period in breast-feeding women. In non-breast-feeding women, ovulatory menstrual cycles usually resume within 2 months postpartum. Breast feeding, however, delays the resumption of normal cyclicity, either by inducing amenorrhea or resulting in hormonally deficient cycles (such as cycles with an inadequate or short luteal phase). Amenorrhea is also observed in patients bearing a PRL-secreting adenoma or after intake of drugs that increase PRL. The occurrence of nonpuerperal breast secretion is termed *galactorrhea,* and the combination of milk secretion and acyclicity is commonly referred to as the *galactorrhea-amenorrhea syndrome.* In general, the duration of the amenorrheic period is correlated to the increase in PRL.

Elevated PRL concentrations have been postulated to suppress the hypothalamic GnRH pulse generator,—and, indeed, in some, but not all, hyperprolactinemic patients, there are reports of decreased pulsatile LH release (Fig. 10–9)—or to affect the ovaries (PRL has been reported to modify ovarian steroidogenesis and corpus luteum function). In most species including the

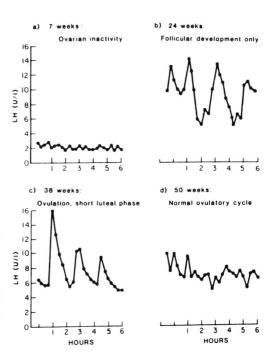

Fig. 10–9. The postpartum and the menstrual cycle. LH pulsatile secretion in a breast-feeding woman in relation to the return of ovarian activity. In this particular patient, normal ovulatory menstrual cycles occur after weaning at 40 weeks, at which time high-frequency and low-amplitude pulses, characteristic of the early follicular phase, reappear. Although pulsatile release is initiated at an earlier stage, pulse patterns are not adequate for a full menstrual cycle. Abbreviations as in Figure 10–1. (From McNeilly AS 1988: In: *The Physiology of Reproduction* [Knobil E, Neill J, eds], Raven Press, NY, chapter 59, 2323) as reproduced from Glasier AF, McNeilly AS, Howie PW (1984). *Clin Endocrinol* 20:415.

human, however, such direct effects of PRL on LH release are minimal, if they occur at all. Thus, although the relationship between elevated PRL secretion and cycle abnormalities is well established, PRL itself is most probably not the *direct* cause of the cyclic disturbance in most instances. In the postpartum period, it is now well established that it is the suckling stimulus itself which, through hypothalamic mechanisms that remain to be uncovered, inhibits GnRH release. Suppression of PRL with a dopamine agonist, such as bromocriptine, does not increase LH if the suckling stimulus is maintained. It is possible that the endogenous opioids are involved in the process since naloxone administration in suckling animals elevates LH secretion. In hyperprolactinemic states other than suckling, such as in the patient with a PRL-secreting adenoma, restoration of normal ovulatory periods typically follows treatment with bromocriptine, a dopamine agonist that lowers PRL. Yet, normal cycles can also be restored by pulsatile GnRH treatment alone, suggesting that the arrest in cyclicity may not uniquely be the result of hyperprolactinemia but be also related to defects in dopaminergic tone. Dopamine is known to be inhibitory to GnRH-LH secretion (see Chapter 2). The apparent discordant effect of treatment with a dopamine agonist may result indirectly for the normalization of PRL levels, which themselves, through the autoregulatory process that links PRL and dopamine, were responsible for excessive hypothalamic dopamine. In hyperprolactinemic states, amenorrhea is then the direct consequence of decreased GnRH pulsatility, absent or deficient follicular development and, therefore, estrogen secretion.

11

Diagnosis of Menstrual Cycle Dysfunction

The normal menstrual cycle is initiated by the recruitment of a new cohort of follicles and their orderly development to maturation, followed by ovulation and menstruation. These processes, as outlined in previous chapters, involve complex feedback interactions between the hypothalamus, the pituitary gland, and the ovaries. Thus, the menstrual cycle may be disrupted by abnormalities occurring at these three critical levels. The ovary produces the most important gonadal steroid, estradiol, and, in turn, this ovarian hormone affects the uterus. Although the patient's uterine status may serve as a bioassay for the presence of estradiol, one should bear in mind that estradiol will of course be ineffective if the uterus is deficient or absent. Thus, the uterus as the end organ must also be considered in the evaluation of menstrual cycle dysfunction.

In this chapter, we will review menstrual dysfunction syndromes resulting from end organ dysfunction, from ovarian disorders, and from dysfunction of the hypothalamic-pituitary unit. [Menstrual dysfunction accompanied by enhanced androgen secretion is reviewed in Chapter 12]. Alterations of menstrual cyclicity may present as *primary amenorrhea* (the patient has never menstruated), or *secondary amenorrhea* (the patient has menstruated before but has stopped menstruating for the last 6 months). Simplified diagnostic approaches to patients in these two categories are outlined in Figure 11–1 (primary amenorrhea) and Figure 11–2 (secondary amenorrhea).

END ORGAN DYSFUNCTION

Conceptually, it is helpful to separate this group into patients who present with primary amenorrhea and those with secondary amenorrhea.

PRIMARY AMENORRHEA

Patients with primary amenorrhea may account for about 40% of cases with end organ dysfunction. They will generally be recognized by a fairly normal pubertal development, but an abnormal physical examination of the lower genital tract. The gonads are usually functioning normally, and normal feedback loops maintain gonadotropin levels within a normal range *(eugonadotropic syndromes).*

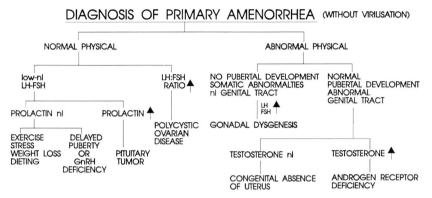

Fig. 11–1. Diagnosis of primary amenorrhea. *FSH,* follicle-stimulating hormone; *GnRH,* gonadotropin-releasing hormone; *LH,* luteinizing hormone.

Complete Androgen Receptor Deficiency

This disorder (previously known as the testicular feminization syndrome) is a form of male pseudohermaphroditism. Patients have an XY karyotype but fail to develop as males because of end organ insensitivity: absence of androgen receptors in target tissue prevents androgen action, even though circulating androgen levels may be elevated (Fig. 11–3). As a result, these individuals, who are genetic males with testes, have a female phenotypic appearance with normal breast development and height; they generally have scanty or complete absence of facial, axillary, and pubic hair. A key to the diagnosis is the presence of a short vagina which ends in a blind pouch. The functioning testes manufacture müllerian-inhibiting factor (MIF) which suppresses the development of the upper

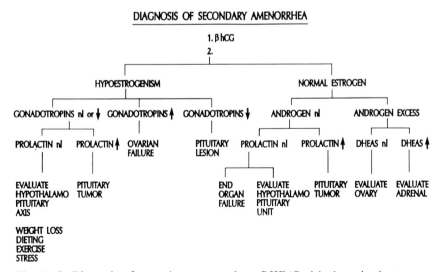

Fig. 11–2. Diagnosis of secondary amenorrhea. *DHEAS,* dehydro-epiandrosterone; *hCG,* human chorionic gonadotropin.

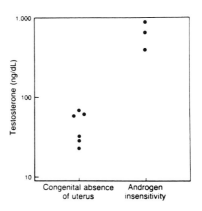

Fig. 11-3. Primary amenorrhea and end organ dysfunction. Serum testosterone levels differentiate the diagnosis in patients with primary amenorrhea and organ deficiency. (From Maschchak CA, Kletzky OA, Davajan V, and Mishell Jr DR 1981: *Obstet Gynecol* 57:715–721. Reprinted with permission from The American College of Obstetricians and Gynecologists.)

third of the vagina, uterus, fallopian tubes, and ovary. Occasionally, the vagina is completely absent. In the complete syndrome, these individuals are always raised as females.

The testes may be palpable in the inguinal canal where hernias are frequent, or may be located intra-abdominally anywhere along the pelvic sidewall. They consist of immature testicular tubules with a normal or increased number of Leydig's cells and secrete normal or even elevated levels of testosterone. The diagnosis is confirmed by measurements of male levels of testosterone and by the karyotype. Estradiol produced by the testis and peripheral conversion of androgens to estrogens cause feminization at puberty; however, the patient classically presents with primary amenorrhea, due to the lack of a uterus. Luteinizing hormone (LH) levels are normal to slightly elevated, due to an active negative feedback loop.

The syndrome of androgen insensitivity is either an X-linked recessive or sex-limited autosomal dominant disorder. Maternal aunts with primary amenorrhea are not uncommon as this syndrome is often transferred through the mother. The dysgenetic intra-abdominal gonad has a high malignant potential and should be removed after adequate feminization, usually after puberty.

Incomplete Androgen Receptor Deficiency

This syndrome may lead to a spectrum of clinical presentations ranging from a female appearance with minimal masculinization of the genitalia to a male appearance with minimal hypospadias. The latter is occasionally referred to as Reifenstein's syndrome.

Congenital Absence of the Uterus

These patients have ovaries and normal hormonal cyclic function with ovulation. Because of normal feedback relationships, they are eugonadotropic; however, due to absence of development of the uterus, they present with primary amenorrhea. There is hypoplasia and failure of fusion of the müllerian anlagen. Commonly, the vagina is also absent (Rokitansky-Küster-Hauser syndrome): the complete failure of the two müllerian anlagen eliminates the natural stimulus for normal canalization of the vagina by upgrowth of urogenital sinus epithelium. Congenital absence of the uterus is often associated with musculoskeletal abnormalities and occasionally with renal anomalies.

Normal ovarian function is confirmed by a biphasic basal body temperature (BBT), ovulatory progesterone levels, and a normal female testosterone level. The latter differentiates this syndrome from androgen insensitivity (Fig. 11–3). Because of normal ovarian function, the physical appearance is normal. When the vagina is absent, the patient is usually treated by vaginal dilatation, or, rarely, by creation of a vagina surgically.

Steroid Synthesis Deficiency

17,20-desmolase or lyase deficiency. Lyase deficiency is an extremely rare condition in which the patient presents with primary amenorrhea and the inability to synthesize sex steroids either in the gonad or the adrenal. The patient lacks the enzyme to convert 17-α-hydroxypregnenolone to dehydroepiandrosterone (DHEA) and 17-α-hydroxyprogesterone to androstenedione (see Fig. 3–1). The one patient described in the literature had abdominal testes, a female phenotype, and lack of breast or uterine development. Gonadotropins may be elevated and testosterone and estradiol levels are low. Diagnosis is confirmed by measuring precursors to the defective enzymatic step.

17-α-hydroxylase deficiency. 17-α-hydroxylase deficiency presents with sexual infantilism, a female phenotype, and a deficiency in manufacturing sex hormones in both adrenals and gonads due to the inability to convert pregnenolone to 17-α-hydroxypregnenolone and progesterone to 17-α-hydroxyprogesterone. This syndrome is extremely rare, having been described usually in boys. Aldosterone secretion is unimpeded and these patients may have hypertension along with primary amenorrhea.

SECONDARY AMENORRHEA

End organ dysfunction and secondary amenorrhea occur in the syndrome of uterine synechiae, usually as a result of an overvigorous dilatation and curretage, or an abortion, particularly a septic one. This syndrome is known as Asherman's syndrome. Patients will report a normal past menstrual record and can usually relate the problem to a specific gynecologic procedure or uterine infection. All hormone tests will be normal (eugonadotropic syndrome), with evidence of good estrogen secretion but no withdrawal bleeding after progesterone alone or cyclic estrogen and progesterone. BBT will show a biphasic curve indicative of ovulation. Diagnosis will be confirmed by an hysterosalpingogram revealing synechiae within the uterus and/or hysteroscopy. The latter procedure is therapeutic when the synechiae are lysed under direct visualization. Endometrial regrowth is enhanced by large doses of estrogen, and occasionally with an intrauterine device left in place to prevent the development of adhesions during endometrial regrowth.

OVARIAN DISORDERS

Cyclic dysfunction due to ovarian disorders is typically characterized by high concentrations of gonadotropins *(hypergonadotropic syndromes)*. This, of course, directly reflects the lack of ovarian steroid production and the consequent deficient long loop negative feedback. Failure of gonadal differentiation or deficient gonadal function during early fetal and neonatal development is the main cause of about 60% of primary amenorrhea cases. Disorders may, however, also present as secondary amenorrhea, as in premature ovarian failure.

GONADAL DYSGENESIS

The classic triad of short stature, primary amenorrhea, and sexual infantilism (Turner's syndrome) was described in 1938 and represents the most frequent error in fetal gonadal differentiation. Patients will fail to have pubertal development. Most patients are less than 150 cm tall and have typical physical abnormalities such as a webbed neck and a shield chest (nipples placed in the anterior axillary line) (Fig. 11-4). Other phenotypic anomalies may include an arched palate, low set ears, low neck hairline, epicanthal folds, a tendency to micrognathia and occasional lymphoedema which may alert the physician in the newborn

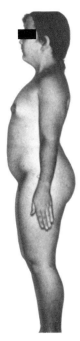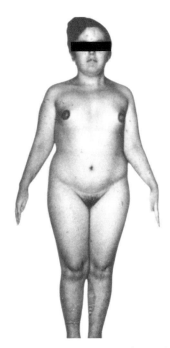

Fig. 11-4. Patient with gonadal dysgenesis (Turner's syndrome). In this syndrome, patients have a 45X karyotype and the gonads fail to develop properly. Symptoms include primary amenorrhea and sexual infantilism. Note the webbed neck, shield chest, increased carrying angle of the arm, as well as short stature.

nursery. Shortening of the fourth or fifth digits may occur and the fourth meta-carpal may be absent; increased pigmented nevi are common. Cardiovascular anomalies, in particular coarctation of the aorta as well as renal anomalies, such as horseshoe kidneys, often accompany the disease. Diabetes mellitus and auto-immune thyroiditis (Hashimoto's disease) are common. There is also a higher than expected incidence of anorexia nervosa for reasons that are unclear.

Gonadal dysgenesis is congenital: the gonads do not develop properly, or germ cells undergo rapid atresia. Patients lack one of the sex chromosomes and are born with a 45X karyotype. As a result, the gonads consist of streaks of white tissue lacking primary follicles and lying adjacent to the fallopian tubes. There is no gonadal sex hormone production at puberty and the patient usually pre-sents with primary amenorrhea with no evidence of estrogen secretion: breasts fail to develop and the vagina remains atrophic. Pubic and axillary hair may be present, as adrenarche occurs normally. Diagnosis is confirmed by a 45X karyo-type and gonadotropin concentrations in the castrate or menopausal level. The buccal smear is also negative.

The X karyotype is thought to be due to nondisjunction or chromosome loss during either spermatogenesis or oogenesis. This may arise at the first cleavage division from anaphase lag during meiosis with cursory loss of a sex chromo-some.

Variants of Gonadal Dysgenesis

Included in this group are mosaicism, structural changes in one of the sex chro-mosomes, mixed gonadal dysgenesis, and the syndrome of pure gonadal dysgen-esis. All of these produce variations of the classical Turner's syndrome.

Two or more cell lines may exist with 46XX/45Y being the most common. Multiple tissues may need to be searched for karyotypic analysis to uncover mosaicism. These patients may also have a variable chromatin count. This may be associated with less pronounced or fewer somatic abnormalities and even normal height with a few follicles in the ovarian streaks and some estrogen secre-tion. Pregnancies, although extremely rare, have been reported; the fetus has a high proportion of congenital and chromosomal anomalies. Other variations include 45X/47XXX/46XX and 45X/46XY. The Y line may be normal or structurally abnormal. The presence of a Y chromosome may be associated with some degree of virilization, ambiguous genitalia, or even phenotypic males. Some testicular tissue may be found within the streak, its amount usually reflect-ing the degree of masculinization. Because of the risk of malignant degeneration (as high as 20%) in the streak containing a Y chromosome, screening for the Y chromosome is extremely important: the gonadal tissue must be removed.

Mixed gonadal dysgenesis refers to the presence of a testis on one side with a streak gonad on the other. This dysgenetic gonad can function, produce testos-terone, and should be removed because of its high malignant potential.

Patients with structural changes in the second chromosome may present with lack of sexual development, partial stigmata of gonadal dysgenesis, but with pos-itive sex chromatin. Particularly common structural abnormalities are deletion of a portion of the X chromosome and an isochromosome for the long arm.

These unusual abnormalities often occur with mosaicism. Deletion of the long arm is associated with normal stature and few of the stigmata of Turner's syndrome. A variety of phenotypes may be associated with structural abnormalities of the Y chromosome but these are rare. Females with no sexual development, normal height, and bilateral streak gonads have been described.

In pure gonadal dysgenesis, patients have a 46XX or 46XY karyotype and streak gonads, like in the Turner's syndrome; however, they are of normal stature and lack the stigmata of the Turner's syndrome. The normal genetic component assures growth, and the patients are tall because the lack of ovarian steroids keeps the epiphyses open. The genetic defect that causes this group of abnormalities is unclear.

PREMATURE OVARIAN FAILURE

Normally, ovarian failure occurs with menopause (see Chapter 9). In 10% of cases of secondary amenorrhea, this process may occur earlier during reproductive life before age 40 years (premature menopause). Patients present with symptoms of hypoestrogenism, including hot flushes and high gonadotropin concentrations. Two different types have been identified: one has generalized ovarian sclerosis with a decrease in the number of follicles, a process similar to that seen in normal menopause, while, in the other, the ovaries contain multiple primordial follicles that fail to develop to the mature antral stage. In the first category are patients who are depleted of ova early on in reproductive life: a timely menarche may be followed by a few normal periods and then progressive menstrual irregularity may set in. Patients with mosaicism and gonadal dysgenesis typically follow this pattern. Some cases may present with incomplete sexual development followed by a few irregular periods and then complete amenorrhea. Premature ovarian failure can occur in association with other endocrine gland dysfunction, in particular thyroid and adrenal. This association may be an autoimmune dysfunction, and thyroiditis with high antibody titers is common. Sometimes, the autoimmune ovarian failure occurs independently. Hypoparathyroidism, mucocutaneous candidiasis, and alopecia can also be seen in association with this disorder. The etiology of the autoimmune dysfunction is unknown, although circulating antibodies to ovarian tissue and to the follicle-stimulating hormone (FSH) receptor have been shown in two women with ovarian failure and myasthenia gravis.

In rare patients, there may be evidence of ovarian resistance to gonadotropins. The ovaries are small, hypoplastic, and appear unstimulated: biopsy reveals unstimulated primordial follicles. This symptom complex is sometimes called the *"resistant ovary syndrome"*. Ovarian enzymatic defects, including $17-\alpha$-hydroxylase, $3-\beta$-ol-dehydrogenase and 17-ketoreductase have been associated with ovarian failure.

Occasionally, surgery or infection appear to be the precipitating cause. Premature ovarian failure has been seen in association with mumps or in patients who have had ovarian cystectomies, usually bilateral for removal of dermoids or endometriomas. This syndrome is also seen in patients treated for tubo-ovarian abscess without surgery, but in which there has been presumably large amounts of tissue destruction by the infection. Irradiation and chemotherapy, especially alkylating agents, may also lead to ovarian failure.

Evaluation includes gonadotropin and estradiol measurements, thyroid function tests and antibodies, a chemistry profile and, if indicated, a 24-hour urinary free cortisol to rule out adrenal failure and associated endocrinopathies. FSH concentrations will usually rise before those of LH. If patients do not menstruate in response to a progesterone withdrawal test, cyclical estrogen-progestin replacement therapy is indicated. Chromosome studies are usually not cost effective as they do not change management but are indicated in some cases in the perimenarchial group or in those patients who present with some of the stigmata of gonadal dysgenesis, especially if a Y cell line is suspected.

Ovarian failure is not always permanent and reinitiation of menstrual cycles and even pregnancy can occur in these groups, even when the classic diagnosis is made in the patient with secondary amenorrhea, hypoestrogenism, and hypergonadotropism, but this is extremely rare. Usually, prognosis for fertility is almost nonexistant and, with the rare exceptions already cited, patients do not respond to ovulation induction therapy. However, new reproductive technologies, such as in vitro fertilization (IVF), egg or embryo donation, have opened new therapeutic avenues for these patients.

HYPOTHALAMIC-PITUITARY DYSFUNCTION

The intimate anatomical and functional relationships of the hypothalamus and pituitary gland cause heterogeneous symptoms that often involve both organs. In general, specific hypothalamic problems are difficult to differentiate clinically from pituitary problems except by initial exclusion of pituitary dysfunction. Thus, the diagnosis of hypothalamic amenorrhea is often made by exclusion. The availability of many of the hypothalamic trophic neurohormones has not fulfilled expectations that pituitary disease can be differentiated from hypothalamic disease on the basis of stimulation studies. Indeed, the pituitary response to the stimulatory or inhibitory neurohormones reveals much overlap between pituitary and hypothalamic disease; this may, in part, be related to pituitary cell atrophy that results from lack of stimulation by releasing factors accounting for the blunted response also seen in hypothalamic disease. Functional abnormalities of the feedback loops may also come into play. Depending on the time of onset, these syndromes may appear as primary or secondary amenorrhea. In general, hypothalamic-pituitary syndromes will be *eugonadotropic* or *hypogonadotropic* and patients will present with decreased ovarian function and/or hypoestrogenism. We will review first disorders that implicate a primary causal origin residing in the pituitary, then discuss the syndrome of hypothalamic amenorrhea.

PITUITARY DYSFUNCTION

Defects in menstrual cyclicity may relate to a number of pituitary conditions that, through the secretion of other hormones, impinge directly or indirectly on the proper secretion of gonadotropins. Overall, these conditions can be classified into two categories: (1) those which relate to the presence of tumors, resulting in hypersecretion of one or more trophic hormones, and (2) those which relate to pituitary lesions that result in trophic hormone deficiency.

Trophic Hormone Excess: Tumors

Pituitary disorders generally present with a cluster of endocrine symptoms that depend on the etiology of the dysfunction. Most commonly, evidence of excessive secretion occurs due to a tumor secreting one of the trophic hormones. Many of these syndromes are accompanied by disruption of pituitary function and amenorrhea. The three best known entities include prolactin hypersecretion causing the amenorrhea-galactorhea syndrome, adrenocorticotropin hormone (ACTH) excess causing Cushing's syndrome, and growth hormone (GH) excess causing acromegaly. Rarely, thyroid-stimulating hormone (TSH), LH, FSH, and β-endorphin adenomas occur.

Prolactin-secreting adenomas. Prolactin-secreting adenomas are the most common types of tumors causing amenorrhea or menstrual cycle dysruption. Secretion of prolactin by the adenoma can result in primary or secondary amenorrhea by affecting the secretion of gonadotropin-releasing hormone (GnRH) and/or by inhibiting the release of LH and FSH, and perhaps also by affecting ovarian synthesis of androgens (see Chapter 10). This syndrome may present with only amenorrhea, or more typically, is accompanied by galactorhea (the amenorrhea-galactorhea syndrome). Most tumors are small (less than 1 cm; microadenoma) and may only be detected by computerized axial tomography or magnetic resonance imagery (MRI) aimed at the sella turcica. Larger tumors may cause dysfunction of other trophic hormones, in particular thyroid and adrenal function. Thus, in the patient with amenorrhea, hyperprolactinemia, and evidence of a pituitary tumor, thyroid studies and a 24-hour urinary free cortisol should also be performed. Visual fields should be obtained as a baseline in case of further growth, or, in the case of a macroadenoma, to rule out impairment of the visual nerves by superior growth of the tumor. Typically, large tumors will produce bitemporal hemianopsia. All prolactin-secreting adenomas should be followed carefully: growth will occur gradually in most cases but occasionally the tumor may enlarge more rapidly, particularly during pregnancy. Other trophic tumors can also secrete prolactin, in particular GH-secreting tumors; if clinically indicated, these should be ruled out. (Other causes of elevated prolactin should also be considered, such as drugs, especially phenothiazines or antidepressants, hypothyroidism, pregnancy, nipple stimulation, and prior chest wall surgery.)

Prolactin-secreting tumors respond well to treatment with dopamine agonists; bromocriptine is commonly used (see Chapter 13). About 80% of patients resume normal menses and ovulatory function. Hyperprolactinemia usually recurs after bromocriptine is withdrawn.

ACTH-secreting adenomas. ACTH-secreting adenomas present with clinical features of glucocorticoid excess (Cushing's syndrome) and menstrual irregularities, usually anovulation. Typical physical changes include abdominal obesity, hypertension, a moon face, chipmonk jowls, buffalo hump, and abnormal striae. There may also be signs of adrenal androgen excess with hirsutism, and aldosterone excess with hyperkalemia. The overnight dexamethasone suppression test (1 mg dexamethasone at 11 P.M. and 8 A.M. cortisol determination) is usually sufficient to rule out the diagnosis. In suspicious cases, a 24-hour urinary free cortisol is the best and easiest screening test. If positive, a dexamethasone suppression test will rule out adrenal hyperplasia and an ACTH level should be drawn. Cushing's syndrome is a serious disorder, which frequently requires transsphenoidal pituitary surgery with a success rate of over 90% reported in a recent series. Other treatments include pituitary radiation (proton or conventional) or bilateral adrenalectomy, which should be reserved for micropituitary surgical failures. (Adrenalectomy carries a 10% risk of development of Nelson's syndrome: compensatory pituitary enlargement with hyperpigmentation.) In general, treatment will result in a return of normal menstrual function, although overproduction of adrenal androgens often produces polycystic-like ovaries and resultant anovulation, which may require treatment even after a cure of the Cushing's syndrome has been established.

GH-secreting adenomas. Acidophilic in nature, GH-secreting adenomas are rare tumors. If they occur in the prepubertal state before closure of the epiphyses, gigantism results. Combinations of extraordinary growth and amenorrhea are, in fact, an unusual occurrence and this syndrome should be suspected in this case. Gonadotropin deficiency probably occurs because of the mass effect of the tumor in the pituitary, but elevated prolactin may also lead to hypogonadotropism. In adult women, acromegaly occurs with associated amenorrhea and prolactin may be elevated. These patients will have a distinctive appearance with enlargement of the skull, a prognathic jaw, and enlargement of the hands and feet. Teeth may become separated and the supraorbital ridges bulge. Skin and subcutaneous tissues become thickened, sinuses enlarge, and voice changes may occur due to modifications in the structure of the larynx. The tongue may enlarge and the speech may thicken. The hair is coarse and hirsutism is present due to an accompanying adrenal androgen increase. Excess sweating and galactorrhea are common as well as glucose intolerance. The diagnosis of a GH-secreting adenoma is easily confirmed by elevated GH levels which do not suppress with a glucose load. Computerized axial tomography (CAT) scan or MRI of the sella turcica may show enlargement due to the presence of a tumor and visual fields may show a temporal field deficit.

TSH-secreting tumors. TSH-secreting tumors and the resultant hyperthyroidism may be accompanied by galactorrhea and amenorrhea because of an increase in prolactin. The tumor may respond to bromocriptine administration. A distinctive syndrome occurs in children who are hypothyroid: enlargement of TSH-secreting cells occurs, while regression is observed with treatment with thyroid hormone. This syndrome may occur rarely in adults. Prolactin is often elevated, so that the hypothyroid patient may present with the symptoms of galactorrhea, a low T4 and a high TSH. This syndrome is thought to be due to a lack of T4 negative feedback on thyroid-releasing hormone (TRH); elevated TRH would then stimulate both TSH and prolactin secretion.

FSH- and LH-secreting adenomas. These tumors are difficult to detect as FSH and LH elevation rarely produces noticeable symptoms.

Trophic Hormone Deficiency
Pituitary lesions may be suspected in the presence of a cluster of symptoms which include hormone deficiency. A list of clinical symptoms appears in Table 11–1; some of these may be age-dependant.

Craniophargyngiomas. Craniophargyngiomas are tumors that occur mainly in the second and third decade of life. They rise from remnants of Rathke's pouch, are usually found along the anterior surface of the infundibulum and pituitary stalk, and may occur above or below the diaphragma sellae; they are often cystic. The syndrome may include visual impairment, amenorrhea, symptoms of GH deficiency in children, adrenal deficiency, and occasionally depressed thyroid function. Prolactin may be elevated, because the tumor may prevent the prolactin-inhibiting hormone dopamine from reaching the pituitary. Occasionally diabetes insipidus may occur. Enlargement of the pituitary fossa is confirmed by radiologic assessment, and treatment is usually surgical excision of the tumor followed by radiation. Other tumors in the region of the hypothalamus and pituitary stalk include meningiomas, hamartomas, gliomas, and metastatic disease usually from the breast.

Sheehan's syndrome. Sheehan's syndrome occurs in conjunction with peripartum or postpartum hemorrhage and shock (postpartum necrosis). During pregnancy, the pituitary is susceptible to ischemic shock as the anterior lobe nearly doubles in size. This growth is due mostly to hypertrophy and hyperplasia of the lactotropes. The patient presents with a failure to lactate, fatigue, loss of vigor,

Table 11–1. Clinical Symptoms of Parasellar Tumors

Age Related	
Prepubertal	Headache, vomiting
Young adult	Sexual infantilism, growth deficiency, impotence, amenorrhea, loss of libido, obesity
Adult	Headache, visual disturbances, hair loss, asthenia, galactorrhea

Age Unrelated	
Frequent	Headache, visual disturbances, oculomotor function, endocrine dysfunction
Less frequent	Seizures, facial pain, disturbance of consciousness, temperature instability, blood pressure instability

Source: Garnica AD, Netzloff ML, Rosenbloom AL 1980: *Ann Clin Lab Sci* 10:474.

hypotension, loss of pubic and axillary hair, delayed reflexes, and amenorrhea. Depending on the extent of trophic hormone deficiency, symptoms of gonadotropin, thyroid, and adrenal hormone deficiency may co-exist. The degree of deficiency is highly variable; partial or complete spontaneous recovery has been reported, although the majority of patients will require long-term replacement of the deficient hormones.

Pituitary apoplexy. Pituitary apoplexy may occur with massive infarction of the pituitary gland often associated with hemorrhage into a tumor. It is a rare but life-threatening condition and the severe headache that accompanies it may be an important sign. Dramatic neurologic symptoms may also occur, usually related to edema. Visual acuity and field defects may be present with impairment of cranial nerves III, IV, V, and VI. Prompt therapy with corticosteroids is indicated to treat deficiency and edema, but early transsphenoidal decompression may be necessary. Occasionally, conservative therapy leads to complete spontaneous neurologic recovery.

Empty sella syndrome. Empty sella syndrome results from a defect in the diaphragma sellae anteriorly. This allows for an extension of the subarachnoid space, which may become filled with cerebrospinal fluid (CSF). This makes the sella appear empty, but pituitary tissue is often found flattened against its side or displaced upward. Most often the problem is idiopathic and occurs in middle-aged obese women with little or no endocrine dysfunction: a ballooned sella is discovered serendipitously on a radiographic study. Occasionally, the patients complain of headache, CSF rhinorrhea, and, rarely, of symptoms due to one or more trophic hormone deficiency. Hypersecretion of trophic hormones can occur rarely, particularly of prolactin. This syndrome may also occur after surgery or radiation therapy. No specific treatment is usually necessary except for trophic hormone replacement when needed.

Primary hypopituitarism of idiopathic etiology. Primary hypopituitarism may occur with multiple or isolated deficiencies of trophic hormones. The most common are associated with GH deficiency and dwarfism if they occur prepubertally. Some of these deficiencies have now been identified as being of hypothalamic etiology (see later).

Other miscellaneous conditions. Occasionally carcinomatosis may involve the pituitary and alter its function. Other conditions include vascular malformations, trauma with or without skull fracture, and surgical or radiotherapy of a pituitary lesion. Hemochromatosis may also replace pituitary tissue.

HYPOTHALAMIC DYSFUNCTION

Hypothalamic disorders are thought to affect the secretion of GnRH by a mechanism that has not yet been well defined. The majority of the disorders described here modify GnRH pulse frequency and/or amplitude, most probably through a direct or indirect effect on the GnRH pulse generator. Because GnRH secretion cannot be directly documented in the human, alterations of GnRH secretion are generally studied by frequent sampling (every 10–15 min) of peripheral LH levels. This method is, of course, too cumbersome for routine examination and is usually reserved for medical research. It may also be that, under some still undefined circumstances, peripheral monitoring of LH may not represent accurately the activity of the GnRH pulse generator. Thus, as a general rule, disorders of hypothalamic function leading to amenorrhea are diagnosed first by eliminating abnormal end organ, ovarian, or pituitary defects. GnRH stimulatory tests are not helpful in diagnosing hypothalamic amenorrhea in most patients.

Patients may present with *primary* or *secondary* amenorrhea. Patients with primary amenorrhea will have normal physical appearance and a normal genital tract, but little or no pubertal development. Patients with secondary amenorrhea will have decreased ovarian function and/or hypoestrogenism. In both cases, gonadotropin concentrations are low to normal and there is no evidence of pituitary dysfunction, such as hyperprolactinemia.

Nutrition or Weight Loss Related Amenorrhea

It is well recognized that weight loss and food restriction can affect the normal menstrual cycle. The insult to the reproductive system occurs in a manner that is related to the percentage of weight loss below the ideal. The fundamental physiologic insult appears to be to the GnRH pulse generator; this is reflected in a decreased number and/or decreased amplitude of both LH and to some extent FSH pulses (see Chapter 10).

The menstrual irregularities which occur in this setting are relatively frequent, but appear to be generally reversible on return to a normal nutrition status. They may present with a spectrum that ranges from a prolongation of the follicular phase, a shortening of the luteal phase, or amenorrhea. We will highlight three important examples of nutrition-associated reproductive deficiency: anorexia nervosa, simple and diet-associated weight loss, and bulimia.

Anorexia nervosa. An extreme example of the nutrition related amenorrhea condition, anorexia nervosa is generally seen in young, predominately white women under the age of 25 years. The condition presents with a classic triad: amenorrhea, weight loss to emaciation, and behavioral changes. While the overall incidence of anorexia nervosa is fairly rare, it differs greatly in population groups and an at-risk population appears to exist. One of every 100 middle class adolescent girl develops the syndrome; professional ballet dancers have an incidence ranging from 1 in 20 to 1 in 5, depending on the competitive level of the company from which the survey originates. The striking incidence of this disorder in the latter population may relate to the rigid standards for thinness as well as the significantly greater number of hours of exercise.

Some recent studies have suggested a metabolic or genetic factor that may predispose the individual to the emergence of anorexia nervosa. For instance, the incidence for a female monozygous twin is as high as 6%. There is an increased incidence in association with gonadal dysgenesis and with diabetes mellitus. The syndrome is rare in men (the male/female ratio is 9:1), although it has been reported in men who are training for competitive activity while restricting their weight. Anorexia nervosa is particularly frequent at puberty, suggesting that the metabolic demands of adolescence may predispose girls to the emergence of the syndrome.

Reproductive endocrinologists have been particularly interested in anorexia nervosa because it represents a prototype of the so-called hypothalamic amenorrhea syndrome, and the reproductive abnormalities are potentially reversible with weight gain. The reproductive and physiologic adjustments appear to be an adaptive phenomenon appropriate for the semistarved state. Amenorrhea, weight loss, and psychiatric disturbance appear to occur together and generally recovery parallels the weight gain. Unfortunately, there is no blood test or specific physical findings which confirms diagnosis of the syndrome. Thus, the clinician must make a diagnosis based on a symptom complex which includes amenorrhea, severe weight loss (usually to less than 80% of ideal body weight), and behavioral changes such as hyperactivity, preoccupation with food, and perceptual changes. In particular, the patient has a distorted view of her body and generally demonstrates an unreasonable concern about being "too fat." Common signs and symptoms of anorexia nervosa are outlined in Table 11–2. Amenorrhea often can be related to the onset of food restriction even if weight loss has been slight. If weight loss occurs prior to menarche, the patient may present with primary amenorrhea. The familiar syndrome that ensues with the onset of the weight loss is a syndrome that has generally been attributed to starvation.

The endocrine profile associated with anorexia nervosa has been studied in depth and provides strong evidence of hypothalamic dysfunction. Low levels of plasma LH and FSH are accompanied by a profound estrogen deficiency. There

Table 11–2. Common Signs and Symptoms of
Anorexia Nervosa

	%	Reported in Starvation
Amenorrhea	100	Yes
Hypotension	86	Yes
Hypothermia	64	Yes
Constipation	62	Yes
Dry skin	62	Yes
Lanugo-type hair	52	Yes
Preoccupation with food	45	Yes
Bradycardia	26	Yes
Edema	26	Yes
Abdominal pain	19	Yes
Intolerance to cold	19	Yes
Systolic murmur	14	No
Petechiae	9	Yes
Vomiting	5	No

Source: Adapted from Warren MP, Vande Wiele RL 1973: *Am J Obstet Gynecol* 117:435.

is a lack of the normal episodic variation of LH secretion, which directly reflects the suppression of activity of the GnRH pulse generator induced by the disease (see Fig. 10–4). In severe cases, a reversion to a prepubertal pattern of low secretory LH activity is seen. A nocturnal, sleep-related increase in LH pulsatility (typical of early puberty) can also be seen in adult anorectics; the appearance of this LH pattern may signal a return to normal function in a previously severe case. When a severely ill anorectic is challenged with GnRH, a prepubertal pattern of response is observed: the FSH response is greater than that of LH (Fig. 11–5). A reversion to an adultlike response pattern generally occurs with weight gain and recovery. The pattern of gonadotropin secretion can be made to revert to a normal adult one by long-term pulsatile GnRH infusion: LH secretion is enhanced and ovulation and menstruation can be induced. The exact hypothalamic mechanism for the suppression of GnRH remains unclear (see also Chapter 10). In some patients, opioid antagonism following naloxone infusion restores LH pulsatility, suggesting that increased endogenous opioid activity may interfere with the function of the pulse generator. This effect, however, is not consistent in all patients with anorexia nervosa.

A number of other abnormalities have been described in anorexia nervosa which suggest a more general hypothalamic dysfunction than one confined to the area of the GnRH pulse generator. These include abnormal thermoregulatory responses to temperature extremes, a deficiency in the handling of a water load (thought to result from a mild diabetes insipidus), and behavioral abnormalities, including altered food intake. These abnormalities are all controlled by mechanisms which most likely engage hypothalamic pathways (Table 11–3). Thyroid metabolism is altered so that the picture of a "euthyroid sick syndrome" is seen. The peripheral deiodination of T4 is diverted from formation of the active T3 to the production of reverse T3, an inactive metabolite. These changes promote a generally reduced metabolic rate and prevent nitrogen loss and muscle catabolism. Replacement with thyroid in fact serves only to accelerate the loss of lean body mass. Clinically, one sees bradycardia, hypothermia, hypotension, slowed relaxation of reflexes, and hypercarotinemia. (A metabolic deficit that appears to occur with dieting prevents the normal metabolism of carotene,

Table 11–3. Abnormalities Suggestive of Hypothalamic Dysfunction in Anorexia Nervosa

Abnormality	Hypothalamic Area
Amenorrhea	Medio basal
Thermoregulation	Anterior-posterior
Water conservation	Supraoptic-paraventricular
Behavioral	Ventromedial
Altered food intake	
Activity	

Source: Adapted from Warren MP 1988: Anorexia nervosa and bulimia. In: *Gynecology and Obstetrics* (Sciarra JW, ed), Harper and Row, Hagerstown, NJ.

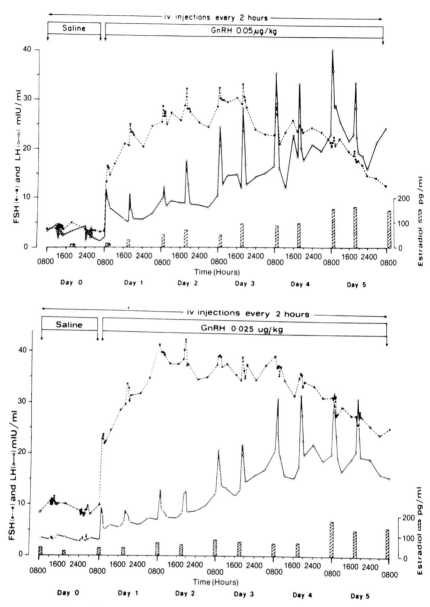

Fig. 11–5. Anorexia nervosa. LH and FSH responses to intravenous *(IV)* GnRH pulses, at 2-hour intervals, in two patients with anorexia nervosa. Note the initial predominance of the FSH response in a typical prepubertal pattern. Abbreviations as in Figure 11–1. (From Marshall JC, Kelch RP 1979: Low dose pulsatile gonadotropin-releasing hormone in anorexia nervosa: a model of human pubertal development: *J Clin Endocrinol Metab* 49:712. Copyright © by The Endocrine Society.)

a precursor of vitamin A. An increase in vegetables intake also may contribute.) Levels of cortisol are elevated, although episodic function and circadian rhythmicity are retained. This change, which is also seen in malnutrition, reflects, in part, the prolonged half-life of cortisol due to reduced metabolic clearance. However, several studies have also suggested that cortisol production rates may be elevated and that there may be a decreased affinity of cortisol-binding globulin for the hormone; thus, bioactive cortisol may be available to tissues of patients with anorexia nervosa in increasing amounts. The failure of these higher levels of cortisol to suppress ACTH suggests that a new set point has been determined by the hypothalamic-pituitary-adrenal axis. Abnormal responses to CRH have also been described. The overall effects of hypercortisolemia, however, increase gluconeogenesis and decrease peripheral glucose utilization.

Dieting and low energy diets have a recognized effect on catecholamine secretion; norepinephrine secretion has been shown to fall, with resultant effects which include a lowering of blood pressure, pulse and resting metabolic rate. A sensitivity to insulin has been shown in anorexia nervosa. This disease has been used as a model to demonstrate changes in the affinity and the binding to the insulin receptor. These changes would presumably alter carbohydrate metabolism in the direction of energy conservation. Increased GH levels may also be present and probably reflect a decrease in the levels of somatomedin C, which exerts a suppressive influence on GH. Although no distinct endocrine target organ for GH action is known, many of its peripheral effects, especially on tissue growth and anabolism, are mediated by the somatomedins. Somatomedin C is a sensitive indicator of nitrogen loss, and with inadequate caloric intake, somatomedins levels fall. A decrease of somatomedin levels thus represents a reflex adaptive response, which protects against protein catabolism and favors nitrogen conversion.

Overall, the anorexia nervosa syndrome appears to be reversible although groups at risk such as ballet dancers may have permanent problems possibly related to the combination of nutritional deprivation and estrogen deficiency during an important period of growth.

Simple weight loss and diet-associated weight loss. Both simple and diet-associated weight loss may produce menstrual dysfunction and amenorrhea which are qualitatively similar to the amenorrheic syndrome seen in anorexia nervosa, although to a lesser degree. LH secretion in particular is affected and a reversal to a 24-hour pubertal secretory pattern, with sleep entrained nocturnal spurting, may occur. Patients may complain of amenorrhea, but a history of weight loss may not be volunteered. Thus, history of a recent diet and amount of weight loss is an important lead to the diagnosis. The FSH:LH ratio is generally decreased, while prolactin levels are normal. Response to GnRH is extremely variable, but estrogen levels are generally low. Patients occasionally may become anovulatory with a positive response to a progesterone challenge, a good prognostic sign. Pituitary disease should be ruled out as part of the workup for this syndrome. The condition usually reverses with weight gain but amenorrhea may persist for prolonged periods even after gain of weight to near normal levels.

Dieting with weight loss can produce a variety of other changes in normal women including a reduction in estradiol levels and anovulation in the face of apparently normal LH concentrations and LH pulse frequency (24-hour circadian studies, however, have not been reported). Changes in circulating LH have also been reported during the process of weight recovery in underweight infertile women.

Qualitative changes in the type of diet may also affect reproductive function. A vegetarian diet, for example, is associated with a higher than expected incidence of reproductive disorders and anovulation; depressed LH and estrogen levels have been documented. A high fiber vegetarian diet may affect estrogen levels by increasing fecal estrogen excretion in a bulky stool and preventing a normal enterohepatic circulation. In general, however, these syndromes have not been well studied.

Bulimic syndrome. Bulimia, although more common in slightly older age groups than anorexia nervosa, is also generally a condition seen in young women and often related to previous anorectic behavior. In this syndrome, individuals gorge themselves and then use artificial means to purge calories: these include vomiting, laxative, or diuretic abuse. Gorging episodes may alternate with periods of severe food restriction. The bulimic's weight may fluctuate but usually not to dangerously low levels. There is often a history of other impulsive behaviors, such as alcohol or drug use (some features of this disorder are not unlike those seen with drug addiction), stealing and shoplifting, as well as unrestrained promiscuity. This is unlike the restrictive anorectic who remains generally asexual. A separate condition known as bulimia nervosa has been described in which the bulimic behavior evolves from the completely restricting anorexia nervosa type pattern.

Bulimics have a wide variety of medical problems which may be superimposed on the anorectic syndrome. These include severe tooth decay, parotid enlargement, stomach rupture, metabolic alkalosis, carpal pedal spasm, hypercarotenemia, and pancreatitis. The bulimic individual may also present with menstrual irregularity, but the incidence is highly variable. These individuals may have adequate estrogen secretion but present with an anovulatory syndrome. This type of problem may be difficult to diagnose because the menstrual disorder and amenorrhea may develop even when the weight remains normal. Bulimic behavior is often secretive and patients will not admit to these patterns even when questioned directly. The behavior is often chronic and increased anxiety, irritability, depression, and poor social functioning are common. Weight may remain within a reasonable range, but protein caloric malnutrition must usually supervene and most likely contributes to the development of the reproductive disorder.

It is thought that, at least in some cases, bulimia may have an organic cause. The association of neurologic abnormalities and bulimia raises the intriguing possibility of underlying neuroendocrine dysfunction as a cause of both the nutritional and the menstrual disorder. Hypothalamic diseases may be associated with excess appetite and lack of satiety inhibition.

Exercise-Related Amenorrhea

The reproductive cycle may be profoundly influenced by strenuous exercise. The exercise-related anovulatory syndrome which may progress to an hypoestrogenic hypogonadotropic pattern is most probably multifactorial in origin: physical activity alone may not be a sufficient factor as a cause of amenorrhea, and other predisposing factors, such as low body weight, changes in diet, weight loss, particularly in subjects who were near their normal weight, or the perceived stress of the activity, must also be accounted for. The syndrome is particularly frequent in elite groups of athletes required to maintain low body weight.

The normal function of the hypothalamic-pituitary unit in exercise is usually altered as suggested by a decrease in the frequency of pulsatile LH secretion and in some cases by a reversion to a pubertal pattern type of LH secretion with nocturnal entrainment, or in severe cases, to a prepubertal pattern (see Fig. 10–2). Small changes in pulsatile patterns usually precede obvious changes in menstrual cycle function. Activation of the hypothalamic-pituitary adrenal axis during exercise can be documented by increased ACTH and cortisol levels. The signals which affect the GnRH pulse generator may also involve key metabolic hormones or substances found in the adaptive state to vigorous exercise. Insulin in particular has been implicated, as have various amino acids, in particular tryptophan, which has been found to be elevated in the brain of exercising animals. However, no conclusive metabolic factors have been identified and much work remains to be done in this area (see also Chapter 10).

A low body fat has been suggested as a primary causal factor by several investigators. Yet, several large-scale studies comparing normal cycling runners to amenorrheic runners have failed to find low body fat as a differential variable. In fact, this paradigm does not appear to be part of the causal mechanism, for menstrual cyclicity can be reinitiated soon after exercise ceases, prior to changes in weight or body composition. Emerging literature suggests that the reproductive alterations may represent an adaptive effect which conserves energy.

Three specific problems are commonly seen with exercise: delayed menarche, secondary amenorrhea, and inadequate luteal phase.

Delayed menarche. In adolescence, the hypothalamic-pituitary axis is immature and weight control may have a greater impact than at other phases of reproductive life. In general, the dieting pattern to maintain a low body weight in association with exercise influences the time of menarche, and thus, delayed menarche is common in athletes (Fig. 11–6). Ballet dancers and skaters, who are required to maintain low body weight, are more likely to have delayed menarche and more negative eating attitude scores than swimmers and nonathletes. Dancers would experience the greater difficulty achieving their desired degree of thinness without significant dieting. The swimmers, by contrast, exhibit little if any dieting behavior, because low weight is not essential and caloric expenditure is relatively high. Overall, weight (or degree of leanness) is a better predictor of age of menarche in athletes while in nonathletes age of menarche is usually best predicted by maternal menarcheal age.

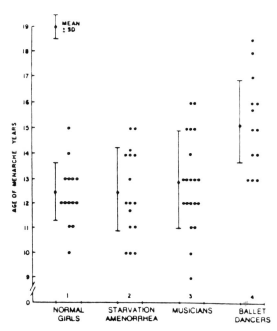

Fig. 11–6. Age at menarche. A delay in menarche is frequently seen in ballet dancers, perhaps reflecting the combination of exercise with stress and dieting. (From Warren MP 1980: The effects of exercise on pubertal progression and reproductive function in girls. *J Clin Endocrinol Metab* 51:1150–1157. Copyright © by The Endocrine Society.)

Physical demands of training may also contribute to delayed menarche. For example, it has been shown that for each year of training prior to the expected age of menarche, menarche may be delayed by 4 months (see, e.g., Fig. 7–6). In another study in fifteen ballet dancers, aged 13–15 years, progression of sexual development and onset of menarche occurred when a decrease in exercise and/ or injury forced rest of at least 2 months duration. Weight gain was minimal or absent in these girls and no significant change in body composition occurred. Progression of puberty, as manifested by breast development and the onset of menarche, was more evident in the leaner girls during periods of rest. In general, dancers are consistently delayed even when they reach the so-called crucial weight for height or body fat; periods of rest, however, often result in striking "catch-up" development.

A remarkable dichotomy in the order of pubertal development is also noted with exercise: pubarche, or the development of body hair, is reached at a nearly normal age, but breast development and other estrogen-related factors are suppressed. The large caloric demands of training may therefore have little impact on central mechanisms triggering pubic hair development or may even advance that process, whereas these demands impair the central mechanism(s) responsible for initiating ovarian estrogen secretion.

Secondary amenorrhea. The incidence of secondary amenorrhea in athletes is extremely variable, from 2–20% in runners and 30% in adult ballet dancers (50% in adolescent ballet dancers). The degree of incidence is generally correlated with the intensity of activity and is definitely higher in elite competition. It is also more common in women with delayed menarche. Body weight correlates negatively with the occurrence of reproductive dysfunction. There is also increasing evidence that the reproductive dysfunction attributed to exercise may be associated with eating disorders.

Exercise-induced amenorrhea may represent an adaptive response to the large energy requirements in a normal to underweight individual. Amenorrheic runners appear to become more energy efficient by lowering their metabolic rate and thermic response to food. One study suggests that this effect may be a previously unrecognized physiologic response to exercise observed in all trained individuals but more prominent in the amenorrheic athlete. Physiologic studies have demonstrated that the thermal response to the physiological progesterone increase in the postovulatory luteal phase costs 500 calories per cycle; anovulation would therefore lower caloric requirements!

Inadeqate luteal phase. More subtle changes in the follicular phase and mid-cycle gonadotropin secretion may occur when initially increasing training intensity. This can result in prolongation of the preovulatory phase with a resulting short or inadequate luteal phase characterized by blunted secretion of progesterone (see Chapter 10 for details on this syndrome). This effect has been reproduced experimentally; it occurs only after a heavy exercise load and is more prominent when weight loss occurs (Fig. 11–7).

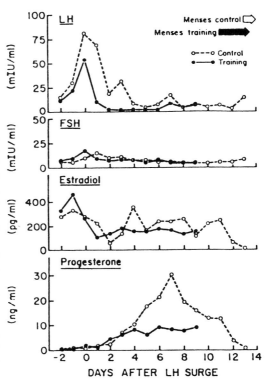

Fig. 11–7. Short luteal phase in a long-distance runner. Abnormal progesterone secretion (short or inadequate luteal phase) may follow deficiencies in gonadotropin secretion and in follicular maturation. In this example, the cycle during training *(solid circles)* is characterized by a short luteal phase. Abbreviations as in Figure 11–1. (From Shangold M, Freeman R, Thysen B, Gatz M 1979: The relationship between long-distance running plasma progesterone, and luteal phase length. *Fertil Steril* 31:130–3. Reproduced with permission of the publisher, The American Fertility Society.)

Stress-Related Amenorrhea

Psychological stress has long been known to cause amenorrhea. Stressful events such as leaving home for school, death of a close relative or friend, or psychological problems are associated with amenorrhea at an incidence ranging from 22–83%. Stress is also thought to contribute to athletic amenorrhea and the amenorrhea of anorexia nervosa and starvation. Cortisol excess and abnormal responses to CRH have been documented in these circumstances.

The precise mechanisms through which stress may influence reproduction are not entirely known; however, as in other syndromes, decreased LH pulsatility is frequently observed. (Stress in postmenopausal women also can dramatically decrease LH secretion.) Recent attention has focused on the inhibitory role that CRH exerts on GnRH secretion (see Chapter 10). In fact, in animals, stress-induced inhibition of pulsatile LH release can be prevented by administration of a CRH antagonist.

The degree of menstrual cyclicity disturbances is very variable, probably reflecting the intensity of the stressful stimulus, and its effect on pulsatile activity of the GnRH pulse generator. Because of the unpredictability of the phenomenon, these patients have been less well studied than those with exercise or starvation-induced amenorrhea.

Congenital Hypothalamic Syndromes

Kallman's syndrome. Congenital hypothalamic hypogonadotropic hypogonadism, known as Kallman's syndrome, is usually associated with anosmia or hyposmia, color blindness, and occasionally nerve deafness. It is known that the olfactory tracts and the GnRH neuronal system develop from similar areas, and when development is incomplete, GnRH deficiency may ensue (see Chapter 2). Women present with lack of sexual development and primary amenorrhea, although there is considerable clinical and laboratory heterogeneity with respect to sexual development. These differences appear to be related to the degree of endogenous GnRH deficiency. The ovaries will respond to induction of ovulation therapies.

Lawrence-Moon-Biedl syndrome. These patients present with obesity, lack of sexual development, stunted growth, diabetes insipidus, mental deficiency, retinitis pigmentosa, polydactylism, and syndactylism. The problem is thought to be due to a congenital defect in the hypothalamus and is inherited as an autosomal recessive.

Noncongenital Hypothalamic Syndromes

Histiocytosis X. Histiocytosis X is an entity encompassing three varieties of histiocytosis: eosinophilic granuloma of bone (infiltration by eosinophiles), Letterer-Siwe disease, and Hans-Schüller-Christian disease (histiocytic proliferation). It has been suggested that the three variants are actually all manifestations of eosinophilic granuloma. All varieties may be associated with diabetes insipidus and may infiltrate the hypothalamus. Diabetes insipidus may be the presenting symptom and may persist for a long time (up to 10 years) before an etiologic diagnosis is made. Although visceral and osseous involvement may occur, the disease in adults seems to have a propensity for the hypothalamic-pituitary region and may also infiltrate the optic chiasm. Paradoxically, the isolated lesions confined to bone almost never involve the sella turcica or sphenoid bone.

Intrinsic and contiguous mass lesions. Lesions involving the hypothalamus are divided into those that do structural damage due to tissue destruction and those that cause damage by triggering inappropriate signals from other parts of the hypothalamus or the C.N.S. Reproductive dysfunction is the most frequent early manifestation of organic hypothalamic disease. Neurologic symptoms usually occur later than endocrine symptoms, although the pattern of presentation and the association with neurological symptoms is an important key. Symptomatology evidently varies with the original location of the tumor (Table 11–4). Lesions arising in the anterior hypothalamus display a wide variety of symptoms including altered food intake and abnormal temperature control. Ventromedial neoplasms have been associated with hyperphagia, rage, and dementia. Tumors of the posterior fossa may cause internal hydrocephalus and hypothalamic symptoms due to pressure in the third ventricle.

Treatment of hypothalamic mass lesions is aimed at the underlying condition. Since the hypothalamus lies in a critical area, surgical treatment is not easy. Some mass lesions are radiosensitive and drug therapy is used for replacement of hormone deficiencies. Antiepileptics are used to treat some behavioral abnormalities and seizures that may occur.

Granulomatous disease. Tuberculomas and sarcoid are the most frequent infectious causes of hypothalamic dysfunction with associated amenorrhea. Sarcoid in particular produces diabetes insipidus associated with amenorrhea.

Table 11–4. Symptomatology of Hypothalamic Lesions

Location	Symptomatology
Preoptic area	Autonomic disturbances, cardiac arrhythmias, bladder incontinence, pulmonary edema
Anterior hypothalamic-preoptic region	Hyperthermia
Anterior hypothalamus	Altered food intake, cachexia
Lateral anterior hypothalamus	Altered food intake, loss of thirst
Ventromedial area	Hyperphagia, obesity, abnormal emotional states
Ventromedial area-median eminence	Diabetes insipidus, hypogonadism, abnormalities of ACTH, GH, and PRL secretion
Lateral hypothalamus	Anorexia, weight loss
Caudal hypothalamus	Disorders of consciousness, somnolence, hypokinesia, hypothermia, poikilothermia

Source: Martin JB, Reichlin S, Brown GM 1977: *Clinical Neuroendocrinology.* FA Davis, Philadelphia.
ACTH, adrenocorticotropin hormone; *GH,* growth hormone; *PRL,* prolactin.

Post "Pill" and Postpartum Amenorrhea

Prolonged suppression of the hypothalamic-pituitary unit with oral contraceptives may cause amenorrhea in a small number of patients when the treatment is discontinued. This has also been observed after a pregnancy. The incidence varies from 1–2% of patients treated with contraceptives and during the postpartum period. The syndrome is thought to be more common if menstruations were irregular to begin with. Generally, normal gonadotropins and normal to low estrogen levels are found and the condition reverses spontaneously. The condition is more common if weight loss has occurred on oral contraceptive pills. Once pregnancy is ruled out, other forms of amenorrhea should be evaluated if the condition has existed for more than 6 months, including hyperprolactinemia and androgen excess.

Pseudocyesis

This syndrome (the so-called false pregnancy from the Greek *cyesis* meaning pregnancy) is a dramatic example of psychogenic amenorrhea. The condition appears to be more common in societies where there is a high premium placed on a woman's fertility. The symptoms are very consistent and include amenorrhea, gradual abdominal enlargement, breast changes, and, occasionally, galactorrhea and alveolar pigmentation. The patient usually experiences nausea and vomiting, perceives fetal movements, and gains weight. (An occasional positive pregnancy test may be obtained.) The distention of the abdomen may be impressive: one patient, for example, underwent a cesarean section for nonproductive labor. Pregnancy is almost always desired and the patient becomes hostile and defensive if challenged about her pregnant state.

Investigations into this syndrome reveal an abnormal hormonal profile which shows elevated LH levels accompanied by elevated prolactin levels (Fig. 11–8). Pulsations of LH appear to be increased as well. The unusual combination of elevated LH and prolactin is particularly intriguing in view of the luteotropic effects of LH (in the human) and of prolactin (in animals). The synergistic effects of elevated LH and prolactin concentrations may be responsible for the emergence of this syndrome which involves very dramatic changes in behavior as well as physiology. The presence of elevated prolactin levels explains the development of galactorrhea.

Exaggerated PRL response to TRH, which has been described in pseudocyesis, is also seen in depression. The drug reserpine which may induce depression by virtue of its biogenic amine depletion effect may also induce pseudocyesis in animals and lactation and amenorrhea in humans. Thus, changes in central neurotransmitter activity, such as seen in depression, may be a causal event in the development of this syndrome and provide the setting for the endocrine dysfunction. Other abnormalities suggestive of hypothalamic-pituitary derangement include abnormal responses to exogenous releasing hormone, in particular increased LH response to GnRH and PRL response to TRH, together with aberrant LH responses to TRH (FSH levels, however, remain normal). With the resolution of the depressive state the rapid reversal of these endocrine patterns is very dramatic, suggesting a causal effect of depression in patients with pseudocyesis (Fig. 11–8).

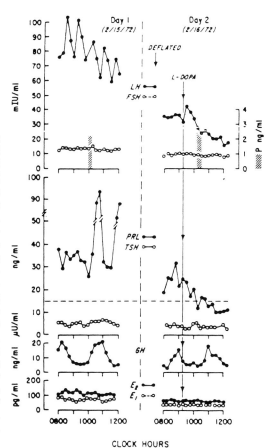

Fig. 11–8. Hormone patterns in pseudocyesis. Note the unusual combination of elevated LH and prolactin *(PRL)* secretion (FSH levels remain unchanged). On day 2, the nature of the problem was explained to the patient. Within 30 minutes, her distended abdomen completely disappeared after passage of large amounts of flatus. Note the lowered LH and PRL levels immediately thereafter. *E1,* estrone; *E2,* estriol; *GH,* growth hormone; *L-DOPA,* a dopamine precursor; *P,* progesterone; *TSH,* thyroid-stimulating hormone; other abbreviations as in Figure 11–1. (From Yen SSC, Rebar RW, Quesenberry W 1976: Pituitary function in pseudocyesis. *J Clin Endocrinol Metab* 43:132–136. Copyright © by The Endocrine Society.)

Patients with pseudocyesis can usually be diagnosed by elevated prolactin and gonadotropin levels and a negative pregnancy test. It may be difficult to convince patients that they are not pregnant and often a sonogram as well as psychotherapy are necessary. The underlying depression should also be treated.

Iatrogenic Hypothalamic Disease

Iatrogenic disease of the hypothalamus should also be considered. Radiation of the head and neck for treatment of nasopharyngeal cancer is associated with endocrine deficiencies, particularly of the thyroid and pituitary. A recent study indicates that some of the latter may be hypothalamic in origin: twelve of fifteen irradiated patients showed hypothalamic abnormalities. Subnormal GH and cortisol response to insulin hypoglycemia was accompanied in some patients by growth failure and delayed bone age and in others by signs of adrenal cortical insufficiency. All of the patients received 5,000 to 8,300 rads to the hypothalamic-pituitary area.

12

Menstrual Cycle Dysfunction: Enhanced Androgen Secretion

In addition to the ovulatory disorders described in Chapter 11, there are pathological states specifically associated with increased production of androgens. Generally, these states are related to a luteinizing hormone (LH)-induced ovarian overproduction of androgens, usually the result of a disturbance in the endocrine feedback loop. Occasionally the adrenals are involved in the androgen pathology. These states are usually referred to as the polycystic ovarian disease or syndrome (PCO). In fact, there is no single pathological entity and several pathological conditions can contribute to the clinical picture of a PCO patient: it is the physician's task to diagnose these and treat accordingly. This is not always possible, however, and often the condition is treated successfully without obtaining a full understanding of the causal factors. We will review the pathogenesis of PCO, its clinical symptoms, and specific therapeutical aspects related to PCO.

THE PATHOGENESIS OF PCO

Since the disease is associated with hyperandrogenism, we will first review androgen metabolism, then discuss the possible causes for the syndrome.

ANDROGEN METABOLISM

The androgens are part of the C-19 androstane series of steroids; they are integral intermediates in the steroidogenic pathways in the adrenal, testis, and ovary (Fig. 12–1). Androgens are mandatory to normal male sexual development. They are normally present in women, but when concentrations exceed normal values, hyperandrogenic symptoms appear.

Testosterone is the most active of the circulating androgens: it is ten times more active than androstenedione and twenty times more active than dehydroepiandrosterone (DHEA). After entering the target cell, testosterone is reduced by 5-α-reductase to dihydrotestosterone (DHT) which is the most active androgen. Approximately 98% of plasma testosterone is bound, mostly to sex hormone binding globulin. Only the free testosterone is biologically active, and

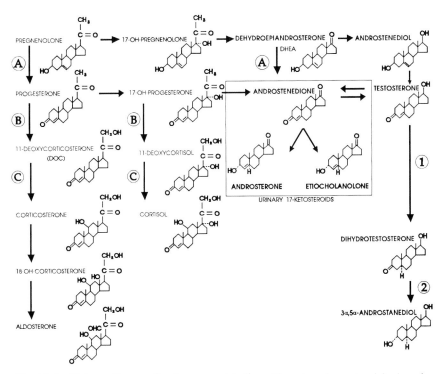

Fig. 12–1. Major pathways of androgen metabolism. The adrenal secretes dehydroepi-androsterone *(DHEA),* but also androstenedione. The ovary secretes testosterone and androstenedione. Measurement of urinary 17-ketosteroids reflects adrenal DHEA secretion mostly. In the target cell, testosterone is metabolized into dihydrotestosterone (1: 5-α-reductase), a much more potent hormone, and to 3-α, 5-α androstanediol (2: 3-α-diol glucuronide). (For further information on steroid biosynthesis, see also Chapter 3.) Enzymes that may be deficient in the general steroid scheme include 3-β-ol-dehydrogenase *(A)*; 21-hydroxylase *(B)*; and 11-β-hydroxylase *(C)*. Accumulation of 17-hydroxy (OH) progesterone signifies B or C enzyme deficiency, while that of 11-deoxycortisol signifies a C deficiency.

therefore factors that affect the level of free testosterone will also affect the degree of androgenicity.

When dealing with hyperandrogenic states in women, it may be important in some patients to distinguish whether the source of increased androgens is ovarian or adrenal, particularly to rule out an ovarian or adrenal androgen-producing neoplasm. The ovary secretes mostly testosterone and androstenedione and very little DHEA and androstenediol. The adrenal secretes mostly DHEA, but also androstenedione in about the same amount as the ovary. Various methods have been used to evaluate the source of androgens. One way to assess androgen production by the adrenal cortex is to measure urinary 17-ketosteroids, the most abundant of which are androsterone, epiandrosterone, and etiocholanolone, usually secreted as sulfates. These steroids are derived mostly from DHEA and DHEA-sulfate (DHEA-S); 80% of DHEA and more than 90% of DHEA-S are secreted by the adrenal cortex. However, testosterone, androstenedione, and cortisol must also be included among a large number of precursors of this group of urinary metabolites. Usually, only about 10% of cortisol metabolism is accounted for as 17-ketosteroids, most of it secreted as tetrahydrocortisol. Testosterone, which is the most active androgen in PCO, is only minimally detected as a 17-ketosteroid. Thus, measurement of 17-ketosteroids may provide an important diagnostic tool and is relatively simple and inexpensive. It must always be remembered, however, that not all 17-ketosteroid measured are androgens. DHEA-S can be used as a convenient measure of adrenal androgen excess. Selective catheterization of adrenal and ovarian veins and measurement of the steroid profiles also yield information on the site of origin of hyperandrogenism. This is a complex and very expensive approach, however, and therefore not used in the routine clinical evaluation. Various ovarian or adrenal stimulation and suppression tests have been used. The problem is that almost all exogenously administered agents may affect both ovary and adrenal and a clear picture is therefore difficult to obtain. Most recently, gonadotropin-releasing hormone (GnRH) agonists have been used to distinguish between ovarian and adrenal sites of androgen origin. By "down regulating" gonadotropin release, GnRH agonists almost completely stop ovarian secretion (see Chapter 13), and thus ovarian androgen secretion reflected by testosterone and androstenedione can be distinguished from adrenal secretion of DHEA and DHEA-S. Because androstenedione is secreted in equal amounts by the ovary and the adrenal, plasma testosterone is a better marker for ovarian androgen production. (About one-third of testosterone is secreted directly by the ovary [0.25–0.35 mg/day] and the remaining two-thirds are derived by peripheral conversion of ovarian and adrenal precursors in about equal proportions.) Thus, under normal conditions, two-thirds of the circulating testosterone is originating from the ovary.) Determinations of free testosterone are expensive and for practical purposes it is adequate to measure total testosterone.

PATHOPHYSIOLOGY

It is difficult to propose a single pathophysiologic explanation for the development of PCO. It is indeed a very heterogeneous syndrome that may have more than one etiological cause. One attractive hypothesis (by no means the only one) is as follows (Fig. 12–2): PCO may be initiated at puberty and involve at first normal but intensified physiological relationships between the hypothalamic-pituitary-adrenal and hypothalamic-pituitary-ovarian axes. At puberty, the adrenals begin to secrete increased amounts of C-19 steroids and their precursors. (This is part of the normal process of *adrenarche* [see Chapter 7]. This androgen increase occurs in the absence of an increase in cortisol.) Androgens are aromatized to estrone at several extraglandular sites, especially the stromal cells of adipose tissue. Estrone, in turn, activates the estrogen long loop negative feedback. Follicle-stimulating hormone (FSH) is more sensitive than LH to this action. If, for some reason, initial adrenal androgen production is abnormally high at puberty, this physiological phenomenon may be accentuated and LH secretion by the pituitary may exceed that of FSH. Increased LH secretion then

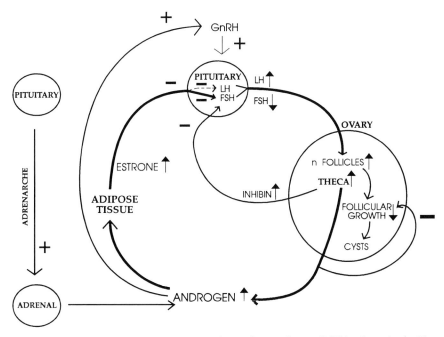

Fig. 12–2. Pathophysiology of the polycystic ovarian syndrome (PCO): a hypothesis. The syndrome may be initiated at adrenarche. An exaggeration of this phenomenon may result in higher than normal androgens, which in turn are converted in peripheral tissues, mainly adipose, into estrone. While androgens may enhance pituitary stimulation by gonadotropin-releasing hormone *(GnRH)*, follicle-stimulating hormone *(FSH)* is more sensitive to the estrogen negative feedback loop than luteinizing hormone *(LH)*. The result is an increased FSH:LH ratio. Excessive LH in turn stimulates theca cells to produce increased androgens, thus establishing a constant *(noncyclic)* source of estrogens: an endocrine vicious circle has been initiated. The ovaries contain numerous tertiary follicles (n: number), but androgens directly inhibit folliculogenesis, leading to arrest of follicular growth and formation of multiple cysts. These may secrete inhibin which may further decrease FSH output.

stimulates ovarian theca cells which become hypertrophied and the secretion of androgens is enhanced. In turn, these androgens are aromatized, and thus a constant *(noncyclic)* source of estrogens is established, sensitizing the gonadotrope to endogenous GnRH. An endocrine vicious circle has been created. Abnormally high concentrations of androgens within the ovary have also been speculated to inhibit the proper process of folliculogenesis directly. This leads to repeated arrests of follicular development resulting in the formation of multiple cystic follicles. Excessive secretion of inhibin from these multiple follicles may suppress FSH secretion and further enhance the LH:FSH ratio. Abnormally fast pulse frequencies have been reported in a small percentage of PCO patients (perhaps induced by the androgens), another possible contributor to a high LH:FSH ratio. In fact, a persistent defect at any part of the physiological system that produces this type of endocrine vicious circle may result in the development of PCO, as has been demonstrated experimentally. Another hypothesis suggests that PCO may arise from hyperfunction of the enzyme responsible for the formation of androgens in the ovarian thecal environment. (It should be pointed out that the functional integrity of the hypothalamic-pituitary-ovarian axis remains intact in PCO patients, since they respond to experimental manipulations of the long loop estrogen positive and negative feedback.)

Of course, the clinical symptoms are long to establish, and by the time the patient consults, the original defect(s), which may or may not be related to that in the hypothesis presented here, may be impossible to trace. However, the endocrine vicious circle can be temporally disrupted by the treatment procedure (discussed later).

Ovaries of PCO patients are usually enlarged, containing numerous tertiary follicles at various stages of development (between 4–7 mm diameter) which involute into cysts (the "polycystic ovary"). This reflects the multiple waves of interrupted folliculogenesis. Expectedly, few corpora lutea are usually seen, the follicles lacking normal maturation and therefore not ovulating. While the number of granulosa cells is decreased and there is evidence for diminished aromatase activity, cells of the theca interna in follicular cysts are usually numerous and hypertrophied, reflecting the process of LH hyperstimulation and excessive androgen production. The ovarian capsule is usually thickened, for reasons not well understood (Fig. 12–3).

Covert congenital adrenal hyperplasia. Late onset or partial congenital adrenal hyperplasia in women may present clinically as PCO. These patients may have partial deficiencies in enzymes involved in the cortisol biosynthetic pathways. The incidence of such deficiencies among PCO patients is not yet known. There may be an ethnic variability in its presentation. These disorders are genetically endowed and family members have been shown to be heterozygous for this disorder either by human leukocyte antigen (HLA) typing or adrenocorticotropin hormone (ACTH) stimulation tests. It is most common in Ashkenazi Jews and certain Eskimo tribes and less common in the northern European population.

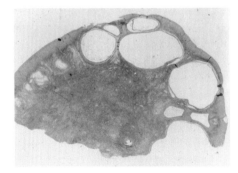 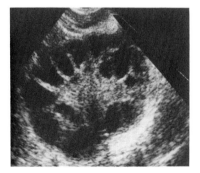

Fig. 12–3. The polycystic ovary. *Left,* ovary after wedge resection. Note the thickened capsule and the multiple follicular cysts. *Right,* ultrasonographic image. Follicles are crowded at the surface of the spherical polycystic ovary. (Sonography from Timor-Tritsch IE, Rottem S 1987: *Transvaginal Sonography,* Elsevier, NY. Reprinted by permission of the publisher).

The three deficient enzymes that may be encountered are 21-hydroxylase (the most common) (*B* in Fig. 12–1), 11-β-hydroxylase (*C*) and 3–β-ol dehydrogenase isomerase (*A*). Measurements of 17-hydroxyprogesterone (17-OHP) after ACTH stimulation can distinguish between PCO and covert congenital adrenal hyperplasia. 17-OHP is markedly elevated when there is 21-hydroxylase or 11-β-hydroxylase deficiency. Measurement of 17-OHP in an early morning blood sample is a good screening test. If levels are elevated or at the upper limits of normal (normal <3 ng/ml), an ACTH stimulation test will confirm the diagnosis. Levels greater than 8 ng/ml are diagnostic of congenital adrenal hyperplasia. In patients with high 17-OHP concentrations, measurement of 11-desoxycortisol will differentiate between 21-hydroxylase deficiency and 11-β-hydroxylase deficiency. In the latter, 11-desoxycortisol will be elevated. It should be mentioned that 11-β-hydroxylase deficiency may be associated with hypertension. Delta-5 and delta-4 steroids need to be measured to diagnose 3-β-ol dehydrogenase deficiency. These patients will have high levels of DHEA-S and normal or low levels of testosterone. ACTH stimulation and marked increases of delta-5 and delta-4 steroid precursors will make a definitive diagnosis.

Although in most instances hirsutism is the most troublesome symptom, many, but not all, of these patients appear as typical PCO patients. In some patients, the primary complaint is infertility.

CLINICAL ASPECTS OF PCO

SYMPTOMS

Most symptoms in PCO patients directly or indirectly reflect the increased rate of androgen production. The prominent clinical features include (1) hirsutism, (2) obesity, and (3) menstrual irregularity and chronic anovulation. In most instances, patients seek treatment for infertility or because of cosmetic concerns.

Hirsutism

Hirsutism and acne are the effect of hyperandrogenism, but they are not a uniform manifestation. Hirsutism appears in about 70% and acne in about 35% of women with PCO. Yet, clinical signs of hyperandrogenicity can vary considerably, depending on the degree and duration of hyperandrogenism and the individual sensitivity of the patient. A young woman can see herself as hairy and unattractive and be emotionally and socially inhibited, while objectively there is only minimal hirsutism, while another individual can be markedly hairy without subjective problem. More overt signs of androgen virilization, such as clitoromegaly, are very infrequent in PCO and should make one suspicious of an androgen producing tumor.

Obesity

Obesity was one of the cardinal symptoms in the classical description of PCO (Stein-Leventhal syndrome). It is not, however, a necessary feature in PCO patients, and only about 40% are obese. In general, free plasma androgen levels are increased in obese women, a result of increased production rate and of a lower level of sex hormone binding globulin. (However, metabolic clearance rates are also increased, keeping the androgen increase modest.) Enhanced conversion of androgen to estrone in adipose tissue may certainly be an important contributor to the menstrual irregularity encountered in obese PCO patients. Increased plasma androstenedione concentrations in obese patients have been found to normalize on weight reduction, and, in some patients, considerable weight loss may revert the cycle irregularity. (Not all obese women have polycystic ovaries, although menstrual dysfunction frequently results from obesity.)

Menstrual Irregularity

Menstrual irregularity may be manifested as oligomenorrhea or amenorrhea. It is the result of the endocrine vicious circle described earlier, and of the presence of a continuous noncyclic source of androgens and estrogens. The resultant anovulatory state is the main reason for infertility in PCO patients. Luteal phase defects have also been observed. Dysfunctional uterine bleeding is quite common due to unopposed estrogenic stimulation of the endometrium. This can lead to endometrial hyperplasia and eventually endometrial carcinoma. Indeed, about 20% of women who develop endometrial carcinoma before age 40 years have evidence of PCO.

ANATOMICAL AND BIOCHEMICAL FEATURES

Ovarian Visualization

The original definition of PCO includes the presence of palpable enlarged ovaries which on exploration have a pearly white, smooth capsule and are histologically polycystic. Recent advances in ultrasound, particularly with the vaginal probe, make the diagnosis of polycystic ovaries easier. Nonetheless, up to 15% of PCO patients undergoing laparotomy have what appear to be normal ovaries, and many patients with what appear to be typical polycystic ovaries have ovulatory cycles and conceive spontaneously. The variability is considerable and there are really no narrowly defined criteria to describe the ovaries in PCO.

Hormone Measurements

Several typical abnormalities in hormone levels have been described in PCO. Nonetheless, not all changes are present in each individual case at all times.

Gonadotropins. Generally, LH concentrations are elevated compared to levels in the normal follicular phase. FSH levels are normal or slightly lower. Typical in many patients is an increased LH:FSH ratio. Still, there may be patients with typical PCO features who have normal LH levels and LH:FSH ratios. In studies using frequent blood sampling, increases in frequency and/or amplitude of LH pulses when compared to the normal follicular phase have been described in some PCO patients (20%). There may also be qualitative differences in LH secretion, in that mean bioactive LH concentrations have been reported to be sometimes higher in PCO women than in controls and bioactive: immunoreactive LH ratio may be elevated.

When tested with GnRH, PCO patients show increased pituitary sensitivity, and the LH response is usually similar to that seen in a normal woman at mid-cycle, the time of maximal sensitivity. This is usually observed in patients with high basal LH levels and is probably the result of constant pituitary priming by estrogens. In contrast, the FSH response is small and compares to that seen in the early follicular phase of a normal cycle.

Estrogen. Estrogen levels are increased in PCO. However, only the levels of estrone are markedly elevated; estradiol concentrations are similar to those seen in the early follicular phase of a normal cycle. As mentioned previously, most of the circulating estrone derives from peripheral conversion of androgens. In addition, PCO patients usually have lower than normal levels of sex hormone binding globulin, due to increased androgens and obesity, and therefore, higher levels of free estrogens.

Androgens. Androgens are generally at the upper level of normal or elevated in PCO patients. However, there are considerable fluctuations in the degree of elevation and there is a marked overlap between PCO patients and normal subjects. Since sex hormone binding globulin is lower in PCO, a greater percentage of testosterone circulates as free hormone, which is responsible for the hyperandrogenic symptoms. The response of hair follicles to androgens is difficult to correlate with peripheral testosterone concentrations, since it depends mostly on their capacity to metabolize the steroid into DHT. This steroid is further reduced to 3-α, 5-α-androstanediol and its glucuronide (Fig. 12–1). Recent studies have shown that skin levels of 5-α-reductase and 3-α-diol-glucuronide show excellent correlation with the degree of hyperandrogenicity.

Although DHEA and its sulfate are mostly adrenal products, at least 50% of patients with PCO have elevated levels. A role for the adrenal in increased androgens and in the pathogenesis of PCO has been proposed but remains controversial. Evidence includes, in some PCO patients, a decreased response after adrenal suppression with glucocorticoids and an increased androgen response to exogenous administration of ACTH or metyrapone. The latter is a drug used in testing pituitary-adrenal reserve. It inhibits 11-β-hydroxylase, which is critical in cortisol biosynthesis, thus decreasing cortisol secretion and inducing compensatory ACTH release, which stimulates adrenal steroid secretion. A standard test of pituitary-adrenal reserve is performed by giving 10 mg metyrapone per kg of ideal body weight every 4 hours for 6 doses. A normal response consists of a two-fold or more increase in total urinary 17-hydroxycorticosteroids on the day of treatment or the subsequent day. Ovarian suppression with GnRH agonists will reduce the ovarian steroids but will not markedly suppress DHEA and DHEA-S.

Prolactin (PRL). Hyperprolactinemia has been reported in about 27% of patients with PCO. In the majority, PRL is at the upper limits of normal or only slightly elevated. These patients show an excessive PRL response to metaclopramide (a dopamine-receptor antagonist) and to thyrotropin-releasing hormone (TRH). Such enhanced responses, however, are most probably caused by the elevated estrogen levels in PCO patients.

PRL may have a direct effect on DHEA-S secretion. Patients with hyperprolactinemia treated with bromocriptine to decrease PRL show a diminished DHEA-S production rate. Whatever the reason for elevated PRL, PCO patients should have a PRL assessment and hyperprolactinemia should be corrected.

Insulin resistance. Insulin resistance has been demonstrated in PCO patients, independent of the degree of obesity: basal insulin secretion and insulin response to glucose tolerance testing are both increased. Hyperinsulinemia may impact on androgen production: insulin binds to ovarian tissue where it may stimulate ovarian androgen production. A positive correlation between fasting insulin and circulating androgen concentrations has been reported. The precise role of insulin in the pathogenesis of PCO is not clear, but hyperinsulinemia may somehow help in promoting androgen overproduction in these patients. Whether insulin action involves its own receptor, or whether it works through the insulin-like growth factor receptor, remains to be determined.

SPECIFIC ASPECTS IN THE TREATMENT OF PCO

There are three major aims in the treatment of PCO: (1) cosmetic alleviation of hirsutism and acne, (2) restoration of fertility, and (3) prevention of hyperplastic changes in the endometrium which can lead to endometrial carcinoma.

TREATMENT OF HIRSUTISM

In women not interested in pregnancy, reduction of androgen production by suppression of ovarian function with oral contraceptives will result in subjective improvement in 65% of patients. The low-dose estrogen (e.g., 35 μg ethinyl estradiol) and progestins with the least androgenic activity (ethynodial diacetate or norethindrone) should be used. Oral contraceptives will suppress LH secretion and thus LH-dependent ovarian androgen production will decrease. In addition, the estrogenic component will increase sex hormone binding globulin and thereby lower free testosterone. Oral contraceptives also have an inhibitory effect on 5-α-reductase and on androgen receptor action.

Cyproterone acetate is an effective antiandrogen. It is used extensively in Europe and Canada in the treatment of hirsutism, but is not available in the United States. It is a progestin which is taken up by fat and released slowly. It inhibits ovulation, and has been administered as a reverse sequential oral contraceptive (100 mg, days 5–15). It provides considerable improvement of hirsutism in about 70% of patients within 9–12 months. Acne and seborrhea are improved in 96 and 89% of cases, respectively.

Recently, ovarian suppression with GnRH analogs has been used to suppress ovarian androgen production. The problem, of course, is that ovarian function is totally suspended with resultant hypoestrogenism. This can be overcome by the concomitant administration of estrogens or oral contraceptives. Experience with these approaches is presently still limited and the reader is referred to the literature for an update.

If fertility is a concern, however, oral contraceptives are obviously contraindicated and only drugs that will not interfere with ovulation and have no known teratogenic effects can be used. Such treatment may include the corticosteroids and cyclic spironolactone.

Some patients benefit from corticosteroid therapy, especially if the adrenals are responsible for the excess androgens. Spironolactone, an aldosterone antagonist, was found to have antiandrogenic properties similar to those of cyproterone acetate with greater antagonism of androgen receptors. It inhibits cytochrome P-450 and thus decreases ovarian testosterone and ovarian and adrenal androstenedione production. It displaces testosterone from sex hormone binding globulin and thus also increases its metabolic clearance rate. Spironolactone has been used effectively for hirsutism in doses of 50–200 mg/day. Usually the higher dose is required. Transient initial diuresis is the main side effect. Marked electrolyte changes have not been observed in healthy women. (Some patients may develop irregular bleeding which can be controlled by the addition of oral contraceptives if pregnancy is not desired.) If a patient is trying to conceive, spironolactone is prescribed for days 1–21 to avoid use in early pregnancy and to avoid potential teratogenic effects. Both approaches can be used in conjunction with ovulation-inducing drugs (discussed later).

Other drugs that have been used experimentally to treat hirsutism include cimetidine, a histamine H2-receptor antagonist that blocks androgen action on its receptor in hair follicles, and cyproheptadine. Treatment with cimetidine has resulted in 50–80% improvement of hirsutism, though experience is still limited.

Topical application of antiandrogens as a cream or lotion has been reported. Progesterone, cyproterone acetate, and spironolactone have been applied with various results. This approach may be useful when hirsutism is localized (mostly facial). It should be kept in mind, however, that these active drugs may be absorbed and therefore possibly interfere with the menstrual cycle.

The medical treatment of hirsutism should be combined with some form of epilation. Electrolysis, if done correctly, is the best adjunct to medical treatment. It is important to impress upon the patient that combined medical treatment as described may not bring noticeable improvement in the pattern of hair growth for 6–12 months. Hirsutism is a lifelong problem, which may start around menarche and remain for the rest of the patient's life. This condition may cause a great deal of psychological distress which in turn may aggravate the problem. It requires long-term medical, cosmetic treatment and a lot of support and reassurance.

RESTORATION OF FERTILITY

Restoration of fertility is much easier to achieve than the treatment of hirsutism. Standard methods of ovulation induction, as discussed in Chapter 13, are all effective. The thickened ovarian capsule in PCO is certainly not a mechanical barrier to ovulation as was once believed, since medical induction of ovulation is quite successful in spite of it. If hyperprolactinemia is present, treatment with bromocriptine may be beneficial.

If medical treatment has failed, and in carefully selected cases that demonstrate the typical polycystic ovary syndrome, ovarian wedge resection may be helpful in restoring spontaneous menstrual cycles and fertility, at least for a limited duration. Wedge resection of the ovaries was originally advocated by Stein and Leventhal as a method to induce ovulation and pregnancy in these women. Although the mechanisms through which the surgical procedure affects the cycle are not well understood, it has been speculated that by removing abnormal hypothalamic-pituitary-ovarian feedback relationships, cyclicity could be restored at least temporarily. Review of the older literature reveals that in typical cases where enlarged, pearly white, smooth ovaries are found, surgery results in regular cyclicity in 85% (6–93%) and pregnancy in 67% (13–95%) of cases. Nevertheless, as can be seen from the range, there is a large variation in response from study to study and with the availability of ovulation-inducing drugs, surgery has become unpopular, particularly with the risk of development of postoperative periovarian adhesions. However, when medical induction of ovulation fails and in properly selected cases, there is still a place for ovarian wedge resection, using more recent microsurgical techniques that decrease the risk and incidence of adhesions.

An alternate experimental therapeutical approach, presently being tested, involves pituitary-ovarian axis suppression with a GnRH analog (see also Chapter 13). Presumably, this treatment interrupts the endocrine vicious cycle characteristic of the syndrome and at the end of the suppression period, spontaneous recovery may occur for a limited period. Results from ongoing experiments appear to indicate, however, that FSH recovery and the initial dominant FSH secretion may be unable to correct the defect in some patients who then remain anovulatory. During this period, however, ovulation can be induced with pulsatile GnRH infusions or other means. The reader is referred to the current literature for a more up to date evaluation.

The treatment of choice in cases of congenital or other types of adrenal hyperplasia is adrenal suppression with glucocorticoids. Prednisone (2.5–7.5 mg/day) or dexamethasone (0.5–0.75 mg/day) will rapidly reduce the elevated androgen levels, restore ovulatory function, and improve hirsutism.

TREATMENT OF ENDOMETRIAL HYPERPLASIA AND ENDOMETRIAL CARCINOMA

Women with PCO can develop endometrial hyperplasia at a relatively young age due to prolonged unopposed estrogen stimulation of the endometrium. To prevent endometrial hyperplasia, cyclic treatment with a progestin is indicated (such as Provera, 10 mg/day for 5 days, every 6–8 weeks). This approach also restores regular menstruation. Usually, patients who develop endometrial carcinoma have well differentiated and localized carcinoma. If diagnosed early and properly treated, the prognosis is excellent.

13

Therapeutic Approaches to Acyclicity

One of the characteristics of childbearing years in women is menstrual cyclicity. Although cycles may be irregular in the perimenarchal and perimenopausal years, menstrual cycles are fairly regular during the fertile years. Appearance of menstrual cycles of irregular length indicates disturbances along the hypothalamic-pituitary-ovarian axis which in most instances cause oligo- or anovulation. In rare cases, irregular menstruation or absence of menstruation may result from the presence of a steroid-producing ovarian or adrenal tumor.

From a clinical viewpoint, whenever an irregular menstrual pattern or menstrual failure develop, the pathophysiologic cause has to be diagnosed (see Chapters 10, 11) and measures taken to correct the situation. In very rare instances, such as central nervous system (C.N.S.), pituitary, ovarian, or adrenal tumors, the underlying cause may be life-threatening. In most cases, the diagnosis is important because infertility may result, or because irregular bleeding is inconvenient or troublesome for the woman. Occasionally, prolonged and/or heavy bleeding can lead to anemia.

Once a potential life-threatening condition has been ruled out, treatment is tailored to the interests of the patient. If the main concern is menstrual irregularity, the cycles can be regulated. If the patient wishes to conceive, ovulation induction is indicated. In the few patients in whom medical and surgical treatment of infertility fails, "assisted reproductive technology" (in vitro fertilization [IVF]) procedures may be applicable.

MANAGEMENT OF MENSTRUAL IRREGULARITY

When a patient consults for irregular or absent menses, there are generally two questions to be asked: why are the cycles irregular and can the problem be corrected? The concern is not menstrual irregularity per se, although in some ethnic groups regular menses are considered important.

Management has to be tailored to the needs of the patient. Usually, reassurance is all that is required. When a patient wants to menstruate and is not interested in pregnancy, cyclicity can be induced by the timely use of progestins at regular intervals (Provera 10 mg P.O. daily for 5–7 days every 6–8 weeks) if there is adequate endogenous estrogenic activity, or by the cyclic use of oral contraceptives or of estrogen–progestin combinations if endogenous estrogen activity is lacking.

Long-term effects of a lack of estrogen is a problem that should be discussed with the patient, particularly in regard to bone metabolism. In adolescents, scoliosis has been reported in ballet dancers, although not in other athletic disciplines. Osteopenia, particularly of trabecular bone, is common among amennorheic athletes where the rate of vertebral bone loss during the first few years of menstrual dysfunction is similar to that associated with menopause. If a decrease in exercise or an increase in weight is not feasible or rejected by the patient, cyclic estrogen and progesterone therapy in a regimen to protect from hypoestrogenism, as used in postmenopausal women (see Chapter 8), may be recommended. The long-term effects of replacement treatment in premenopausal women, however, remains to be investigated.

INDUCTION OF OVULATION

When the patient wants to conceive, ovulation can be induced by various methods. Medical induction of ovulation has been one of the most successful treatments in gynecologic endocrinology in the last 30 years, and is used extensively. With increased understanding of the physiology of the menstrual cycle, our choice of medications has grown. Most importantly, patients have to be reassured that the condition is usually benign and that successful treatment is available. At present, there are three major approaches to induce ovulation; a fourth one is reserved for patients with hyperprolactinemia. These are:

1. indirect stimulation of the hypothalamic-pituitary unit by clomiphene citrate;
2. direct stimulation of the pituitary gonadotrope by gonadotropin-releasing hormone (GnRH);
3. direct stimulation of the ovaries by gonadotropins;
4. suppression of prolactin (PRL) secretion by bromocriptin.

A general step-by-step procedural outline is sketched in Figure 13–1. Before starting treatment, a complete fertility workup should be carried out and any reason for infertility except for anovulation ruled out. It is particularly important to exclude premature ovarian failure through blood follicle-stimulating hormone (FSH) measurements. If FSH falls in the menopausal range, end organ (ovarian) failure is present, and ovulation induction treatment will, of course, be ineffective. Hyperprolactinemia must also be ruled out, as the treatment modality in this circumstance will be specific. Finally, sterility may be related to the inadequate luteal phase syndrome, in which case the treatment will be different.

CLOMIPHENE

Clomiphene citrate is a nonsteroidal, mild estrogen of the triarylethylene series of compounds. Its chemical name is 2-[4-(2 chloro-1,2-diphenyl ethenyl) phe-

THERAPY OF ANOVULATION

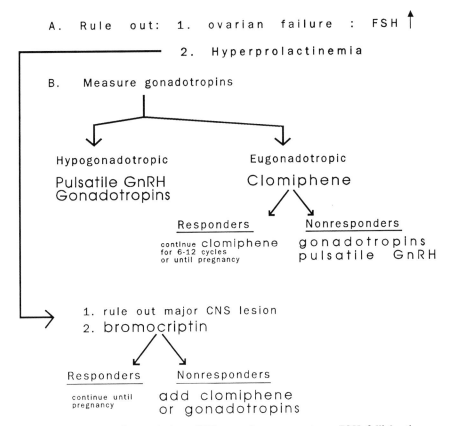

A. Rule out: 1. ovarian failure : FSH ↑

2. Hyperprolactinemia

B. Measure gonadotropins

Hypogonadotropic

Pulsatile GnRH
Gonadotropins

Eugonadotropic

Clomiphene

Responders

continue clomiphene
for 6-12 cycles
or until pregnancy

Nonresponders

gonadotropins
pulsatile GnRH

1. rule out major CNS lesion
2. bromocriptin

Responders

continue until
pregnancy

Nonresponders

add clomiphene
or gonadotropins

Fig. 13–1. Therapy of anovulation. *CNS*, central nervous system; *FSH*, follicle-stimu-lating hormone; *GnRH*, Gonadotropin-releasing hormone.

noxy] ethanamine (Fig. 13–2). After extensive and careful clinical trials, the drug was approved by the Food and Drug Administration (FDA) for induction of ovulation in 1967 and has been widely used ever since.

Mode of Action

Clomiphene binds to high-affinity estradiol receptors and acts as a competitive inhibitor of estradiol in several tissues. Thus, although clomiphene is a mild estrogen on its own, its major action is most probably antiestrogenic since, through competitive binding, it prevents endogenous estradiol from exerting its effects. Although the possibility of an action of clomiphene on ovarian steroido-genesis cannot be entirely discounted, the most probable mode of action of clo-miphene requires clomiphene binding to the hypothalamic and/or pituitary estradiol receptor, thereby inactivating the long loop estradiol negative feedback.

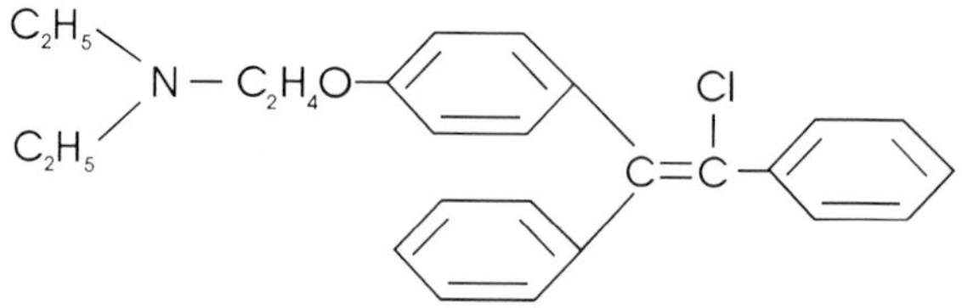

CLOMIPHENE

Fig. 13–2. The structure of clomiphene. Clomiphene is a nonsteroidal compound which, although possessing mild estrogenic activity, acts primarily as a competitive inhibitor of estradiol.

The consequence is a rise in gonadotropin secretion, stimulation of folliculogenesis, and an increase in estradiol secretion, the result of follicular maturation (Fig. 13–3).

Patient Selection

In view of its mode of action, clomiphene is best used in patients with an intact hypothalamic-pituitary-ovarian axis and normal genital organs. Oligo-ovulatory patients and amenorrheic women with evidence of endogenous estrogenic activity who respond with withdrawal bleeding to progestins may all be candidates for clomiphene. By far the largest group of women treated with clomiphene are those with the polycystic ovary syndrome. (Recently, clomiphene has also been used for induction of superovulation in assisted reproductive technology.) It is important to emphasize that, understandably, clomiphene is *not* effective in patients lacking endogenous estrogen production.

Clomiphene has also been used extensively to treat ovulatory women with normal menstrual cycles but with unexplained infertility. There is no objective evidence that such use of clomiphene is effective.

Administration and Dosage

Clomiphene citrate is water soluble, easily absorbed orally, cleared by the liver, and excreted in the feces. Studies in monkeys reveal that its half-life after intravenous injection is about 48 hours and that 83–90% of it is excreted by 6.3 days.

Clomiphene citrate is administered orally, beginning on the 3d–5th day of the menstrual cycle. If there are no spontaneous menstruations, withdrawal bleeding is induced with progestins prior to treatment (see Chapter 9). Clomiphene therapy is started at 50 mg/day for 5 days, and the ovulatory response is assessed by the basal body temperature (BBT) curve, midluteal phase serum progesterone values, and/or premenstrual endometrial biopsy. Patients are advised to have intercourse every other day starting 5 days after the last dose of clomiphene citrate, for a period of 10 days. If ovulation does not occur, the dose is increased by 50 mg/day in subsequent cycles up to a maximum of 200 mg/day. Patients are seen monthly, usually before initiation of a new cycle in order to monitor ovar-

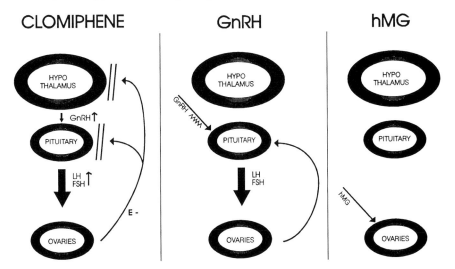

Fig. 13–3. Contrasting modes of action of clomiphene, GnRH, and hMG. Clomiphene acts as an antiestrogen and blocks the long loop estradiol negative feedback (E−). As a result, gonadotropin concentrations rise and folliculogenesis is initiated. Thus, clomiphene will be effective only in patients with endogenous estrogen secretion. Therapy lasts 5 days, after which endogenous feedback mechanisms carry on the cycle.

Pulsatile GnRH stimulates luteinizing hormone *(LH)* and FSH secretion and, hence, folliculogenesis. Because the estradiol negative feedback is in effect at least at the pituitary level, the risk of ovarian hyperstimulation is limited.

Human menopausal gonadotropins *(hMG),* a mixture of LH and FSH, directly stimulate the ovary. There is no internal feedback control, and ovarian hyperstimulation is sometimes difficult to avoid. Abbreviations as in Figure 13–1.

ian size and evaluate the ovulatory response. However, once a patient ovulates and several cycles are uneventful with minimal side effects, such close follow-up can be discontinued. Although the maximal dose of clomiphene is 1 g/cycle, the patient's weight has to be considered. In very obese patients, the dose of clomiphene may be increased to 250 mg/day for 5–8 days.

Results of Treatment

Ovulation rates, as judged by the indirect criteria outlined here, are 70–80%, with a total pregnancy rate of 30–40% and a multiple pregnancy rate of about 7%. The reasons for the discrepancy between the apparent ovulation and pregnancy rates are not clear. Speculations include a high percentage of luteinized unruptured follicles and abnormal luteal phase function. An increased spontaneous abortion rate has also been reported in pregnancies following clomiphene treatment, although the data are controversial.

Side Effects and Complications

Generally, clomiphene is a safe drug with few side effects. These may include ovarian enlargement (14%), vasomotor flushes (10%), lower abdominal pain and discomfort (7.5%), nausea (2%), and breast tenderness (2%). In a few instances and particularly at the higher doses, patients may develop visual symptoms, such as flashes of light, blurred vision and spots. These symptoms are usually temporary and always revert to normal; they are therefore not an indication to discontinue treatment. Rare side effects include headaches, dizziness, and depression.

Clomiphene in Combination With Other Drugs

Various combinations of drugs have been tried for the induction of ovulation when patients fail to conceive after clomiphene alone. Clomiphene treatment has been combined with human chorionic gonadotropin (hCG), human menopausal gonadotropin (hMG) and hCG, estrogens, corticosteroids, or bromocriptin.

The addition of hCG may occasionally induce ovulation in patients who fail to ovulate on clomiphene alone. This may be useful in patients with adequate follicular development but an inadequate luteinizing hormone (LH) surge. The injection of hCG, however, must be accurately timed to avoid the demise of the selected follicle and to occur within the ovulability window (see Chapter 4). With the use of estrogen measurement or ultrasonography to assess follicular development, the injection of hCG can be more accurately timed (discussed later). Follicles greater than 15 mm are mature and ready to ovulate. Usually 10,000 IU of hCG are given intramuscularly. Repeat injections of 2,500–5,000 IU of hCG at 3–4 day intervals may stimulate the corpus luteum and help in maintaining the luteal phase.

Clomiphene has been combined with estrogens when there appears to be a negative effect of the compound on the cervical mucus. The effect of clomiphene on the quality of cervical mucus has been controversial, but since clomiphene is mildly antiestrogenic, it may adversely affect cervical mucus properties. Yet, this is not necessarily so. In various studies, the incidence of a negative effect on cervical mucus varied from 15–50%. Short-term treatment with estrogens around the time of ovulation may improve cervical mucus, although there is no good evidence that pregnancy rates improve.

The addition of corticosteroids to clomiphene treatment may be beneficial where there is adrenal hyperandrogenicity and elevated levels of dehydroepiandrosterone sulfate (DHEA-S) and testosterone. These conditions have to be documented, however, before clomiphene is started (see Chapter 13).

The success rate of these combination therapies is hard to establish since there are no large, controlled studies proving their effectiveness. Overall, it is probably quite low, although occasionally, as outlined earlier, a combination treatment will be very effective in a particular patient.

GnRH

Isolation, identification, and synthesis of GnRH was a major achievement in reproductive endocrinology. It is now available commercially. The compound is a decapeptide, able to release both LH and FSH in most species (see Chapter 2). The first reports of successful induction of ovulation and pregnancy with pulsatile infusions of GnRH appeared in 1980 and since then many successful pregnancies have been induced by GnRH treatment.

Mode of Action

In regard to the use of GnRH as an ovulation-inducing agent, the first results were quite disappointing. The reasons for this became clear only after extensive physiological studies in animals which established that, physiologically, the peptide is released in a pulsatile fashion and that this mode of release is essential for the normal gonadotropin response. Thus, to be maximally effective, GnRH is administered in a pulsatile infusion: this will provoke the release of LH and FSH and, provided a proper pulse frequency is respected, gonadotropin release will in turn stimulate folliculogenesis. In contrast to gonadotropin therapy, GnRH treatment allows for partial operation of the long loop negative feedback, which maintains gonadotropin and ovarian steroid secretion within the normal range (Fig. 13–3).

Patient Selection

Successful treatment with GnRH depends to a large extent on the selection of the patient. Although generally the indications are similar to those for gonadotropin treatment, the ideal patient for pulsatile GnRH treatment is the one with hypogonadotropic hypogonadism who lacks endogenous GnRH secretion. In this patient, the GnRH pulsatile infusion must not compete with endogenously released GnRH pulses. Other groups, such as patients with the polycystic ovary syndrome who failed to respond to clomiphene and patients with a short luteal phase, may also benefit from the treatment, although with a lesser success rate. GnRH has also been given to women undergoing IVF procedures in an attempt at superovulation (see later).

Administration and Dosage

The decapeptide has a short half-life and cannot be administered orally because of degradation in the gastrointestinal tract. GnRH has been given by intravenous, subcutaneous, intramuscular, intranasal, and sublingual routes. For the purpose of induction of ovulation, the intravenous route is generally the most commonly used and effective. The subcutaneous route presents problems of variability of absorption depending on the location of the needle and, although adequate in some patients, in general is a less desirable approach. After an intravenous pulse of GnRH, LH blood levels begin to rise rapidly and peak within 20–30 minutes. The peak of plasma LH concentration and the duration of the LH increase are closely related to the dose of GnRH. In most studies, the dose of GnRH is 10–20 μg/pulse, although lower or higher concentrations have been used.

The development of small portable infusion pumps has made it possible to deliver GnRH pulses at predetermined intervals over long periods of time. There are several infusion pumps on the market. GnRH comes as a lyophylized powder and must be dissolved in sterile saline before it is loaded into the pump. The frequency used most often is 1 pulse/90 min. Since pumps are relatively expensive and must be used for long periods of time, they are usually leased out to patients as needed. This helps to cut expenses for the patient.

Patients are monitored by blood estradiol levels, timed ultrasonography sessions, BBT, and clinical follow-up. The pulsatile GnRH infusion is usually continued for 2 weeks. Once plasma estradiol concentrations reach 800–1,000 pg/ ml and there are follicles over 15 mm in diameter, a single injection of 10,000 IU hCG is given intramuscularly to trigger ovulation (although in a few patients, an endogenous LH surge may occur spontaneously in response to the increase in estradiol). Patients are advised to have intercourse for 3 consecutive days after hCG is given. In order to maintain a normal luteal phase, three injections of 2,500 IU hCG each may be given at 3-day intervals after the first injection of hCG. An alternative method is to continue the GnRH infusion for 2 more weeks throughout the luteal phase to allow for continuing LH stimulation on which the corpus luteum is dependent for survival. In general, however, most programs discontinue GnRH once ovulation has occurred and maintain luteal function with hCG supplementation. When the patient fails to menstruate and the BBT remains elevated for more than 14 days, a β-hCG blood level is determined. Once pregnancy is established, no additional treatment is required. If the patient is not pregnant, another cycle of GnRH treatment may be started.

Results of Treatment

GnRH therapy is relatively recent and, therefore, there are no published large long-range series allowing for comparisons of success rates with other therapies. Most probably, GnRH therapy will compare favorably with gonadotropin treatment in the same type of patient: it elicits similar results, but with fewer complications and at less cost. In properly selected cases, ovulation rates range from 80–100%, with pregnancy rates of 40–60% and spontaneous abortion rates of 27–35%. The incidence of congenital malformations following GnRH treatment is the same as in the general population. As mentioned previously, best results are obtained in hypogonadotropic hypogonadal patients. Generally, the success rate is considerably less with other diagnoses.

Side Effects and Complications

Overall, there are few side effects to the GnRH treatment. Although mild to moderate ovarian hyperstimulation has been reported and the incidence of multiple gestations is higher than in the normal population, these side effects are much less frequent than those following treatment with gonadotropins. An important contrast between the two therapies is that during the GnRH treatment long loop steroid inhibitory feedback mechanisms remain in action and can moderate the amounts of endogenous gonadotropin that are released in response to pituitary stimulation by GnRH. There have, however, been a few reports of twins, triplets, and quadruplets following GnRH treatment.

If an intravenous route of injection is chosen, the site must, of course, be inspected frequently. Care must be taken to clean the site and insert the needle in a sterile fashion. If precautions are taken, infections are rare and the needle can stay in place for up to 1 week. If there are signs of infection, the site must be changed immediately.

Patients must also pay attention to the function of the pump. If it stops, batteries have to be checked and/or changed or the pump replaced. Any clinical service should have several extra pumps available in order to replace a malfunctioning one rapidly so as to preserve the integrity of the cycle.

GONADOTROPINS

The use of hMG in combination with hCG was introduced in the 1960's for the treatment of anovulation caused by disorders along the hypothalamic-pituitary-ovarian axis. This therapy has been used extensively and very successfully, particularly since the introduction of sophisticated and rapid methods for estrogen determination and of ultrasound for the assessment of follicular development, both of which allow for easy and close monitoring.

Mode of Action

Since the growth and development of ovarian follicles depend on proper amounts of the two gonadotropins, treatment with gonadotropins will of course induce folliculogenesis, stimulate steroidogenesis, and result in ovulation, bypassing a role for endogenous brain or endogenous pituitary hormones (Fig. 13–3). Thus, ovulation can be induced in a variety of patients, including hypophysectomized women, who lack endogenous gonadotropins.

Patient Selection

The sole indication for gonadotropin treatment is induction of ovulation. The ideal candidates are patients with hypogonadotropic hypogonadal amenorrhea. However, normogonadotropic, oligo-ovulatory patients who fail to respond to clomiphene, or hyperprolactinemic patients who fail to respond to bromocriptin and clomiphene, are also candidates for gonadotropin treatment. Recently, gonadotropins have also been used extensively to superovulate normally ovulating women undergoing IVF (discussed later).

Administration and Dosage

Human pituitary gonadotropins (hPG) are isolated from cadaver pituitaries; these preparations are not recommended for human use because of potential viral contamination and are not available commercially. hMG is isolated from urine of postmenopausal women. hMG is a mixture of LH and FSH in a ratio of approximately 1:1. Each hMG vial is standardized and contains 75 IU FSH and 75 IU LH. Vials of 150 IU are also available. hMG is supplied as a lyophylized powder which is dissolved in normal saline before use and injected intramuscularly every 24 hours, starting on day 3 of the menstrual cycle. It is necessary to give hMG parenterally: gonadotropins are rapidly destroyed when given orally. Injections should preferably be given at a consistent time of the day, so that adequate gonadotropin levels will be maintained over the 24-hour period. The patient herself or her partner can be taught to administer the injections.

hCG is derived from urine of pregnant women and has an LH-like activity; it is used to trigger ovulation once there are mature follicles.

A follow-up examination is scheduled 1 week after initiation of hMG treatment. The patient is then seen every 2–3 days until hCG is given. Careful monitoring of these patients is essential not only to improve pregnancy rates but also to prevent ovarian hyperstimulation (see later). The use of several monitoring techniques will assure maximal results and optimal patient safety. Monitoring has three components: (1) clinical examination in order to assess cervical mucus properties and ovarian size and a postcoital test prior to hCG administration to ascertain the presence of active sperm; (2) measurement of blood estradiol or of total estrogen levels which reflect follicular development and maturation. Ovulation should be triggered with hCG when the estradiol level is about 1,000 pg/ml; and (3) ultrasonographic evaluation of follicular development, particularly with use of the vaginal probe. Mature preovulatory follicles are about 15–20 mm in diameter or more. When several such follicles are present and correlate with appropriate estrogen levels, the patient is ready for hCG administration. On the other hand, even in the presence of adequate estrogen levels, folliculogenesis is inadequate if only small follicles, with no dominant one, are observed. In this case, the patient will not ovulate or will have an inadequate luteal phase, and it is useless to inject hCG.

After hCG administration, patients are advised to have intercourse daily for 3 days. The luteal phase itself can be assessed through BBT, a midluteal phase progesterone measurement and appropriately timed uterine bleeding, indirectly indicative of ovulation. Unless hyperstimulation is suspected, further examination of the patient is then unnecessary. In general, during a treatment course, patients are seen about three times, blood estrogen levels are determined two to three times, and ultrasound examination is performed one to two times. This should be sufficient to monitor the patient adequately and economically.

The dose of hMG varies from patient to patient, and sometimes from cycle to cycle in the same patient. On the average, two vials/day (150 IU) are given for 10–15 days. If the response is inadequate, the amount is increased by one to two vials/day until an adequate response is observed. Thus, the usual dosage is two to four vials/day for 10–12 days, but it is not unusual to give six vials/day and the use of as much as twelve vials/day for 24 days has been reported. The standard ovulatory dose is 10,000 IU.

Recently, a "pure FSH" preparation that lacks most of the LH biological activity of hMG has become available. Each vial contains 75 IU of FSH and it is administered the same way as hMG. Theoretically, administration of a pure FSH preparation early in the cycle alone or as an adjunct to hMG may better simulate physiological conditions that characterize this early part of the follicular phase, at which time the FSH:LH ratio decidely favors FSH (see Chapter 1). Thus, it has been proposed that addition of pure FSH early in the cycle may enhance follicular development and allow for the recruitment of more follicles. Double blind, controlled studies have yet to be carried out and for the time being, the value of this therapy remains to be determined. This approach may possibly be particularly advantageous in women with the polycystic ovary syndrome in which a high LH:FSH ratio usually predominates.

Results of Treatment

In the proper population, ovulation following gonadotropin therapy occurs in 90–100% of the patients. Overall pregnancy rate is 65–70%, with pregnancy per treatment cycle at 22–25%, and an overall abortion rate of 27%. The multiple pregnancy rate with hMG is about 21%, with more than 50% of these twin conceptions.

It is of interest to note that, contrary to initial findings, the chances of conception do not decline significantly as the number of treatment cycles increases. Therefore, it is justified to encourage patients to continue treatment beyond the first 3–6 cycles.

The spontaneous abortion rate of 27% is higher than in the general population. This increase is due to the greater incidence of multiple gestations, and to the close follow-up for early diagnosis of pregnancy, leading to detection of abortions which otherwise might not have been detected.

Side Effects and Complications

No toxic effects have been reported following hMG or hCG injection, except for occasional, mild febrile reactions. There are, however, two major complications of gonadotropin treatment: (1) ovarian hyperstimulation and (2) multiple gestations.

Ovarian hyperstimulation. The ovarian hyperstimulation syndrome is a serious complication of treatment with gonadotropins. Although this syndrome has been described following clomiphene, GnRH, or pure FSH administration, it is relatively uncommon in those cases. During hMG therapy, however, normal feedback mechanisms which physiologically control endogenous gonadotropin release and thus the degree of ovarian stimulation are not functioning (Fig. 13–3) and hyperstimulation, as evidenced by the multiple pregnancy rate, is common. Hyperstimulation can be prevented, however, by careful monitoring of follicular maturation. hCG administration must be withheld if estrogen levels are too high (> 2,000–2,500 pg/ml). It is important to keep in mind that the hyperstimulation syndrome cannot be prevented once hCG has been given.

There are three degrees of hyperstimulation: mild, moderate, and severe. The first two are quite common and of little concern. Severe hyperstimulation, which occurs in about 0.9% of gonadotropin-treated cycles, is a serious condition that may become life-threatening.

The pathogenesis of the hyperstimulation syndrome is not completely understood. For instance, it is not known why some patients develop hyperstimulation while others with similar estrogen levels do not become hyperstimulated. There is experimental evidence indicating that high estrogen concentrations increase capillary permeability, which would explain ascites formation. However, high estrogen levels by themselves do not produce hyperstimulation; only after ovulation and corpus luteum formation does this syndrome appear. Therefore, additional unknown factors must be involved.

Hyperstimulation symptoms appear 4–5 days after hCG administration. The overstimulated ovaries become extremely enlarged and can be easily palpated abdominally. They are studded with multiple follicular and corpora lutea cysts and stromal edema is present. Massive ascites and resulting hypovolemia are the cardinal events in the development of this syndrome. Ascites may occasionally be accompanied by pleural effusion. The diminished intravascular volume accounts for the hemoconcentration (the hematocrit may reach the high 40s and 50s), decreased central venous pressure, low blood pressure, and tachycardia. Diminished renal perfusion, caused by decreased intravascular volume, stimulates the proximal renal tubules to reabsorb salt and water and is manifested clinically by oliguria and electrolyte imbalance. Due to the low urinary flow, there is an increase in reabsorption of urea leading to a rise in blood urea nitrogen (BUN). Creatinine, on the other hand, is not reabsorbed by the proximal tubule and therefore remains normal or only slightly elevated. Clinically, this results in an elevation of BUN which is disproportionate to that of creatinine. The retained fluid and sodium accumulate as ascitic fluid. Because of fluid retention, there is considerable weight gain, usually more than 5 kg during the severe stages of hyperstimulation.

Therapy is symptomatic. It is important to reiterate that the syndrome can be prevented by *withholding hCG administration.* When estrogen levels are too high and hCG is given nonetheless, a full blown picture of severe ovarian hyperstimulation may develop and there is very little that can be done. In severe cases, patients are hospitalized to guard against hypovolemia and its complications. Hospitalized patients are on complete bedrest with strict monitoring of intake and output, daily weight, and vital signs. Baseline blood studies are done, including coagulation parameters. Fluid is replaced, with special care to avoid hyperhydration. In order to improve hypovolemia and increase renal perfusion, serum albumin or plasma expanders may be given as needed. Diuretics are contraindicated since they will cause additional loss of fluid from the intravascular space and the extravascular fluid is not available for diuresis. As conditions improve, patients will diurese the extra fluid and gradually return to normal. In the absence of pregnancy, improvement is very rapid after the onset of menses, and within 7–10 days, patients return to normal. When patients are pregnant—and many of the hyperstimulated women are pregnant—endogenous hCG prevents rapid recovery, with only gradual improvement over a period of 6–8 weeks. In extreme cases, pregnancy can be terminated resulting in rapid improvement.

Recently, with advances in ultrasonography, paracentesis has been performed under sonographic guidance and large amounts of ascitic fluid removed. Although this is not curative and the ascitic fluid will reaccumulate, this procedure may give temporary relief to patients. As long as urinary output is adequate, ovarian hyperstimulation is self-limiting. If urinary output falls to dangerous levels and the patient becomes severely oliguric or anuric, more drastic measures, such as dialysis, are necessary.

The possibility of ovarian rupture with hyperstimulation should always be considered, and pelvic examinations, if done at all, should be most gentle to avoid iatrogenic rupture. A crucial question is whether there is intraperitoneal bleeding. Surgery should be avoided, if possible, since it is difficult to resect large, cystic and friable ovaries. If the ovary is bleeding, however, oophorectomy may be necessary. Fortunately, such complications are very rare.

Multiple gestations. Multiple gestations are a complication of induction of ovulation with gonadotropins. Since the feedback loops are not operational, the physiological mechanisms that account for the selection of a single follicle to become the dominant one (see Chapter 5) are overtaken: multiple follicles mature leading to multiple ovulations with resultant multiple fertilizations and conceptions. There is no correlation between the degree of hyperstimulation, as evidenced by the preovulatory estrogen level or the number of mature follicles seen on ultrasonography, and the number of embryos conceived. With our present knowledge, it is difficult to control the number of fertilized eggs. Attempts at decreasing the degree of ovarian stimulation may result in a lowering of the incidence of multiple gestations, but it may also reduce the general pregnancy rate. Once pregnancy is established, ultrasound is done routinely at 6 weeks gestation in order to determine the number of fetuses. Some patients may choose to have fetal reduction. When there are three or more fetuses, fetal reduction may be induced by transvaginal injection of potassium chloride into the embryo at 8–10 weeks gestation. Although this procedure is new, it is quite effective, though it carries an abortion rate of around 10–15%.

Other complications. Another very serious, but fortunately very rare, complication of gonadotropin therapy is thrombosis. In 1965, two cases were reported in which one woman died as a result of thrombosis of the internal carotid artery and another had her left leg amputated due to thrombosis of the femoral artery. Since then, at least two deaths have occurred because of extensive pulmonary embolism. Fluid shifts, blood hyperviscosity, and increase in many coagulation factors can cause such complications. Generally, prevention of severe hyperstimulation will reduce the incidence of these complications.

Last, but not least, the psychological aspects of induction of ovulation can be overwhelming, especially when the treatment continues over long periods of time.

GONADOTROPINS IN COMBINATION WITH GnRH AGONISTS

Superovulation with gonadotropins has also been used extensively in normally ovulating women with idiopathic infertility or undergoing IVF. Because the hypothalamic-pituitary-ovarian axis is intact and normal feedback mechanisms are operational in these women, the increase in estradiol levels during gonadotropin treatment may activate the long loop estradiol positive feedback and trigger a premature LH surge; this, in turn, may result in damage to the growing follicle, premature ovulation, or luteinization of unruptured follicles. In assisted reproduction programs, as many as 20–30% of gonadotropin-induced cycles may have to be cancelled because of such circumstances. Clinically, this may be manifested by a poor rise or an outright drop in estradiol concentrations before hCG administration, a smaller number of oocytes retrieved, decreased fertilization rates, and a reduced pregnancy rate.

In these situations, it has been proposed to precede the gonadotropin treatment with a GnRH analog therapy. While the native GnRH decapeptide molecule has a very short half-life, enhanced ability to withstand rapid degradation has been obtained by substituting amino acids at the sites of enzymatic cleavage. Such GnRH *agonists* are able to stimulate LH and FSH. However, because of their longer half-life, the initial period of enhanced gonadotropin release is followed by down regulation of the gonadotrope, the result of *continuous* receptor stimulation (see Chapter 2), and an arrest in gonadotropin secretion. There are several GnRH agonists available presently (Fig. 13–4). Thus, administration of a GnRH agonist results in a suppression of LH and FSH, inducing an hypogonadotropic hypogonadal state that lasts as long as the compound is administered. When the patient has become hypogonadotropic, ovulation is induced with gonadotropins. This treatment appears to result in improved follicular recruitment, retrieval of an increased number of oocytes, and better pregnancy rates. There is also some evidence that it may improve pregnancy rates in patients with the polycystic ovary syndrome who have higher risks of ovarian hyperstimulation. This combined approach is presently being tested in larger groups of patients and the reader is referred to the literature for current evaluation of success rates and of the optimal treatment regimens. A current regimen starts with 1 mg of leuprolide given subcutaneously during the midluteal phase (day 6–7 after BBT rise), to be continued daily for 10 days. On the 10th day, blood estradiol concentrations are measured and an ultrasound is performed to assess follicular development. If estradiol level is under 35 pg/ml and there are no follicles over 10 mm in diameter, hMG is started. At that time, the dose of leuprolide is reduced to 0.5 mg. Generally, the amount of hMG required after leuprolide suppression may be somewhat higher. Patients are followed every 2–3 days by measuring blood estradiol levels and on ultrasound. Once estradiol level reaches 1,000 pg/ml and follicles are over 15 mm in diameter, hCG (10,000 IU) is given and leuprolide is discontinued. This regimen considerably reduces spontaneous ovulation and luteinization, though it is not clear at this time whether the pregnancy rate improves significantly.

In the future, a new generation of GnRH analogs may be used for this purpose. These are compounds that inhibit gonadotropin secretion presumably by competing with endogenous GnRH for its receptor on the pituitary gland. These compounds, presently being tested experimentally, are referred to as GnRH *antagonists*. Because of the mode of action, these compounds allow for an immediate suppression of gonadotropin secretion without the initial stimulatory effect. Research on these antagonists was delayed because of allergic reaction (histamine release) to the first generation of compounds. Amounts of histamine released by second-generation compounds—for example, (Nal-glu)-

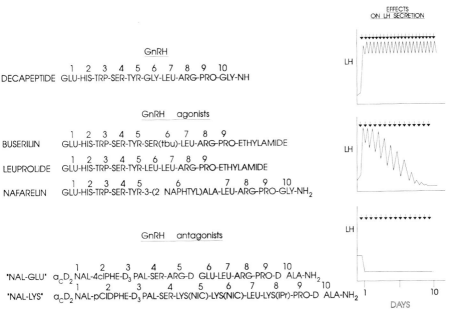

Fig. 13–4. GnRH analogs. Enhanced biologic activity of the GnRH decapeptide is obtained by substituting amino acids at the sites of enzymatic cleavage, rendering the compound more resistant to degradation (GnRH *agonist*). Although GnRH agonists initially release LH and FSH with resultant gonadal stimulation, paradoxically, these stimulatory effects are not sustained, and soon, gonadotropin secretion is suppressed (down regulation). Hence, these compounds can be used in patients in whom endogenous gonadotropin secretion must be inhibited. The GnRH molecule can also be manipulated in such a way that it yields GnRH *antagonists,* thought to compete with endogenous GnRH for its receptor. These compounds suppress gonadotropin release, without the initial stimulation. *Natural amino acids:* Ala: alanine, arg: arginine, glu: glutamine, gly: glycine, his: histidine, leu: leucine, lys: lysine, pro: proline, ser: serine, trp: tryptophan, tyr: tyrosine. *Unnatural amino acids:* ser (tbu): serine ((tertiary-butyl), D2Nal: 3-(2 naphthyl)-D-alanine, D4ClPhe: 4-chloro-D-phenylalanine, D3Pal: 3-(3-pyridyl)-D-alanine, lys (NIC): lysine (nicotinyl), lys (ipr): lysine (isopropyl). AC: acetylated.

GnRH)—was significantly less, while third-generation compounds—for example, (Nal-lys)—appear to be largely devoid of allergic problems (Fig. 13–4).

DOPAMINE AGONISTS

Hyperprolactinemia is seen occasionally in women with menstrual dysfunction and infertility. Although hyperprolactinemia in itself does not cause any symptoms except for occasional galactorrhea, the accompanying anovulation and infertility may be a problem. Drugs that reduce prolactin (PRL) secretion have proven effective in restoring ovulatory cycles and fertility.

Mode of Action

PRL secretion is mainly under the inhibitory influence of dopamine. Thus, administration of dopamine or of ergot alkaloids that are dopamine agonists, will reduce PRL concentrations not only in normal women but also in hyperprolactinemic patients. The treatment will usually be followed by a restoration of normal cyclicity and fertility. Whether this is the result only of the reduction in PRL levels, or whether modifications in dopamine tone are also important remains to be elucidated (see Chapter 10).

Patient Selection

The incidence of hyperprolactinemia in women with secondary amenorrhea is 15–30% and is less in oligomenorrhea (8%). Therefore, any patient with menstrual irregularity should have PRL determinations. The normal range of PRL is 1–25 ng/ml. When PRL is found to be elevated, a computerized axial tomography (CAT) scan of the pituitary fossa should be done since approximately 20% of amenorrheic hyperprolactinemic women have pituitary tumors. Most tumors are very small, typically microadenomas of less than 10 mm in diameter. These are confined within the pituitary fossa, grow very slowly, if at all, and are symptomless. Some tumors are larger than 10 mm (macroadenomas) and may be accompanied by visual field and cranial nerve function defects. When this occurs, patients should be referred to a neurologist or neurosurgeon for definitive treatment.

In hyperprolactinemic amenorrheic patients not interested in pregnancy, the problem is hypoestrogenism with resulting osteoporosis. It is beneficial to treat these patients with bromocriptine, restore ovulatory cycles and ovarian steroid production and thus prevent osteoporosis. If the patient is sexually active and not interested in pregnancy, an effective contraceptive should be used.

Patients with moderately elevated PRL, who object to taking medication, should be followed with yearly PRL levels and CAT scans every 2–3 years to rule out the emergence of a pituitary tumor. If osteoporosis becomes an issue, estrogen replacement therapy should be considered (see Chapter 8).

In hyperprolactinemic patients interested in pregnancy, bromocriptine is a treatment of choice.

Administration and Dosage

Alpha-ergocryptine mesylate (bromocriptine) is a semisynthetic ergot alkaloid that is a dopamine receptor agonist and was specifically developed to inhibit prolactin secretion. Oral administration of bromocriptine results in 28% absorption from the gastrointestinal tract. The compound is usually administered orally at a dose of one tablet (2.5 mg) t.i.d. After 4 weeks of treatment, blood PRL levels are determined. If the level is still above normal, bromocriptine may be increased. Generally, however, 7.5–10 mg/day will normalize PRL levels in most hyperprolactinemic patients. In a few patients, it may be necessary to increase the dose to 40–50 mg/day, but this is rare. Patients are advised to maintain a menstrual calendar and to monitor BBT to determine whether ovulation has occurred. Once pregnancy is confirmed, the medication is discontinued.

Pergolide mesylate, a new ergot derivative, has a considerably longer duration of action, perhaps because of its greater affinity to the dopamine receptor. Thus, this drug need only be given once a day.

Results of Treatment

Bromocriptine is extremely effective in normalizing plasma PRL levels, suppressing galactorrhea, and restoring menstruation in about 90% of patients. Ovulation resumes in 80%, and of these, 80–85% will conceive spontaneously. Return to normal menstrual function may occur within 1 month of bromocriptine therapy. In general, most women on this therapy will conceive within six treatment cycles.

In cases where ovulation does not occur spontaneously in spite of normalization of PRL levels, ovulation-inducing drugs (clomiphene or gonadotropins) can be used in conjunction with bromocriptine. Most of these patients ovulate and conceive.

More recently, dopamine agonists have also gained favor as the primary treatment for PRL-secreting macroadenomas or as a prelude to surgery; indeed, these compounds not only reduce PRL secretion but also induce substantial shrinkage of the adenoma, as assessed by CAT scan and improvement of visual fields.

Side Effects and Complications

The most common side effects of bromocriptine are nausea and orthostatic hypotension, which occur primarily at initiation of the treatment. These side effects may be minimized by beginning therapy with 1.25 mg/day (half a tablet) taken at bedtime with food; medication can then be gradually increased every 3 days until the full therapeutic dose is achieved. Constipation is also a frequent side effect. Evaluation of pregnancies after bromocriptine treatment indicates that there is no increase in the rate of congenital anomalies. Despite this reassurance, it is recommended that bromocriptine treatment be discontinued once pregnancy is confirmed.

Follow-Up of the Pregnant Hyperprolactinemic Patient

When a hyperprolactinemic patient is pregnant, she has to be followed closely for the possible emergence of a pituitary tumor which may cause neurological symptoms. The great majority of patients (around 98%) will have uneventful pregnancies, but some may develop enlargement of pituitary tumors, causing visual or other symptoms. Blood PRL levels are of no value since PRL increases physiologically during pregnancy. A careful history of headaches and visual disturbances and sequential determinations of visual field are sufficient for follow-up. There is no need for routine skull x-rays. If symptoms emerge, more precise evaluation and CAT scan of the pituitary fossa will substantiate the diagnosis. In the majority of cases, treatment with high doses of bromocriptine (20–30 mg/day) will control symptoms until after delivery. In cases where there is rapid deterioration of vision or other alarming symptoms, surgical decompression of the pituitary fossa is mandatory. Generally, these patients do very well.

Pregnancy in hyperprolactinemic patients is not a contraindication to breast feeding. Women with pituitary tumors who had uneventful pregnancy can safely nurse without deleterious effects on the tumor.

TREATMENT OF THE INADEQUATE LUTEAL PHASE

Since the major problem, a lack of sufficient amounts of progesterone to sustain implantation, occurs in the luteal phase (see Chapter 11), the treatment should start in the cycle during which pregnancy occurs. The goal is to facilitate normal implantation and early embryonic development. The logical treatment of choice is the substitution and supplementation of the missing hormone, progesterone. Many practitioners supplement progesterone after ovulation has occurred in the form of injectable progesterone or progesterone suppositories given vaginally or rectally. Synthetic progestagens are contraindicated, since most are derivatives of testosterone and may be luteolytic, may interfere with progesterone secretion, and may cause masculinization of female fetuses.

Another approach to the treatment of the inadequate luteal phase is to start therapy early on in the follicular phase in order to improve on follicular maturation and development, since deficiencies in corpus luteum activity usually reflect prior defects in the follicular development process. The various ovulation-inducing therapies have been used for this purpose, with varying results. Because a double blind controlled study has not been conducted yet, it is not possible at present to assess the efficacy of these therapeutical approaches in this particular syndrome. Once this treatment is given, however, it is important to document that normal luteal function has been restored, usually by a timed endometrial biopsy, which should be in phase.

ASSISTED REPRODUCTION

When medical and surgical treatment of infertility fails, what other options are available? In 1978, the first baby was born after conception by IVF and embryo transfer. Since then, what is generally referred to as "assisted reproductive technology" has expanded markedly. Technology has improved, procedures have been simplified and with advanced developments in ultrasound, IVF has become an office procedure. Gamete intrafallopian tube transfer (GIFT), zygote intrafallopian tube transfer (ZIFT), donor embryos, donor sperm, donor eggs, cryopreservation, and microfertilization are all variants of the same approach. Despite much activity in the field, however, the success rate of these techniques is still low and, at the time of writing, the live birthrate after IVF does not exceed 15–18% in the best centers. No doubt, continuing research in the field will be required to determine what the optimal conditions for this technique are. Thus, a detailed description of an optimal protocol for IVF is out of the scope of this text and only a cursory review of the general steps is given at this time.

In Vitro Fertilization

Patient Selection

When initially introduced by Steptoe and Edwards, the IVF approach was used in women whose fallopian tubes were absent or not functioning. Since then, the indications have been broadened to include all infertility cases that fail to result in pregnancy by other methods. This includes idiopathic infertility, endometriosis, male factor, and immunologic infertility.

In most clinics, the cutoff age for IVF is 40 years old, since very few pregnancies occur after that age.

Procedures

There are four basic steps in IVF: (1) induction of superovulation, (2) oocyte retrieval, (3) fertilization, and (4) embryo transfer.

Induction of ovulation. In the first IVF case, the oocyte was retrieved during a natural menstrual cycle. However physiological this approach may be, difficulties in pinpointing the exact time of ovulation, logistic problems in organizing retrieval around that time, and the retrieval of only one oocyte have made most clinicians abandon this approach. Instead, ovulation-inducing drugs are used to achieve superovulation and optimize the time of retrieval. Basically, all methods for induction of ovulation have been used, although most approaches use the gonadotropins. Once mature follicles are present, as determined by blood estrogen levels and ultrasound, a single injection of 10,000 IU hCG is given and retrievals are done 34 hours later, usually during the morning hours.

Oocyte retrieval. At present, the method most commonly used for oocyte retrieval is an ultrasound-guided transvaginal approach. The patient is lightly sedated and through a vaginal ultrasound probe with a guide the follicles are punctured with a long #20-22 needle. Using gentle vacuum suction and a culture medium-containing trap, the follicles are aspirated and the oocytes collected. In the laboratory, the oocytes are identified under a dissecting microscope, transferred to a culture medium, and incubated.

Fertilization. When the oocytes are removed from the aspirate and transferred to the culture medium, their stage of maturation is assessed using morphological criteria. Appearance of the granulosa cells surrounding the oocyte (cumulus oophorus) is used: a tightly clustered cumulus indicates immaturity, while a loosely expanded cumulus is typical of maturity. Unfortunately, at present there are no very precise criteria to better assess oocyte maturity. Mature oocytes are incubated for 6–8 hours and immature ones for 24–36 hours before spermatozoa are added.

While the oocytes are being incubated, the semen specimen is obtained. The spermatozoa are washed in a special medium to separate them from the seminal plasma. About 100,000 spermatozoa are added to the culture medium containing the oocyte and incubation is continued for 48–72 hours. After the spermatozoum enters the cytoplasm, the oocyte completes its second meiotic division and the second polar body is extruded (see Chapter 6). The next day (16–18 hours after insemination), the oocytes are checked under the dissecting microscope. If fertilization is completed, two pronuclei are usually seen. This stage is followed by cleavage. Development to the four cell stage takes about 48 hours, at which time the embryos are transferred to the uterus.

Embryo transfer. Transfer of the embryos into the uterus is the simplest part of IVF. The patient is placed in lithotomy position. A speculum is placed in the vagina and the vagina and cervix are cleaned with sterile saline. A special sheath is gently advanced into the cervical canal up to the level of the internal os. The embryos are loaded into the tip of a thin catheter in a small amount of culture medium (20 μl). The catheter is then threaded through the sheath until it is within 1 cm of the uterine fundus and the embryos are injected into the uterine cavity. The catheter is held in place for about 30 seconds and then removed. If any embryos remain in the catheter, the same procedure is repeated. The speculum is then removed and the patient transferred to a bed where she remains lying on her back for 6 hours after which she is released. Patients are advised to stay in bed for 48 hours. Progesterone in oil (50 mg/day) is given from the time of embryo transfer until a pregnancy test is positive or menstruation begins.

Results of Treatment

Because of variations in reporting of results and in selection of patients, it is difficult at present to obtain accurate and reliable pregnancy rates from the published literature. Generally, superovulation is very successful and multiple oocytes are retrieved in more than 90% of patients. More than 80% of oocytes are successfully fertilized, but once the embryos are transferred into the uterus, the "take" is not more than 20–25%, a portion of which will be chemical pregnancies and early abortions. It is important to remember that, in the natural cycle of the human, only about 31% of potential fertilizations will actually produce a viable offspring while the other 69% will be lost, usually within the first month of pregnancy. Thus, theoretically, a 31% success rate with IVF would be the maximal one that could be expected. Overall, the present success rate is much lower, ranging from 10–18% live birthrates per oocyte retrieval procedure in the larger and more experienced centers, and lower rates in other centers.

Side Effects and Complications

Since in most IVF cases, multiple embryos are transferred, the incidence of multiple gestation is higher. There is also a higher incidence of ectopic pregnancies, as some of the embryos may migrate into the fallopian tubes. The incidence of congenital anomalies is equal to the general population. Recent psychological and developmental studies on children born after IVF reveal that they are not different than the general population.

GAMETE INTRAFALLOPIAN TRANSFER (GIFT)

The transfer of gametes into the fallopian tubes is an alternative to routine IVF. In this procedure, the first two steps (superovulation and oocyte retrieval) are the same as in IVF, but, instead of fertilization in vitro, the spermatozoa and oocytes are placed into the fimbriated end of the fallopian tubes, generally during laparoscopy. Usually no more than two oocytes are introduced into each fallopian tube. Candidates for GIFT must have at least one normal fallopian tube.

Pregnancy rates appear to be slightly higher with GIFT than IVF, but so are ectopic pregnancy rates. Recently, experiments were carried out to perform

GIFT under ultrasonographic guidance without the need of laparoscopy. If successful, this will simplify this procedure.

DONATED OOCYTES, EMBRYOS, AND SPERMATOZOA

The new reproductive technology enables pregnancy and motherhood for women who never imagined such a possibility. Oocyte donation, fertilization with donated spermatozoa, and even embryo donation are possible and practical. The details of such procedures are beyond the scope of this text. In addition to the medical problems, such procedures involve moral, ethical, and legal issues which in the majority of states have not been resolved yet.

14

Hormonal Contraceptives

Before the 1960s, couples desiring to limit the number of progeny had few efficient choices to consider. Since then, however, alternatives for means of contraception in the female have significantly broadened to include hormonal and intrauterine contraceptives, as well as new techniques for sterilization using laparoscopy and minilaparotomy. Since the normal ovulatory menstrual cycle and successful fertility are the results of interactions between several organs, there is of course a multitude of potentially vulnerable sites that can be influenced with contraception as a goal. Perhaps because of their potential to act at multiple sites, steroid hormones, the so-called *oral contraceptives,* have become the most effective contraceptive approach on the market short of sterilization. We will review the chemistry and mechanism of action of the steroid contraceptives, the metabolic and potential side effects of steroid contraceptives, and other potential approaches to hormonal contraceptives.

CHEMISTRY AND MODE OF ACTION OF STEROID CONTRACEPTIVES

CHEMISTRY

Three types of oral contraceptives have been used: combined progestin/estrogen, sequential estrogen/progestin, and continuous progestin. The *combined* type is the most widely used at present, as it is consistently more effective. The estrogen is given daily for 21 days together with a progestin, followed by 7 days off therapy. In the monophasic regimen, a single dose of progestin is used, while, in the biphasic regimen, two doses of progestin are used within a cycle. In the newer multiphasic regimen, the dose of progestin changes every 7 days. Common regimens are shown in Table 14–1. The *sequential* type has been abandoned in many areas, although new formulations containing lesser amounts of estrogen still offer a potentially reasonable approach. The *continuous* type, progestin alone, has been of more limited use because of the high incidence of intermenstrual bleeding associated with it, although the Food and Drug Administration (FDA) recently approved long-term progestin subcutaneous implants.

The estrogenic component of the commonly used oral contraceptives consists of ethinyl estradiol or mestranol, two synthetic orally active estrogens. These two

Table 14–1. Currently Available Oral Contraceptives

Product	Estrogen (μg)	Progestogen (mg)
Multiphasic		
Ortho 7/7/7	EE 35	NE 0.5/0.75/0.5
Tri Norinyl	EE 35	NE 0.5/1/0.5
Triphasil, Tri-Levien	EE 30/40/30	LN 0.05/0.075/0.125
Biphasic		
Ortho 10/11	EE 35	NE 0.5/1
Monophasic		
Loestrin	EE 20	NEA 1
Norinyl 1/50	ME 50	NE 1
Ortho-Novum 1/50		
Genora 1/50		
Nordette	EE 30	LN 0.15
Levien		
Lo-Ovral	EE 30	NG 0.3
Loestrin 1.5/30	EE 30	NEA 1.5
Ovcon 35	EE 35	NE 0.4
Brevicon	EE 35	NE 0.5
Modicon		
Norinyl 1/35	EE 35	NE 1
Ortho Novum 1/35		
Genora 1/35		
Demulen 1/35	EE 35	ED 1
Ovcon 50	EE 50	NE 1
Norlestrin 1	EE 50	NEA 1
Norlestrin 2.5	EE 50	NEA 2.5
Ovral	EE 50	NG 0.5
Demulen 1/50	EE 50	ED 1

ED, ethynodiol diacetate; *EE*, ethinyl estradiol; *LN*, levonorgestrel; *ME*, mestranol; *NE*, norethindrone; *NEA*, norethindrone acetate; *NG*, norgestrel.
    Source: Derman R: Oral contraceptives: a reassessment. *Obstet Gynecol Surv* 44:662.
© and reproduced by permission of Williams & Wilkins, 1989.

compounds are closely related chemically (Fig. 14–1) and, in fact, the biological activity of mestranol is related to its conversion to ethinyl estradiol.

The progestin usually consists of a compound that belongs to one of two groups: the 19-nor steroids (Fig. 14–2) or a derivative of 17-α-hydroxyprogesterone (Fig. 14–3). 19-nor refers to the absence of a methyl group on C-10; the absence of this group not only enhances biological activity but also confers a more complex activity to the steroid. These steroids are derived from testosterone and, thus, most have some androgenic action. They have some estrogenic activity as well, related to a small degree of conversion to ethinyl estradiol but possibly also to some inherent estrogenic activity of the molecule. Of course, they are also powerful progestins.

Derivatives of 17-α-hydroxyprogesterone are increasingly used for contraceptive purposes. This steroid is a naturally occurring intermediate in the biogenesis

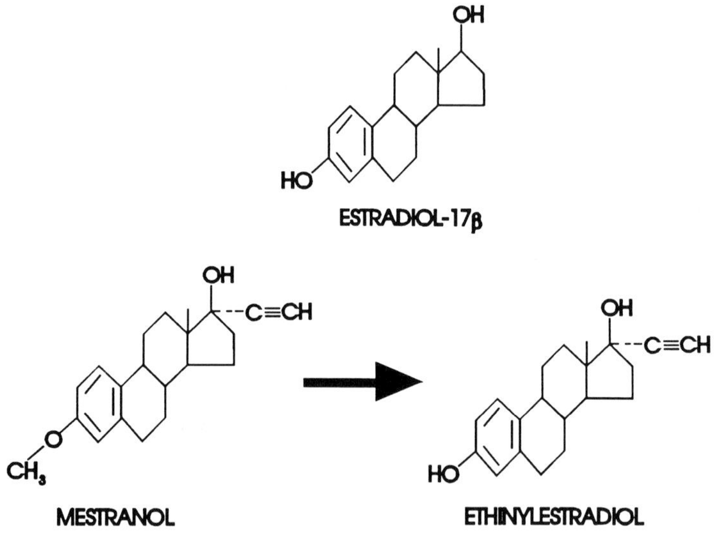
OH
HO
ESTRADIOL-17β
OH
C≡CH
CH_3
O
MESTRANOL
OH
C≡CH
HO
ETHINYLESTRADIOL

Fig. 14–1. Chemical structure of natural and synthetic estrogens. Estradiol-17β, the natural estrogen, is rapidly degraded in the gastrointestinal tract. Synthetic estrogens are therefore used in hormonal contraception. Shown here are the two most used estrogen components in the "pill."

of steroids (see Fig. 3–1); it has little biologic activity on its own, but esterified derivatives are highly active progestins (Fig. 14–3).

MODE OF ACTION OF STEROID CONTRACEPTIVES

Potentially, oral contraceptives can exert their effects at multiple sites (Fig. 14–4). It is usually difficult to pinpoint with precision *one* site of action, as it may

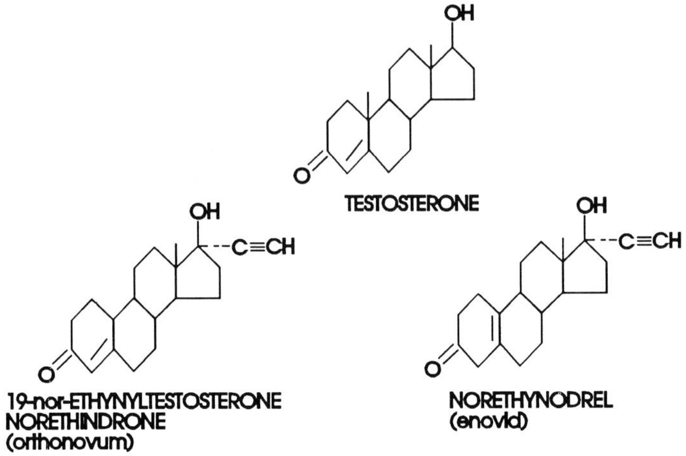
OH
O
TESTOSTERONE
OH
C≡CH
O
19-nor-ETHYNYLTESTOSTERONE
NORETHINDRONE
(orthonovum)
OH
C≡CH
O
NORETHYNODREL
(enovid)

Fig. 14–2. Chemical structure of the 19-nor steroids. These derivatives of testosterone exert a powerful progestinic effect. They also possess some androgenic as well as estrogenic activities.

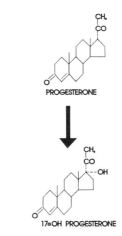

Fig. 14–3. Chemical structure of 17-α-hydroxyprogesterone derivatives. 17-α-hydroxyprogesterone has little biological activity on its own, but its esters are powerful progestins.

vary with each individual hormonal regimen and as more than one site may be affected simultaneously.

One of the main sites that can potentially be affected is the hypothalamic-pituitary unit. In general, estrogen–progesterone combinations inhibit follicle-stimulating hormone (FSH) and luteinizing hormone (LH) secretion and prevent ovulation. This action may reflect interferences with the proper secretion of gonadotropin-releasing hormone (GnRH) by the hypothalamus. In some cases, the inhibitory effect can be overcome by the administration of GnRH. Many studies, however, report a lack of response to GnRH, suggesting potential direct inhibitory effects on the pituitary as well; this is more pronounced in formulations containing a more potent progestin. Inhibition of ovulation is not necessary to obtain satisfactory contraception; for example, with continuous progestin therapy, ovulatory surges of gonadotropins may persist. In these cases, the contraceptive effect can be achieved by affecting (1) cervical mucus: the progestins inhibit mucorrhea to some degree or another and hinder sperm penetration through the cervical mucus; (2) tubal physiology: oral contraceptives may affect the morphology and function of the fallopian tube epithelium, tubal secretion and tubal contraction, thereby disrupting proper ovum transport; (3) uterine morphology: steroidal contraceptives can affect myometrial and endometrial histology, and thereby alter functional activity of the uterus. Marked alterations of various endometrial enzymes occur under oral contraceptives. These uterine changes may interfere with the proper implantation process; and (4) ovarian function: contraceptives may affect ovarian function not only indirectly through

PUTATIVE SITES OF ACTION OF HORMONAL CONTRACEPTIVES

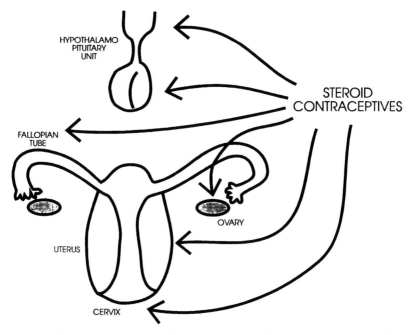

Fig. 14–4. Mode of action of steroid contraceptives. Sites with the potential of being affected by hormonal contraceptives are multiple. Different hormonal regimens may affect each site differentially, and therefore, it is usually difficult, if not impossible, to pinpoint the one and only site of action of a particular "pill."

their inhibitory action on gonadotropin secretion, but also directly perhaps by disturbing the delicate hormonal environment of the developing follicle, thereby interfering with its development or the maturation of the oocyte, or by affecting the steroidogenic function of the corpus luteum.

GENERAL EFFECTS OF STEROID CONTRACEPTIVES

METABOLIC EFFECTS

In addition to affecting the reproductive axis at different levels, oral contraceptives may exert various metabolic effects, which, in some instances, have the potential of producing adverse clinical symptoms. It is important to note that the potential for adverse impact has significantly decreased with the newer combinations and lower doses. Nevertheless, these adverse effects must always be kept in mind.

Effects on Lipid Metabolism

Contraceptive estrogens and progestins (particularly the derivatives of 19-nortestosterone which possess significant androgenic activity) have opposite effects on lipoprotein metabolism. Estrogens elevate plasma very low-density lipoprotein (VLDL) and triglycerides as well as high-density lipoprotein (HDL) cholesterol (mostly of the steroid-sensitive subfraction HDL_2) levels, while they decrease low-density lipoprotein (LDL) cholesterol concentrations. These changes in LDL and HDL are associated with decreased cardiovascular risks. In contrast, with a steady low-estrogen preparation, progestins decrease triglycerides and HDL, while increasing LDL, in a dose responsive manner. The plasma triglyceride effect of estrogens is the result of increased production of VLDL, while androgenic steroids stimulate the removal of plasma triglycerides. The estrogen-induced HDL increase results both from the suppression of hepatic lipase activity, causing reduced conversion of HDL_2 into HDL_3 and the increased synthesis of apolipoprotein A. Androgenic progestins stimulate hepatic lipase activity and suppress the synthesis of apolipoprotein A. The mechanism for the alteration of LDL is not entirely clear.

Since most contraceptive treatments depend on combination preparations, the relative potencies of the estrogenic and progestinic components will, of course, determine the net effect on lipid metabolism. The negative impact can be related to the androgenicity of the progestin. Specifically, levonorgestrel and norgestrel, two 19-nor steroids, have been associated with a more negative impact on lipids than other progestins. These two steroids are significantly more potent than other 19-nor steroids as progestins (10–20 times for levonorgestrel and 5–10 times for norgestrel). Levonorgestrel has also greater androgenicity than other progestins, independent of dose or clinical potency. Whether these metabolic changes have a clinical effect on cardiovascular disease (discussed later) remains controversial. In general, low-dose formulations should be used; perhaps, in the future, nonandrogenic preparations will be found that may have a more beneficial effect on lipids.

Effects on Glucose Metabolism

Glucose tolerance, which depends on several factors the most important of which are insulin secretion and action, is unfavorably altered by oral contraceptives. The precise mechanism of decreased glucose tolerance in contraceptive users is still unknown, but may in part relate to increased peripheral insulin resistance perhaps caused by a postreceptor defect. Several studies have shown that formulations containing potent progestins have the greatest adverse effect on carbohydrate metabolism. Although studies have shown no difference in the frequency of clinical diabetes mellitus in nonusers and users of high-dose combination contraceptives (about 4%), women with previous gestational diabetes are at a much greater risk (44%). The use of low-dose oral contraceptives is accompanied by a lower, but not insignificant, frequency of impaired glucose tolerance, even in women at risk. Although recent epidemiologic studies also indicate a low cardiovascular disease risk in low-dose oral contraceptive users, women with diabetes may still be at an increased risk. Older women (over 35 years of age), obese women, women with a history of stillbirth or a large infant, women with demonstrated glucose intolerance or with a close diabetic relative should be tested for glucose tolerance prior to oral contraceptive use.

Effects on Protein Metabolism

Estrogens increase plasma proteins which bind steroids. These include cortisol-binding globulin, sex hormone binding globulin, and thyroid-binding globulin. Plasma proteins which bind iron and copper are also increased. These factors are particularly important to remember when diagnostic tests require measurements of these substances. Usually, bound as well as unbound fractions are measured, thus yielding falsely elevated levels.

Drug Interaction

A number of medications will interfere with oral contraceptive effectiveness by a number of mechanisms, including inhibition of microsomal enzymes, increased metabolism, or changes in enterohepatic circulation (Table 14–2).

POTENTIAL SIDE EFFECTS OF STEROID
CONTRACEPTIVES

Cardiovascular Risk

Cardiovascular risk may be venous or arterial in origin. In the former category are venous thrombosis and pulmonary emboli, which are related to the estrogen component. This component in high-dose oral contraceptives affects the hemostatic system and induces an increase in procoagulant factor activities and a simultaneous decrease in the levels of the naturally occurring coagulation inhibitor, antithrombin III. Myocardial infarction and cerebral vascular accidents of arterial origin are more specifically related to problems with lipid metabolism and glucose intolerance. With the introduction of low-dose estrogen and pro-

Table 14–2. Clinically Important Drug Interactions with Oral Contraceptives

Drug	Mechanism
Agents that reduce oral contraceptive effect	
Anticonvulsants	↑ Metabolism through
Barbiturates	enzyme induction
Carbamazepine	
Phenytoin	
Primidone	
Griseofulvin	Enzyme induction
Rifampin	Enzyme induction
Tetracycline	↓ Urinary, ↑ fecal excretion
Agents antagonized by oral contraceptives	
Anticoagulants	↑ Synthesis of clotting factors
Diazepam	↓ Clearance
Folic acid	↓ Metabolism
Imipramine	↑ Metabolism
Insulin	Impaired glucose tolerance
Theophylline	↓ Clearance

Source: Derman R: Oral contraceptives: a reassessment. *Obstet Gynecol Surv* 44:662, © and reproduced by permission of Williams & Wilkins, 1989.

gestin combinations, the cardiovascular risk has been greatly reduced; however, associated risk factors remain important. These include smoking, obesity, hypertension, hyperlipidemia, and diabetes.

Oral contraceptives, particularly the estrogen component, cause an increase in hepatic production of several globulins. Increased levels of globulin angiotensinogen may cause an increase in angiotensin II, and thus aldosterone. In the majority of subjects, excessive vasoconstriction is prevented by a compensatory decrease in plasma renin concentrations. Only a few patients develop hypertension even though changes occur in all subjects. The development of high blood pressure may also increase the risk of cardiovascular problems in these patients. Again, reduced formulation dosage increases the safety effect, although blood pressure should be monitored in all patients on oral contraceptives, since a transient increase may occur.

Cancer

Oral contraceptives are potent hormones and their potential association with cancer is a persistent concern for patients taking these medications. Multicenter reports, however, have repeatedly cited a reduced risk for endometrial and ovarian cancer. At present, the majority of evidence shows no increased risk for either cervical or breast cancer, although the latter association remains the most controversial.

Endometrium. Data from several epidemiological studies indicate that women users are less likely to develop endometrial cancer than nonusers. Frequency may be reduced by 50% after 1 year of oral contraceptive use, especially in multiparous women (Fig. 14–5). The "protective" effect may persist for 10–15 years after discontinuation. The decrease in risk is most probably related to the progestin, which blocks the estrogen receptor and thereby prevents this hormone's growth-promoting action.

Ovary. Risk of ovarian cancer can also be reduced by oral contraceptives, with the greatest reduction occurring in nulliparous women starting within 1 year of treatment and persisting for 10–15 years, with a larger reduction with duration of treatment (Fig. 14–5). After 10 years on oral contraceptives, all women experience a reduction. The mechanism is not well understood, but a decrease in the degree of gonadotropin stimulation or in the number of ovulations may play a role.

Cervical dysplasia. Some reports on users of oral contraceptives have indicated that the risk of cervical dysplasia may increase after prolonged use. These results are conflicting, however, as oral contraceptive users tend to have earlier sexual relations, more frequent intercourse, more partners, and better gynecologic screening. A slightly higher risk of dysplasia may persist when adjusting for these factors. Yet, the association of papilloma virus and cervical cancer suggests that sexual practices may be more likely to parallel cervical dysplasia than oral contraceptives use.

Effect of OC Use on Risk of Endometrial and Ovarian Cancer

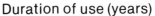

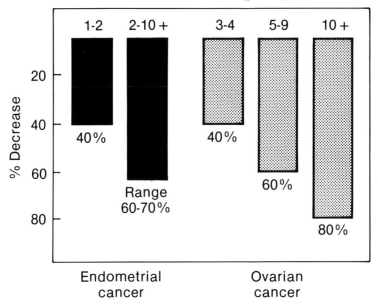

Fig. 14–5. Steroid contraceptives and risk of endometrial and ovarian cancer. (From Speroff L 1990: *Women's Health Consensus. Program Handbook.* Health Learning Systems Inc., Littlefalls, NJ.)

Breast. The incidence of breast cancer has been increasing throughout the world, and, in North America, incidence runs from 1:9 to 1:10 women. The vast majority of studies show no relationship between breast cancer and oral contraceptives. However, three of the twenty-six studies do suggest an increased risk. Thus, all women over 35 years of age as well as those at high risk from family history should be carefully screened by physical examination and mammogram before therapy and at intervals thereafter. Undoubtedly, if cancer is present before initiation of therapy, there may be a greatly increased risk of accelerated growth depending on the estrogen receptivity of the tumor. It should be noted that these observations and association in certain subgroups have been shown for the high-dose oral contraceptives. The newer low-dose oral contraceptives have not been reported to be associated with increased risk.

Liver and Gallbladder Disease

The occasional occurrence of jaundice and liver malfunction in patients on oral contraceptives have led to studies regarding steroid effects on hepatic function. Oral contraceptives, primarily the estrogen component, reduce the excretory capacity of the liver for certain organic anions, such as bromosulfphtalein, and the active transport of biliary components. Decreased hepatic excretion of bromosulfphtalein is not associated with hyperbilirubinemia and mimics what is seen in the last trimester of pregnancy (recurrent jaundice of pregnancy). Thus, these changes are usually benign and reversible. Estrogens have well-documented effects on various hepatic enzymatic processes and affect hepatic lipid and lipoprotein formation as well as intermediary carbohydrate metabolism. Occasionally, there appears to be a nondose related idiosyncratic bile secretory failure, due to sensitivity to the drug through an unknown mechanism. Other patients develop jaundice in pregnancy, with recurrence if challenged later with oral contraceptives. The cholestasis of pregnancy and the estrogen-sensitive group are probably representative of the same phenomenon. Others may have a preexisting defect of bile excretion, which is accentuated by oral contraceptives. It seems reasonable, therefore, to advise caution in patients with a history of liver disease and to discontinue oral contraceptives if signs of hepatic disease develop.

An increase in risk of gallbladder disease, especially cholelithiasis, is observed following oral contraceptives. In these patients, estrogen is thought to alter bile salts and the solubility of the bile acids, predisposing to a cholesterol saturation state. Such an association is not apparent with the low-dose contraceptive.

Reducing Risks of Oral Contraceptive Use

Overall, oral contraceptives remain the safest and most effective form of contraception. Nonetheless, there are absolute contraindications to their use. These risk factors include smoking, thromboembolic disorders and phlebitis, cerebrovascular disease, coronary occlusion, impaired liver function, estrogen-dependent neoplasia such as endometrial carcinoma, undiagnosed vaginal bleeding, and carcinoma of the breast. Pregnancy should be ruled out.

A risk score form, such as one developed by Spellacy, can be used to determine who should not use the "pill". After excluding women with an absolute contraindication for oral contraceptive use, women at greatest risk for cardiovascular problems are those with a family history of hyperlipidemia, gestational or overt diabetes, and hypertension. Pills should be used with caution in patients over 35 years of age. Current knowledge of risk factors permits a reduction of exposure to oral contraceptive-related mortality by 86%.

Oral contraceptives using less potent steroids with lower doses of both estrogen and progestin have become more popular as the importance of minimizing metabolic side effects have been recognized. The first oral contraceptives contained as much as 150 μg of estrogen and 10 mg of a progestin. These were, as it turned out, unnecessarily large doses, and, at present, these amounts have been reduced to 30–35 μg of estrogen and 0.5–1 mg of progestin. The newer contraceptives now reproduce levels of estrogen in the peripheral circulation which resemble those found in the early follicular phase of the normal cycle. The progestin dose has been further reduced with the newer formulations using a multiphasic dosage regimen. Data have shown a trend toward reduction in cardiovascular risk with the use of low-dose preparations oral contraceptives. The disadvantages of low-dose preparations revolve mainly around the increased incidence of breakthrough bleeding, particularly in the first few months. This is due to shedding of a relatively unstimulated endometrium. This problem is minimized with time, and, in the long term, a high incidence of amenorrhea characterizes low-dose preparations. Again, this is due to the lack of endometrial stimulation by estrogen and endometrial atrophy.

Continuous dose of progestin without estrogen are also used for oral contraception (the "mini pill"). The drug is taken daily without interruption and the contraceptive effect is due to inhibition of ovulation and possibly other effects such as on cervical mucus. This approach appears to circumvent the harmful side effects which are primarily due to the estrogen component and, indeed, a lower incidence of adverse metabolic effects are seen with no increase in blood pressure, less hepatotoxicity, less change in coagulation factors, and no increased risk of thromboembolic problems. Nausea and breast tenderness are also eliminated. The disadvantages are the high frequency of amenorrhea and abnormal bleeding patterns, a higher failure rate (2–8% per year) and possibly a higher ectopic pregnancy rate associated with these failures.

Recently, a new continuous progestin contraceptive has been introduced in the form of levonorgestrel implants placed under the skin. A low continuous dose of the hormone is, thus, released into the body preventing pregnancy through a combination of inhibition of ovulation and changes in cervical mucus. The capsules are placed in a fanlike pattern under the skin of the arm, through a small incision using a local anesthetic. This type of contraceptive has the advantage of lasting for 5 years without requiring patient compliance, but the implant can be removed at anytime. The main side effect is amenorrhea and/or irregular menstrual bleeding, although some patients continue to have some monthly bleeding. The levonorgestrel in the implant is also the most potent progestin with reference to adverse lipid and lipoprotein changes. However, the dose released is low and changes have not been observed. Medroxyprogesterone acetate (Depo-Provera) consisting of a progesterone in oil given by injection is a highly effective progestin-only contraceptive; however, at the present time it is not approved for contraceptive use in the United States despite its wide use elsewhere. The hormone is slowly released from the injection site. An injection of 150 mg usually lasts 3 months or longer.

OTHER HORMONAL CONTRACEPTIVES

GnRH ANALOGS

GnRH, when given by constant infusion, will cause a profound suppression of FSH and LH secretion (see Chapter 2). Using this principle, GnRH agonists, which remain in the circulation for a longer time (see Fig. 13–4), are being studied for use as hormonal contraceptives. Experimental GnRH antagonists, which prevent the action of endogenous GnRH, are also under investigation. While these compounds are very successful in suppressing gonadotropin secretion and, therefore, in interfering with the ovulatory process, their major drawbacks are hypoestrogenism and associated symptoms (hot flushes, amenorrhea, potential loss of bone mass) that may accompany their use.

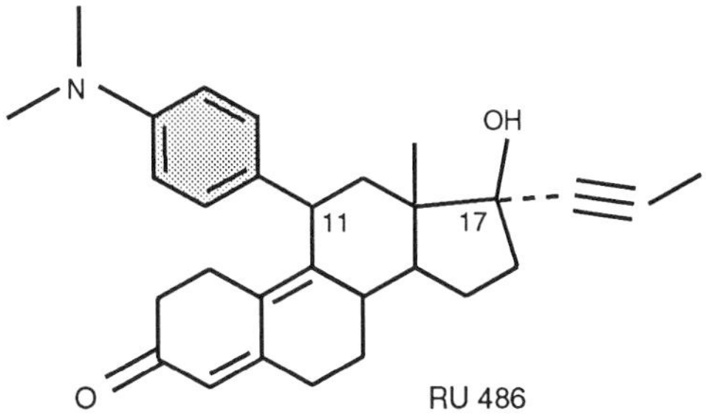

Fig. 14–6. The structure of RU 486. RU 486 is a steroid derived from progesterone, which, because of a supplementary nucleus on C-11, possesses important antiprogesterone activities.

RU 486

This compound is an antagonist of progesterone which acts by blocking the progesterone receptor (it also blocks the cortisol receptor, but to a much lesser degree) (Fig. 14–6). In combination with prostaglandins, RU 486 has a very high success rate in inducing early therapeutical abortions, because it prevents the supportive role of progesterone on the pregnant uterus. Treatment is by oral medication, followed by a prostaglandin vaginal suppository. RU 486 may also have a potential as a contraceptive pill by blocking progesterone effects on the endometrium, thereby preventing maintenance of the secretory endometrium essential for implantation. RU 486 may also become useful in the treatment of progesterone receptor-bearing tumors.

15

The Premenstrual Syndrome

The premenstrual syndrome (PMS) is a recurrent cyclic disorder consisting of an intriguing symptom complex which includes moderate to distressing luteal phase-related changes in physiology, mood, and/or behavior. This syndrome, also referred to as the late luteal phase dysphoric disorder by the American Psychiatric Association, is felt to be reproducible enough to be accorded diagnostic criteria in the *Diagnostic and Statistical Manual of Mental Disorders.* In general, it is thought that biological changes, such as perhaps the large hormonal fluctuations that accompany the menstrual cycle, are related to the intensity of the physical and psychological symptoms, and that environmental factors and individual coping mechanisms may contribute to the development of the symptoms. Most women experience only mild cyclic symptoms that do not affect physical and emotional functioning, however, as many as 30–40% of women report perimenstrual symptoms that are troublesome enough to temporarily interfere with normal functioning. In 5%, the symptoms are frankly disruptive. We will discuss the pathophysiological aspects, the symptomatology and clinical assessment, and the treatment of PMS.

PATHOPHYSIOLOGY OF PMS

The specific etiology of PMS remains unknown, although many theories have been proposed. In time, PMS has been related to a progesterone deficiency during the late luteal phase, an abnormal estrogen: progesterone ratio in the late luteal phase, a too rapid withdrawal of estrogen and progesterone at the end of the luteal phase, hyperprolactinemia, increased aldosterone or renin-angiotensin activity, subclinical hypoglycemia, vitamin B6 deficiency, allergy to endogenous hormones, aberrant prostaglandin metabolism, as well as others. Up to now, investigative endocrine studies have been inconclusive and sometimes conflicting. Most likely, PMS is multifactorial and probably also involves changes in neurohormones and neurotransmitters, which cannot be easily documented in the human.

There is, however, convincing evidence that the PMS syndrome *is* related to the cyclic hormonal rhythmicities of the menstrual cycle. Indeed, (1) PMS improves or resolves when ovarian secretions are abolished. For instance, the syndrome disappears during periods of hypogonadotropic amenorrhea and during treatment with gonadotropin-releasing hormone (GnRH) analogs; (2) the syndrome does not appear prepuberally, when the reproductive axis is inactive; (3) PMS is not present or disappears at menopause (it can, however, reappear with estrogen-progesterone replacement therapy); and (4) PMS persists after hysterectomy if surgery does not include oophorectomy. Furthermore, there is a temporal relationship between symptom intensity and hormonal phase of the cycle, with the lowest intensity in the mid–late follicular phase, a rise in the early luteal, and a peak in the late luteal phase. Thus, a comprehensive theory must take this cyclic relationship into account.

An attractive hypothesis, suggested by Reid and co-workers, would link PMS to the endogenous opioid peptides. These peptides are widely distributed throughout the central nervous system (C.N.S.) and are well known to affect a large variety of functions, which include not only analgesia but also mood, behavior, appetite, sleep, temperature regulation, and bowel function. There is good evidence from nonhuman primate work that brain β-endorphin, a major endogenous opioid peptide, is controlled by ovarian steroids and that its concentrations fluctuate with the menstrual cycle (see Chapter 2 for further details). Present technologies do not allow for brain opioid peptide measurements in the human, but indirect evidence obtained with the use of naloxone, an opiate antagonist, suggests that similar fluctuations in endogenous opioid peptides occur in the human. This direct correlation of brain endogenous opioid peptides to cyclic ovarian activity would, according to this hypothesis, provide a direct link between the cyclic nature of the syndrome and the diversity of symptoms observed. It is possible that in some women, sensitivity to the cyclic exposure to and withdrawal from endogenous opioid peptides (Fig. 15–1, see also Fig. 2–8) may be heightened and thereby elicit the manifestations attributed to PMS. Further work in this area is needed to substantiate this interesting hypothesis. Environmental factors may also contribute to the development of the symptoms. Increased stress or a depressive state are thought to be predisposing factors.

CLINICAL ASPECTS OF PMS

SYMPTOMS

Symptoms of PMS have been defined as falling into one of four temporal patterns according to their onset and duration in relation to the menstrual cycle (Fig. 15–2). In most patients, the symptoms are confined to the luteal phase and terminate rapidly at menstruation. The most common physical symptoms include bloating, abdominal discomfort, change in appetite, breast tenderness, and headache. Behavioral changes include fatigue, depression, anxiety, irritability, anger, confusion, and social withdrawal.

Subtypes with clusters of symptoms have been reported but the data remain controversial. One explanation has been that the varied cyclic manifestations may represent individual differences in the expression of a pathophysiologic process that has not yet been identified. Studies in the 2 weeks preceding menstruation reveal a common evolution of symptoms in many women, with specific problems predominating. Breast swelling and tenderness together with lower

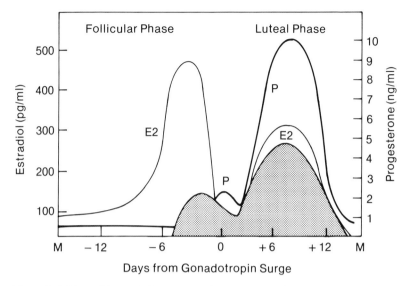

Fig. 15-1. Opioid peptides and the menstrual cycle. Dramatic changes in central opi-atergic activity occur during the menstrual cycle. A significant opiate withdrawal period characterizes the end of the luteal phase and approaching menstruation (*M*). Several symptoms of the premenstrual syndrome resemble acute opiate withdrawal, and, thus, endogenous opiate fluctuations may be related to the expression of the syndrome in women who may be particularly sensitive to them. Presumed changes in the hypotha-lamic opiate tone during the cycle are represented by the *shaded area*. *E2*, estradiol-17β; *P*, progesterone.

abdominal bloating are particularly common and may require looser clothing. These symptoms have been attributed to fluid retention and may sometimes be accompanied by weight gain; they may also occur in the absence of weight gain, suggesting that local fluid shifts may be more important. Also common are a dramatic increase in appetite and unusual cravings such as for chocolate or salty foods. The common occurrence of these symptoms may signal impending menstruation to some patients.

The behavioral symptoms may be particularly troublesome. Fatigue, depression, and emotional lability are common. Crying or emotional outbursts over trivial matters may also herald menstruation. Sometimes there may be severe withdrawal or even suicidal psychotic behavior or combativeness.

CLINICAL ASSESSMENT

Clinical assessment of PMS is often difficult, because diagnosis is based on a symptom complex. As the primary task in the formulation of the diagnosis, how-ever, it is essential to establish that the physiologic and psychologic dysfunctions vary with the menstrual cycle. The diagnosis of PMS should be made only if the criteria, as proposed in the *Diagnostic and Statistical Manual of Mental Disor-ders* (Table 15-1) are met. At present, unfortunately, these standard diagnostic criteria underemphasize the physical symptoms. These, however, are an impor-

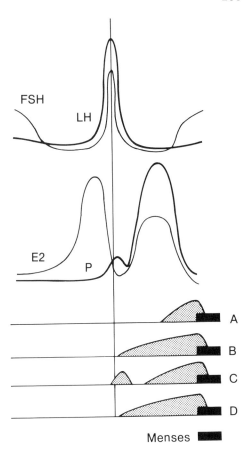

Fig. 15–2. Variability in onset and duration of premenstrual symptoms. Schematic representation of the variability in the onset and duration of premenstrual syndrome (PMS). Most patients experience patterns *A* or *B*. (Symptoms are confined to the luteal phase and terminate rapidly at menstruation.) *FSH,* follicle-stimulating hormone; *LH,* luteinizing hormone; other abbreviations as in Figure 15–1. (Adapted from Reid RL, Yen SSC 1983: *Clin Obstet Gynecol* 26:710.)

tant part of the syndrome as well and most probably have a real physiological origin reflecting the drastic hormonal changes occurring in the luteal phase of the cycle.

It is important to separate patients who meet these criteria from those who have exacerbations of somatic or psychiatric disorders during the luteal phase as well as from others who show fluctuations that are not related to the menstrual cycle. A standardized assessment form is not commonly used by practitioners, although some retrospective questionnaires can be useful. An example is the *Premenstrual Assessment Form* by Halbreich, Endicott, and Schecht. It is best to document the physical symptoms and the major mood disturbances that are hallmarks of the syndrome prospectively. The clinical evaluation should also include a careful history and gynecologic examination to rule out hormonal or gynecologic disorders that can be associated with or confused with PMS, including thyroid disorders, syndromes associated with elevated prolactin secretion, endometriosis, and ovarian cysts. Medication, and drug, alcohol, caffeine, or tobacco use should be reviewed as well as psychiatric history in addition to the general medical examination.

Table 15–1. Diagnostic Criteria for Late Luteal Phase Dysphoric Disorder

1. For most menstrual cycles during the past year, symptoms in 2 occurred during the last week of the luteal phase and remitted within a few days after the onset of the follicular phase. In menstruating females this corresponds to the week prior to menses, and a few days after the onset of menses. In nonmenstruating females who have had a hysterectomy, the timing of luteal and follicular phases may require the measurement of circulating reproductive hormones.

2. At least five of the following symptoms were present for most of the time during each symptomatic periluteal phase; at least one of the symptoms was (a), (b), (c), or (d):
   a. Marked affective lability (e.g., suddenly sad, tearful, irritable, or angry)
   b. Persistent and marked anger or irritability
   c. Feeling extremely anxious, tense, keyed up, or on edge
   d. Markedly depressed mood, marked pessimism, or self-deprecating thoughts
   e. Decreased interest in usual activities (e.g., work, friends, hobbies)
   f. Easily tired or lack of energy
   g. Subjective sense of difficulty concentrating
   h. Marked change in appetite, overeating, or specific food cravings
   i. Hypersomnia or insomnia
   j. Other physical symptoms (e.g., breast tenderness or swelling, headaches, joint or muscle pain, sensation of "bloating," weight gain)

3. The disturbance seriously interferes with work or with usual social activities or relationships with others.

4. The disturbance is not merely an exacerbation of the symptoms of another disorder, such as major depression, panic disorder, dysthymia or a personality disorder, although it may be superimposed on any of these disorders.

5. Criteria 1, 2, 3, and 4 are confirmed by prospective daily self-ratings of at least two symptomatic cycles. The diagnosis may be made provisionally prior to this confirmation.

Source: American Psychiatric Association: Diagnostic and Statistical Manual of Mental Disorders, Third Edition, Revised, Washington, DC, American Psychiatric Association, 1987.

TREATMENT OF PMS

Since the etiology of PMS remains unknown, no established treatment exists. Many studies show the same improvement rate in placebo as in treated groups (30%), although, expectedly, treatments that abolish ovarian hormone secretion are usually associated with amelioration. A general therapeutical outline appears in Figure 15–3.

Intervention may at first include such measures as reduction in exposure to stress, as a relation exists between stress level and intensity of symptoms. Dietary modification including reduction of salt, alcohol, and beverages containing methylxanthine (coffee, tea, and cola drinks) may affect fluid retention, mood, and breast tenderness, respectively.

Pharmacologic intervention is commonly used, particularly progesterone therapy. Progesterone is a known C.N.S. sedative; the rationale for its use is that women with PMS sometimes have a deficient luteal production of progesterone and, therefore, an increased estrogen/progesterone ratio. Progesterone doses

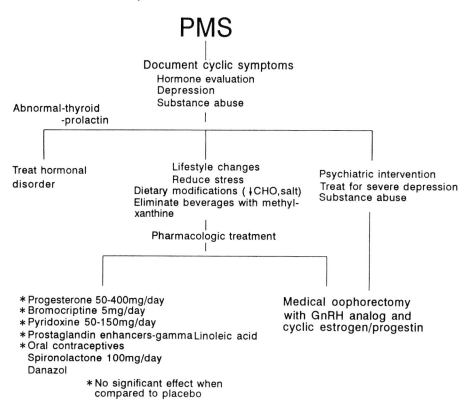

Fig. 15–3. General therapeutical outline for premenstrual syndrome *(PMS)*. *GnRH,* gonadotropin-releasing hormone.

range from 50–400 mg/day, often given vaginally to provide an immediate entry into the blood stream. Generally, however, progesterone therapy has not been found to be more effective than placebo, although it continues to be widely used.

Suppression of the hypothalamic-pituitary-ovarian axis with a GnRH analog or with danazol has been found effective when compared to placebo groups. Both drugs have side effects, however: GnRH analogs are associated with hot flushes and the risk of bone loss due to hypoestrogenism; danazol has androgenic effects and causes fluid retention and weight gain. Recent studies have shown that GnRH agonist treatment reduces PMS symptoms by 75%. The addition of conjugated estrogen and progestin cyclically to the GnRH agonist regimen maintains improvement (60%), although some deterioration is observed. This deterioration, however, is no greater than that of placebo addition to the GnRH regimen, suggesting that the anticipation of steroid replacement, rather than the steroid itself, accounts for the majority of symptoms. This combined regimen represents an important new tool in the treatment of this disorder.

The efficacy of oral contraceptives in the treatment of PMS has been questioned as placebo-controlled trials fail to demonstrate effectiveness. The supression of ovulation that accompanies contraception has been thought to be associated with an improvement in symptoms; thus, oral contraceptives have been commonly used, but further studies are necessary.

Bromocriptine, the dopamine receptor agonist, may reduce breast swelling but may have unpleasant side effects including orthostatic hypotension, nausea, and vomiting. Pyridoxine (vitamin B6), a coenzyme in the metabolism of dopamine, serotonin, and norepinephrine, has also been used, the idea being that defects in these neurotransmitters may be causal to PMS. Low pyridoxine may lead to low dopamine levels, which may in turn elevate prolactin concentrations. Daily doses of 50–150 mg of pyridoxine, however, are not more effective than placebo. Prostaglandin enhancers and prostaglandin inhibitors have also not been found effective. An essential fatty acid precursor of PGE, gamma-linoleic acid, in the form of evening primrose oil, is a popular treatment, but its effectiveness has not been proven.

Diuretics have been widely used in the treatment of PMS, particularly since fluid retention is a common symptom. Again, beneficial effects have not been documented, perhaps because the perceived fluid retention is due instead to bowel distention or local fluid shifts within the breast and bowel. The majority of studies do not provide consistant documented evidence for weight increase or fluid retention. However, sudden weight gain has been documented in the course of PMS; this must be related to fluid retention, although the pathogenesis is not well understood. Dietary factors have been implicated, as sudden carbohydrate increases or salt retention can cause a weight gain of up to 3 kg. For this reason, restriction of salt and carbohydrates is often recommended, and diuretics may be beneficial in the management of patients with sudden premenstrual weight gain.

Various studies have documented a premenstrual elevation of aldosterone, although this is not a consistant finding, even in patients complaining of bloating and weight gain. Most diuretics will cause secondary aldosteronism and potential cyclic edema and/or dependancy. Interest in spironolactone has stemmed from its action as an aldosterone antagonist. Although the data on the use of this drug have been conflicting, it appears to have a role in the management of PMS and its physical and psychological symptoms, particularly bloating. The advantages to using this drug appear to be mainly theoretical.

An experimental therapeutical approach involves the administration of naloxone or naltrexone, with the idea that these compounds would block the addicting potentials of the endogenous opioid peptides. The effectiveness of the approach is under study.

References

CHAPTER 1. THE REPRODUCTIVE CYCLE: AN OVERVIEW

REVIEWS

Freeman ME 1988: The ovarian cycle of the rat. In: *The Physiology of Reproduction* (Knobil E, Neill JD eds), Raven Press, NY, 1893–1928.

Karsch FJ, Bittman EL, Foster DL, Goodman RL, Legan SJ, Robinson JE 1984: Neuroendocrine basis of seasonal reproduction. *Recent Prog Horm Res* 40:185–232.

Ramirez VD, Beyer C 1988: The ovarian cycle of the rabbit: its neuroendocrine control. In: *The Physiology of Reproduction* (Knobil E, Neill JD eds), Raven Press, NY, 1874–1892.

Ross GT, Cargille CM, Lipsett MB, Rayford PL, Marshall JR, Strott CA 1970: Mechanisms regulating the menstrual cycle of women. *Recent Prog Horm Res* 26:63–95.

ARTICLES

Abraham GE, Odell WS, Swerdloff RS, Hopper R 1972: Simultaneous radioimmunoassays of plasma FSH, LH, progesterone, 17-OH progesterone and estradiol during the menstrual cycle. *J Clin Endocrinol Metab* 45:312–318.

Aedo AR, Langren BM, Cekan Z, Diczfalusy E 1976: Studies on the pattern of circulating steroids in the normal menstrual cycle. *Acta Endocrinol (Copenh)* 82:600–616.

Goodman AL, Descalzi CD, Johnson DK, Hodgen GD 1977: Composite pattern of circulating LH, FSH, estradiol and progesterone during the menstrual cycle in cynomolgus monkeys. *Proc Soc Exp Biol Med* 155:479–481.

Hoff JD, Quigley ME, Yen SSC 1983: Hormonal dynamics at midcycle: a reevaluation. *J Clin Endocrinol Metab* 57:792–796.

Mais V, Cetel NS, Muse KN, Quigley ME, Reid RL, Yen SSC 1987: Hormonal dynamics during luteal-follicular transition. *J Clin Endocrinol Metab* 64:1109–1114.

Monroe SE, Atkinson LE, Knobil E 1970: Patterns of circulating luteinizing hormone and their relation to plasma progesterone levels during the menstual cycle of the rhesus monkey. *Endocrinology* 87:453–455.

Pauerstein CJ, Eddy CA, Croxatto HD, Hess R, Siler-Khodr TM, Croxatto HB 1978: Temporal relationships of estrogen, progesterone, and luteinizing hormone levels to ovulation in women and infrahuman primates. *Am J Obstet Gynecol* 130:876–884.

Treloar AE, Boynton RE, Benn BG, Brown BW 1967: Variation of human menstrual cycle through reproductive life. *Int J Fertil* 12:77–126.

Vande Wiele RL, Bogumil J, Dyrenfurth I, Ferin M, Jewelewicz R, Warren M, Mikhail G, Rizkallah T 1970: Mechanisms regulating the menstrual cycle in women. *Recent Prog Horm Res* 26:63–103.

Wayne NL, Malpaux B, Karsch FJ 1988: How does melatonin code for daylength in the ewe: duration of nocturnal melatonin release or coincidence of melatonin with a light-entrained sensitive period. *Biol Reprod* 39:66–75.

Weick RF, Dierschke DJ, Karsch FJ, Butler WR, Hotchkiss J, Knobil E 1973: Periovulatory time courses of circulating gonadotropic and ovarian hormones in the rhesus monkey. *Endocrinology* 93:1140–1147.
WHO Task Force Investigators 1980: Temporal relationships between ovulation and defined changes in the concentration of plasma estradiol-17β, luteinizing hormone, follicle-stimulating hormone and progesterone I Probit analysis. *Am J Obstet Gynecol* 138:383–390.

CHAPTER 2. THE NEUROENDOCRINE COMPONENT: THE HYPOTHALAMIC-PITUITARY UNIT

REVIEWS

Chin W 1986: Glycoprotein hormone genes. In: *Genes Encoding Hormones and Regulatory Peptides* (Habener JF ed), Humana Press, Clifton, NJ.
Crowley WF, Filicori M, Spratt DI, Santoro NF 1985: The physiology of gonadotropin-releasing hormone (GnRH) secretion in men and women. *Recent Prog Horm Res* 41:473–531.
Hazum E, Conn PM 1988: Molecular mechanisms of GnRH action. *I*. The GnRH receptor. *Endocr Rev* 9:379–386.
Huckle WR, Conn PM 1988: Molecular mechanisms of GnRH action. *II*. The effector system. *Endocr Rev* 9:387–395.
Kalra SP, Kalra PS 1983: Neural regulation of LH secretion in the rat. *Endocr Rev* 4:311–351.
Knobil E 1980: The neuroendocrine control of the menstrual cycle. *Recent Prog Horm Res* 36:53–88.
Lincoln DW, Fraser HM, Lincoln GA, Martin GB, McNeilly AS 1985: Hypothalamic pulse generators. *Recent Prog Horm Res* 41:360–419.
Page RB 1988: The anatomy of the hypothalamo-hypophyseal complex. In: *The Physiology of Reproduction* (Knobil E, Neill JD eds), Raven Press, NY, 1161–1233.
Pierce JG, Parsons TF 1981: Glycoprotein hormones: structure and function. *Annu Rev Biochem* 50:465–495.
Silverman AJ 1988: The gonadotropin-releasing hormone (GnRH) neuronal systems: immunocytochemistry. In: *The Physiology of Reproduction* (Knobil E, Neill JD eds), Raven Press, NY, 1283–1304.

ARTICLES

The Hypothalamic-GnRH System

Allen LC, Crowley WR, Kalra SP 1987: Interactions between neuropeptide Y and adrenergic systems in the stimulation of LH release in steroid-primed ovariectomized rats. *Endocrinology* 121:1953–1959.
Antunes JL, Louis K, Cogen P, Zimmerman EA, Ferin M 1980: Section of the pituitary stalk in the rhesus monkey. *I*. Anatomical studies. *Neuroendocrinology* 30:76–82.
Berga SL, Loucks AB, Rossmanith WG, Kettel LM, Laughlin GA, Yen SSC 1991: Acceleration of LH pulse frequency in functional hypothalamic amenorrhea by dopaminergic blockade. *J Clin Endocrinol Metab* 72:151–156.
Carmel PW, Araki S, Ferin M 1976: Pituitary stalk portal blood collection in rhesus monkeys: evidence for pulsatile release of gonadotropin-releasing hormone (GnRH). *Endocrinology* 99:243–248.

Chen WP, Witkin J, Silverman 1990: Sexual dimorphism in the synaptic input to GnRH neurons. *Endocrinology* 126:695–702.

Clark IJ, Cummins JT 1982: The temporal relationship between GnRH and LH secretion in ovariectomized ewes. *Endocrinology* 111:1737–1739.

Daniel PM, Prichard MM 1975: Studies of the hypothalamus and the pituitary gland, with special reference to the effects of transection of the pituitary stalk. *Acta Endocrinol (Copenh)* 80 (suppl 201):1–216.

Dierschke DJ, Bhattacharya AN, Atkinson LE, Knobil E 1970: Circhoral oscillations of plasma LH in the ovariectomized rhesus monkey. *Endocrinology* 87:850–853.

Gambacciani M, Melis GB, Paoletti AM, Cagnacci A, Mais V, Petacchi FD, Fioretti P 1987: Pulsatile LH release in postmenopausal women: effect of a chronic bromo-criptin administration. *J Clin Endocrinol Metab* 65:465–468.

Gibson MJ, Perlow MJ, Charlton HM, Zimmerman EA, Davies TF, Krieger DT 1984: Preoptic area brain grafts in hypogonadal (hpg) female mice abolish effects of con-genital hypothalamic gonadotropin releasing hormone (GnRH) deficiency. *Endocrinology* 114:1938–1942.

Jarry H, Perschl A, Wutke W 1988: Further evidence that preoptic anterior hypothalamic GABAergic neurons are part of the GnRH pulse and surge generator. *Acta Endocrinol* (Copenh) 118:573–579.

Kaufman JM, Kesner JS, Wilson RC, Knobil E 1985: Electrophysiological manifestation of LHRH pulse generator activity in the rhesus monkey: influence of α-adrenergic and dopaminergic blocking agents. *Endocrinology* 116:1327–1333.

Kaufman JM, Vermeulen A 1989: Lack of effect of the α-adrenergic agonist clonidine on pulsatile LH secretion in a double blind study in men. *J Clin Endocrinol Metab* 68:219–222.

King J, Anthony ELP, 1984: LHRH neurons and their projections in humans and other mammals: species comparisons. *Peptides* 5 (suppl 1):195–207.

Kokoris GJ, Lam NY, Ferin M, Silverman AJ, Gibson MJ 1988: Transplanted gonado-tropin-releasing hormone neurons promote pulsatile luteinizing hormone secre-tion in congenitally hypogonadal (hpg) male mice. *Neuroendocrinology* 48:45–52.

Krey LC, Butler WR, Knobil E 1975: Surgical disconnection of the medial basal hypo-thalamus and pituitary function in the rhesus monkey I gonadotropin secretion. *Endocrinology* 96:1073–1087.

Leranth C, Segura LMG, Palkovits M, McLusky MG, Shanabrough F, Naftolin F 1985: The LH-RH-containing neuronal network in the preoptic area of the rat: dem-onstration of LH-RH-containing nerve terminals in synaptic contact with LH-RH neurons. *Brain Res* 345:332–336.

Levine JE, Duffy MT 1988: Simultaneous measurement of LHRH, LH and FSH release in intact and short term castrate rats. *Endocrinology* 122:2211–2221.

Manson AJ, Hayflick JS, Zoeler RT, Young WS, Phillips HS, Nikoliks K, Seeburg P 1986: A deletion truncating the GnRH gene responsible for hypogonadism in the hpg mouse. *Science* 234:1366–1371.

McCormack JT, Plant TM, Hess DL, Knobil E 1977: The effect of LHRH antiserum administration on gonadotropin secretion in the rhesus monkey. *Endocrinology* 100:663–667.

Pau KY, Hess DL, Kaynard AH, Wei-Zhi J, Gliessman PM, Spies HG 1989: Suppression of mediobasal hypothalamic GnRH and plasma LH pulsatile patterns by phen-tolamine in ovariectomized rhesus macaques. *Endocrinology* 124:891–898.

Plant TM, Krey LC, Moossy J, McCormack JT, Hess DL, Knobil E 1978: The arcuate nucleus and the control of gonadotropin and prolactin secretion in the female rhe-sus monkey (Macaca mulatta). *Endocrinology* 102:52–62.

Rangaraju NS, Xu JF, Harris RB 1991: Progonadotropin-releasing hormone protein is processed with hypothalamic neurosecretory granules. *Neuroendocrinology* 53:20–28.

Schwanzel-Fukuda M, Pfaff DW 1989: Origin of LHRH neurons. *Nature* 338:161–164.

Seeburg PH, Adelman JP 1984: Characterization of cDNA for precursor of human LHRH. *Nature* 311:666–668.

Silverman AJ, Antunes JL, Abrams G, Nilaver G, Thau R, Robinson JA, Ferin M, Krey LC 1982: The luteinizing hormone-releasing pathways in the rhesus (Maccaca mulatta) and pigtailed (Maccaca nemestrina) monkeys: new observations using thick unembedded sections. *J Comp Neurol* 211:309–317.

Terasawa E, Krook C, Hei DL, Gearing M, Schultz NJ, Davis GA 1988: Norepinephrine is a possible neurotransmitter stimulating pulsatile release of LHRH in the rhesus monkey. *Endocrinology* 123:1808–1816.

Thind KK, Goldsmith PC 1988: Infundibular GnRH neurons are inhibited by direct opioid and autoregulatory synapses in juvenile monkeys. *Neuroendocrinology* 47:203–216.

Van Vugt DA, Diefenbach WP, Ferin M 1985: GnRH pulses in third ventricular cerebrospinal fluid of ovariectomized rhesus monkeys: correlation with LH pulses. *Endocrinology* 117:1550–1558.

Vaughan L, Carmel PW, Dyrenfurth I, Frantz AG, Antunes JL, Ferin M 1980: Section of the pituitary stalk in the rhesus monkey. *I.* Endocrine studies. *Neuroendocrinology* 30:70–75.

Wilson RC, Kesner JS, Kaufman JM, Vemurat, Akema T, Knobil E 1984: Central electrophysiological correlates of pulsatile luteinizing hormone secretion in the rhesus monkey. *Neuroendocrinology* 39:256–260.

Yang-Feng TL, Seeburg PH, Francke U 1986: Human LHRH gene is located on the short arm of chromosome 8. *Somatic Cell Mol Genet* 12:95–100.

The Anterior Pituitary Gland

Aiyer MS, Chiappa SA, Fink G 1974: A priming effect of luteinizing hormone releasing factor on the anterior pituitary gland in the female rat. *J Endocrinol* 62:573–588.

Belchetz PE, Plant TM, Nakai J, Keogh EG, Knobil E 1978: Hypophysial responses to continuous and intermittent delivery of hypothalamic GnRH. *Science* 202:631–633.

Childs GV, Unabia G, Tibolt R, Lloyd JM 1987: Cytological factors that support nonparallel secretion of LH and FSH during the estrous cycle. *Endocrinology* 121:1801–1813.

Haisenleder DJ, Ortolano GA, Dalkin AC, Ellis TR, Paul SJ, Marshall JC 1990: Differential regulation of gonadotropin subunit gene expression by GnRH pulse amplitude in female rats. *Endocrinology* 127:2869–2875.

Haisenleder DJ, Dalkin AC, Ortolano GA, Marshall JC, Shupnik MA 1991: A pulsatile gonadotropin-releasing hormone stimulus is required to increase transcription of the gonadotropin subunit genes: evidence for differential regulation of transcription by pulse frequency in vivo. *Endocrinology* 128:509–517.

Kazer RR, Liu CH, Yen SSC 1987: Dependence of mean levels of circulating LH upon pulsatile amplitude and frequency. *J Clin Endocrinol Metab* 65:796–800.

Kessel B, Dahl KD, Kazer RR, Liu CH, Rivier J, Vale W, Hsueh AJW, Yen SSC 1988: The dependency of bioactive FSH secretion on GnRH in hypogonadal and cycling women. *J Clin Endocrinol Metab* 66:361–366.

Leung K, Kaynard AH, Negrini BP, Kim KE, Maurer RA, Landefeld TD 1987: Regulation of gonadotropin subunit mRNA's by GnRH pulse frequency in ewes. *Mol Cell Endocrinol* 1:724–728.

Lewis CE, Morris JF, Fink G, Johnson M 1986: Changes in the granule population of gonadotrophs in hypogonadal and normal female mice associated with the priming effect of LHRH in vitro. *J Endocrinol* 109:35–44.

Lloyd JM, Childs GV 1988: Differential storage and release of LH and FSH from individual gonadotropes separated by centrifugal elutriation. *Endocrinology* 122:1282–1290.

Lumpkin MD, McDonald JK, Samson WK, McCann SM 1989: Destruction of the dorsal anterior hypothalamic region suppresses pulsatile release of FSH but not LH. *Neuroendocrinology* 50:229–235.

Phifer RF, Midgley AR, Spicer SS 1973: Immunohistologic and histologic evidence that follicle stimulating hormone and luteinizing hormone are present in the same cell type in the human pars distalis. *J Clin Endocrinol Metab* 36:125–141.

Samuels MH, Veldhuis JD, Henry P, Ridgeway EC 1990: Pathophysiology of pulsatile and copulsatile release of TSH, LH, FSH and α subunit. *J Clin Endocrinol Metab* 71:425–432.

Urban RJ, Veldhuis JD, Dufau ML 1991: Estrogen regulates the GnRH-stimulated secretion of biologically active LH. *J Clin Endocrinol Metab* 72:660–668.

Wang CF, Yen SSC 1975: Direct evidence of estrogen modulation of pituitary sensitivity to luteinizing hormone releasing factor during the menstrual cycle. *J Clin Invest* 55:201–204.

Wang CF, Lasley BL, Lein A, Yen SSC 1976: The functional changes of the pituitary gonadotrophs during the menstrual cycle. *J Clin Endocrinol Metab* 42:718-728.

Weiss J, Jameson JL, Burrin JM, Crowley WF Jr 1990: Divergent responses of gonadotropin subunit mRNA's to continuous vs pulsatile GnRH in vitro. *Mol Cell Endocrinol* 4:557–561.

Wildt L, Hausler A, Marshall G, Hutchinson JS, Plant TM, Belchetz PE, Knobil E 1981: Frequency and amplitude of GnRH stimulation and gonadotropin secretion in the rhesus monkey. *Endocrinology* 109:376–385.

Yuan QX, Swerdloff RS, Bhasin S 1988: Differential regulation of rat LH α and β subunits during the stimulatory and down-regulatory phases of GnRH action. *Endocrinology* 122:504–510.

The Endogenous Opioid Peptides and Other Neuropeptides

Ferin M, Wehrenberg WB, Lam NY, Alston EF, Vande Wiele RL 1982: Effects and site of action of morphine on gonadotropin secretion in the female rhesus monkey. *Endocrinology* 111:1652–1656.

Kaynard AH, Pau KYF, Hess DL, Spies HG 1990: Third-ventricular infusion of neuropeptide Y suppresses LH secretion in ovariectomized rhesus macaques. *Endocrinology* 127:2437-2444.

Kesner J, Kaufman JM, Wilson RC, Kuroda G, Knobil E 1986: The effect of morphine on the electrophysiological activity of the hypothalamic LH-RH pulse generator in the rhesus monkey. *Neuroendocrinology* 43:686–688.

Krieger DT 1983: The multiple faces of pro-opiomelanocortin, a prototype precursor molecule. *Clin Res* 31:342–353.

Quigley ME, Yen SSC 1980: The role of endogenous opiates on LH secretion during the menstrual cycle. *J Clin Endocrinol Metab* 51:179–181.

Reid RL, Hoff JD, Yen SSC 1981: Effects of exogenous β-endorphin on pituitary hormone secretion and its disappearance rate in normal human subjects. *J Clin Endocrinol Metab* 52:1179–1184.

Reid RL, Quigley ME, Yen SSC 1983: The disappearance of opioidergic regulation of gonadotropin secretion in postmenopausal women. *J Clin Endocrinol Metab* 57:1107–1110.

Ropert JF, Quigley ME, Yen SSC 1981: Endogenous opiates modulate pulsatile luteinizing hormone release in humans. *J Clin Endocrinol Metab* 52:583–585.

Shoupe D, Montz FJ, Lobo R 1985: The effects of estrogen and progestin on endogenous opioid activity in oophorectomized women. *J Clin Endocrinol Metab* 60:178–183.

Sutton SW, Toyama TT, Otto S, Plotsky PM 1988: Evidence that neuropeptide Y released into the hypophysial-portal circulation participates in priming gonadotropes to the effects of GnRH. *Endocrinology* 123:1208–1210.

Van Vugt D, Bakst G, Dyrenfurth I, Ferin M 1983: Naloxone stimulation of LH secretion in the female monkey: influence of endocrine and experimental conditions. *Endocrinology* 113:1858–1864.

Wardlaw SL, Wehrenberg WB, Ferin M, Antunes JL, Frantz AG 1982: Effect of sex steroid on β-endorphin in hypophyseal portal blood. *J Clin Endocrinol Metab* 55:877–881.

Wehrenberg WB, Wardlaw SL, Frantz AG, Ferin M 1982: β-endorphin in hypophyseal portal blood: variations throughout the menstrual cycle. *Endocrinology* 111:879–881.

Wehrenberg WB, Corder R, Gaillard RC 1989: A physiological role for neuropeptide Y in regulating the estrogen-progesterone induced LH surge in ovariectomized rats. *Neuroendocrinology* 49:680–682.

CHAPTER 3. THE OVARIAN COMPONENT

REVIEWS

Anderson E, Little B 1985: The ontogeny of the rat granulosa cell. In: *Proceedings of the Fifth Ovarian Workshop* (Toft DO, Ryan RJ eds), Ovarian Workshops, Champlain, 203–225.

Baird DT 1977: Synthesis and secretion of steroid hormones by the ovary in vivo. In: *The Ovary* (Zuckerman S, Weir BJ eds), Academic Press, NY, vol. 2, 305–358.

Erickson GF, Magoffin DA, Dyer CA, Hofeditz C 1985: The ovarian androgen producing cells: a review of structure/function relationships. *Endocr Rev* 6:371–379.

Guraya SS 1971: Morphology, histochemistry and biochemistry of human ovarian compartments and steroid hormone synthesis. *Physiol Rev* 51:785–807.

Hall PF 1984: Cellular organization of steroidogenesis. *Int Rev Cytol* 86:53–95.

Leibfreid-Rutledge ML, Florman HM, First NL 1989: The molecular biology of mammalian oocyte maturation. In: *The Molecular Biology of Fertilization* (Schatten H, Schatten G eds), Academic Press, NY, 259–301.

Lemaire WJ, Curry TE, Morioka N, Brannstrom M, Clark MR, Woessner JK, Koos RD 1987: Regulation of ovulatory processes. In: *The Primate Ovary* (Stouffer RL ed), Plenum Publishing Corp, NY, 91–106.

Lieberman S, Greenfield NJ, Wolfson A 1984: A heuristic proposal for understanding steroidogenic processes. *Endocr Rev* 5:128–148.

Masui J, Clark H 1979: Regulation of oocyte maturation. *Int Rev Cytol* 57:185–282.

Merchant Larios H 1976: The role of germ cells in the morphogenesis and cytodifferentiation of the rat ovary. In: *Progress in Differentiation Research* (Muller-Berat N ed), Elsevier, Amsterdam, 453–462.

Miller WL 1988: Molecular biology of steroid hormone synthesis. *Endocr Rev* 9:295–318.

Richards JS 1980: Maturation of ovarian follicles: actions and interactions of pituitary and ovarian hormones on follicular cell differentiation. *Physiol Rev* 60:51–89.

Richards JS, Hedin L 1988: Molecular aspects of hormone actions in ovarian follicular development, ovulation and luteinization. *Annu Rev Physiol* 50:441–463.

Tonetta S, Dizerega C 1989: Intragonadal regulation of follicular maturation. *Endocr Rev* 10:205–229.

Tsafiri A 1985: The control of meiotic maturation in mammals. In: *Biology of Fertilization* (Hetz C, Monroy A eds), Academic Press, NY, 221–252.

Wassarman P 1983: Oogenesis: synthetic events in the developing egg. In: *Mechanism and Control of Animal Fertilization* (Hartmann J ed), Academic Press, NY, 1–54.

ARTICLES

The Ovarian Steroids

Armstrong DT, Papkoff H 1976: Stimulation of aromatization of exogenous and endogenous androgens in ovaries of hypophysectomized rats in vivo by follicle stimulating hormone. *Endocrinology* 99:1144–1151.

Baird DT 1977: Evidence in vivo for the two-cell hypothesis of oestrogen synthesis by the sheep graafian follicle. *J Reprod Fertil* 50:183–185.

Evans G, Dobias M, King GJ, Armstrong DT 1981: Estrogen, androgen and progesterone biosynthesis by theca and granulosa of preovulatory follicles in the pig. *Biol Reprod* 25:673–682.

Florensa E, Sommerville IF, Harrison RF, Johnson MW, Youssefnejadian E 1976: Plasma 20 α-dihydroprogesterone, progesterone and 17-hydroprogesterone: daily and four-hourly variations during the menstrual cycle. *J Steroid Biochem* 7:769–777.

Gore-Langton RE, Dorrington JH 1981: FSH induction of aromatase in cultured rat granulosa cells measured by a radiometric assay. *Mol Cell Endocrinol* 22:135–151.

Hillier SG, Van Den Bogaard AJM, Reichert LE Jr, Van Hall EV 1981: Control of preovulatory follicular estrogen biosynthesis in the human ovary. *J Clin Endocrinol Metab* 52:847–856.

McNatty KP, Makris A, Degrazia C, Osathonondh R, Ryan KJ 1979: The production of progesterone, androgens and estrogens of human granulosa cells in vitro and in vivo. *J Steroid Biochem* 11:775–779.

Ryan KJ, Petro Z 1966: Steroid biosynthesis by human granulosa and thecal cells. *J Clin Endocrinol Metab* 26:46–52.

Strauss JF, Schuler LA, Rosenblum MF, Tanaka T 1981: Cholesterol metabolism by ovarian tissue. *Adv Lipid Res* 18:99–157.

Folliculogenesis

Adashi EY 1989: Cytokine-mediated regulation of ovarian function: encounters of a third kind. *Endocrinology* 124:2043–2045.

Adashi EY, Hsueh AJW 1982: Estrogens augment the stimulation of ovarian aromatase activity by follicle-stimulating hormone in cultured rat granulosa cells. *J Biol Chem* 257:6077–6083.

Adashi EY, Resnick CE, Resnick CE, Brodie AMH, Svoboda ME, Van WYK JJ 1985: Somatomedin C-mediated potentiation of follicle-stimulating hormone induced aromatase activity of cultured rat granulosa cells. *Endocrinology* 117:2313–2320.

Adashi EY, Resnick CE, Hernandez ER, Svobada ME, Van Wyk IJ 1989: Potential relevance of insulin-like growth factor I to ovarian physiology: from basic science to clinical application. *Semin Reprod Endocrinol* 7:94–100.

Albertini DF, Anderson E 1974: The appearance and structure of intercellular connections during the ontogeny of the rabbit ovarian follicle with particular reference to gap junctions. *J Cell Biol* 63:234–250.

Bagnato A, Moretti C, Frajese G, Catt KJ 1991: Gonadotropin-induced expression of receptors for growth hormone releasing factor in cultured granulosa cells. *Endocrinology* 128:2889–2894.

Baird DT 1983: Factors regulating the growth of the preovulatory follicle in the sheep and human. *J Reprod Fertil* 69:343–352.

Chikazawa K, Araki S, Tamada T 1986: Morphological and endocrinological studies on follicular development during the human menstrual cycle. *J Clin Endocrinol Metab* 62:305–313.

Erickson GF, Garzo VG, Magoffin DA 1989: Insulin-like growth factor-I regulates aromatase activity in human granulosa and granulosa-luteal cells. *J Clin Endocrinol Metab* 69:716–724.

Evans G, Dobias M, King GJ, Armstrong DT 1981: Estrogen, androgen and progesterone biosynthesis by theca and granulosa of preovulatory follicles in the pig. *Biol Reprod* 25:673–682.

Hirshfield AN, Midgley AR Jr 1978: The role of FSH in the selection of large ovarian follicles in the rat. *Biol Reprod* 19:606–611.

Hoage TR, Cameron IL 1976: Folliculogenesis in the ovary of the mature mouse: an autoradiographic study. *Anat Rec* 184:699–710.

Lindner HR, Amsterdam A, Salomon J, Tsafiri A, Nimrod A, Lamprecht SA, Zor U, Koch J 1977: Intraovarian factors in ovulation: determinants of follicular response to gonadotropins. *J Reprod Fertil* 51:215–235.

McNatty KP 1981: Hormonal correlates of follicular development in the human ovary. *Aust J Biol Sci* 34:249–268.

McNatty KP, Moore Smith D, Makris A, Osathonondh R, Ryan KJ 1979: The microenvironment of the human antral follicle: interrelationships among the steroid levels in antral fluid, the population of granulosa cells, and the status of the oocyte in vivo and in vitro. *J Clin Endocrinol Metab* 49:851–860.

Mondschein JS, Canning SF, Miller DQ, Hammond JM 1989: Insulin-like growth factors as autocrine/paracrine regulators of granulosa cell differentiation on growth: studies with a neutralizing monoclonal antibody to IGF-1. *Biol Reprod* 41:79–85.

Nakano R, Mizuno T, Katayama K, Tojo S 1975: Growth of ovarian follicles in the absence of gonadotropins. *J Reprod Fertil* 45:545–546.

Osman P 1985: Rate and course of atresia during follicular development in the adult cyclic rat. *J Reprod Fertil* 73:261–270.

Peluso JJ, Delidow BC, Lynch J, White BA 1991: Follicle-stimulating hormone and insulin regulation of 17β-estradiol secretion and granulosa cell proliferation within immature rat ovaries maintained in preinfusion cultures. *Endocrinology* 128:191–196.

Skinner MK, Coffey RJ 1988: Regulation of ovarian cell growth through the local production of transforming growth factor-a by theca cells. *Endocrinology* 123:2632–2638.

Woodruff TK, Lyon RJ, Hansen SE, Rice GC, Mather JF 1990: Inhibin and activin locally regulate rat ovarian folliculogenesis. *Endocrinology* 127:3196–3205.

Zamboni L 1974: Fine morphology of the follicle wall and follicle cell-oocyte association. *Biol Reprod* 10:125–149.

Zeleznik AJ, Schuler HM, Reichert LE Jr 1981: Gonadotropin-binding sites in the rhesus monkey ovary: role of the vasculature in the selective distribution of human chorionic gonadotropin in the preovulatory follicle. *Endocrinology* 109:356–362.

Oogenesis

Buccione R, Schroeder AC, Eppig JJ 1990: Interactions between somatic cells and germ cells throughout mammalian oogenesis. *Biol Reprod* 43:543–547.

Chiquoine A 1960: The development of the zona pellucida of the mammalian ovum. *Am J Anat* 106:149–170.

Chouinard L 1975: A light- and electron- microscope study of the oocyte nucleus during development of the antral follicle in the prepubertal mouse. *J Cell Sci* 17:589–615.

Dunbar B, Wardrip N, Hedrick J 1980: Isolation, physiochemical properties and macromolecular composition of zona pellucida from porcine oocytes. *Biochemistry* 19:356–365.

Eddy E, Clark J, Gong D, Fenderson B 1981: Origin and migration of primordial germ cells in mammals. *Gamete Res* 4:333–362.

Gilula N, Epstein M, Beer SW 1978: Cell-to-cell communication and ovulation: a study of the cumulus cell-oocyte complex. *J Cell Biol* 78:58–75.

Kang Y 1974: Development of the zona pellucida in the rat oocyte. *Am J Anat* 139:535–566.

Shimuzu S, Tsuji M, Dean J 1983: In vitro biosynthesis of three sulfated glycoproteins of murine zonae pellucidae by oocytes grown in follicle culture. *J Biol Chem* 258:5858–5863.

Sorensen R, Wassarman P 1976: Relationship between growth and meiotic maturation of the mouse oocyte. *Dev Biol* 50:531–536.

Tsafiri A, Dekel N, Bar-Ami S 1982: The role of oocyte maturation inhibitor in follicular regulation of oocyte maturation. *J Reprod Fertil* 64:541–551.

Weakly BS 1966: Electronmicroscopy of the oocyte and granulosa cells in the developing ovarian follicles of the golden hamster. *J Anat* 100:503–534.

Weiss L 1971: Additional evidence of gradual loss of germ cells in the pathogenesis of streak ovaries in Turner's syndrome. *J Med Genet* 8:540–544.

The Ovulatory Process

Aguado LI, Ojeda SR 1984: Ovarian adrenergic nerves play a role in maintaining preovulatory steroid secretion. *Endocrinology* 114:1944–1946.

Armstrong DT 1981: Prostaglandins and follicular functions. *J Reprod Fertil* 62:283–291.

Bahr JM, Ben-Jonathan N 1985: Elevated catecholamine in porcine follicular fluid before ovulation. *Endocrinology* 117:620–623.

Beers WH 1975: Follicular plasminogen and plasminogen activator and the effect of plasmin on ovarian follicle wall. *Cell* 6:379–386.

Bjersing L, Cajander S 1974: Ovulation and the mechanism of follicle rupture. *VI.* Ultrastructure of theca interna and the inner vascular network surrounding rabbit graafian follicles prior to induced ovulation. *Cell Tissue Res* 153:31–44.

Brännström M, Janson PO 1989: Progesterone is a mediator in the ovulatory process of the in-vitro perfused rat ovary. *Biol Reprod* 40:1170–1178.

Bronson RA, Bryant G, Balk M, Emanuels N 1979: Intrafollicular pressure within preovulatory follicles of the pig. *Fertil Steril* 31:205–213.

Burden HW 1972: Adrenergic innervation in ovaries of the rat and guinea pig. *Am J Anat* 133:455–462.

Capps ML, Lawrence IE Jr, Burden HW 1981: Cellular functions in perifollicular contractile tissue of the rat ovary during the preovulatory period. *Cell Tissue Res* 219:133–141.

Ichikawa S, Ohta M, Morioka H, Murao S 1983: Blockage of ovulation in the explanted hamster ovary by a collagenase inhibitor. *J Reprod Fertil* 68:17–19.

Knecht M 1986: Production of cell-associated and secreted plasminogen activator by cultured granulosa cells. *Endocrinology* 118:348–353.

Krishna A, Terranova PF 1985: Alterations in mast cell degranulation and ovarian histamine in the proestrous hamster. *Biol Reprod* 32:1211–1217.

Lau IF, Saksena SK, Chang MC 1974: Prostaglandins F and ovulation in mice. *J Reprod Fertil* 40:467–469.

Lemaire WJ, Marsh JM 1975: Interrelationships between prostaglandins, cyclic AMP and steroids in ovulation. *J Reprod Fertil* 22 (suppl):53–74.

Ny T, Bjersing L, Hsueh AJW, Loskutoff DJ 1985: Cultured granulosa cells produce two plasminogen activators, each regulated by gonadotropins. *Endocrinology* 116:1660–1668.

Pool WR, Lipner H 1965: Inhibition of ovulation in the rabbit by actinomycin D. *Nature* 203:1385–1387.

Reich R, Miskin R, Tsafriri A 1985: Follicular plasminogen activator: involvement in ovulation. *Endocrinology* 116:516–521.

The Corpus Luteum

Anderson W, Kang J, Perotti ME, Bramley TA, Ryan RJ 1979: Interactions of gonadotropins with corpus luteum membranes. *III.* Electron microscopic localization of [^{125}]-hCG binding to sensitive and desensitized ovaries seven days after PMSG-hCG. *Biol Reprod* 20:362–376.

Fitz TA, Mayan MH, Sawyer HR, Niswender GD 1982: Characterization of two steroidogenic cell types in the ovine corpus luteum. *Biol Reprod* 27:703–711.

Hanson FW, Powell JE, Stevens VC 1971: Effects of hCG and human pituitary LH on steroid secretion and functional life of the human corpus luteum. *J Clin Endocrinol Metab* 32:211–215.

Niswender GD, Reimers TJ, Diekman MA, Nett TM 1976: Blood flow: a mediator of ovarian function. *Biol Reprod* 14:64–81.

Rodgers RJ, O'Shea JD, Bruce NW 1984: Morphometric analysis of the cellular composition of the ovine corpus luteum. *J Anat* 138:757–769.

Van Lennys EW, Madden LM 1965: Electromicroscopic observations of the involution of the human corpus luteum of menstruation. *A Zellf Mikrosk Anat* 66:365–380.

CHAPTER 4. HYPOTHALAMIC-PITUITARY-OVARIAN
COMMUNICATION

REVIEWS

Dizerega G, Hodgen GD 1981: Folliculogenesis in the primate ovarian cycle. *Endocr Rev* 2:27–44.

Gindoff PR, Ferin M 1987: Brain opioid peptides and menstrual cyclicity. *Semin Reprod Endocrinol* 5:125–134.

Goodman RL, Knobil E 1981: The sites of action of ovarian steroids in the regulation of LH secretion. *Neuroendocrinology* 32:57–63.

Goodman AL, Hodgen GD 1983: The ovarian triad of the primate menstrual cycle. *Recent Prog Horm Res* 39:1–67.

Knobil E 1974: On the control of gonadotropin secretion in the rhesus monkey. *Recent Prog Horm Res* 30:1–46.

Rotchild I 1981: The regulation of the mammalian corpus luteum *Recent Prog Horm Res* 37:183–298.

Vande Wiele RL, Bogumil RJ, Dyrenfurth I, Ferin M, Jewelewicz R, Warren M, Mikhail G, Rizkallah T 1970: Mechanisms regulating the menstrual cycle in women. *Recent Prog Horm Res* 26:63–103.

Ying SY 1988: Inhibins, activins and follistatins: gonadal proteins modulating the secretion of FSH. *Endocr Rev* 9:267–293.

ARTICLES

Hypothalamic-Pituitary Control of the Ovaries

Araki S, Chikazawa K, Akabori A, IJima K, Tamada T 1983: Hormonal profile after removal of the dominant follicle and corpus luteum in women. *Endocrinol Jpn* 30:55–70.

DiZerega G, Hodgen GD 1982: The interovarian progesterone gradient: a spatial and temporal regulator of folliculogenesis in the primate ovarian cycle. *J Clin Endocrinol Metab* 54:495–499.

Ellinwood WE, Resko JA 1983: Effect of inhibition of estradiol synthesis during the luteal phase on function of the corpus luteum in rhesus monkeys. *Biol Reprod* 28:636–644.

Fisch B, Margara RA, Winston RML, Hillier SG 1989: Cellular basis of luteal steroidogenesis in the human ovary. *J Endocrinol* 122:303–312.

Galway AB, Lapolt PS, Tsafiri A, Dargan CM, Boime I, Hsueh AJW 1990: Recombinant FSH induces ovulation and tissue plasminogen activator expression in hypophysectomized rats. *Endocrinology* 127:3023–3028.

Goodman AL, Hodgen GD 1982: Antifolliculogenic action of progesterone despite hypersecretion of FSH in monkeys. *Am J Physiol* 243:E387–E397.

Hoff JD, Quigley ME, Yen SSC 1983: Hormonal dynamics at midcycle: A reevaluation. *J Clin Endocrinol Metab* 57:792–796.

Hoffman DI, Lobo RA, Campeau JD, Tsai HM, Holmberg EA, Ono T, Frederick JJ, Platt LD, Dizerega GS 1985: Ovulation induction in clomiphene-resistant anovulatory women: differential follicular response to purified urinary FSH vs purified urinary FSH and LH. *J Clin Endocrinol Metab* 60:922–927.

Hutchison JS, Zeleznik AJ 1984: The rhesus monkey corpus luteum is dependent on pituitary gonadotropin secretion throughout the luteal phase of the menstrual cycle. *Endocrinology* 115:1780–1786.

Hutchison JS, Zeleznik AJ 1985: The corpus luteum of the primate menstrual cycle is capable of recovering from a transient withdrawal of pituitary gonadotropin support. *Endocrinology* 117:1043–1049.

Hutchison JS, Nelson PB, Zeleznik AJ 1986: Effects of different gonadotropin pulse frequencies on corpus luteum function during the menstrual cycle of rhesus monkeys. *Endocrinology* 119:1964–1971.

Hutchison JS, Kubik CJ, Nelson PB, Zeleznik AJ 1987: Estrogen induces premature luteal regression in rhesus monkeys during spontaneous menstrual cycles, but not in cycles driven by exogenous GnRH. *Endocrinology* 121:466–474.

McLachlan RI, Cohen NL, Vale WW, Rivier JE, Burger HG, Bremner WJ, Soules MR 1989: The importance of LH in the control of inhibin and progesterone secretion by the human corpus luteum. *J Clin Endocrinol Metab* 68:1078–1085.

McNatty KP, Hillier SG, Vanden Boogaard AMJ, Trimbos-Kemper TCM, Reichert LE, Van Hall EV 1983: Follicular development during the luteal phase of the human menstrual cycle. *J Clin Endocrinol Metab* 56:1022–1031.

Mizumachi M, Voglmayr JK, Washington DW, Chen CLC, Bardin CW 1990: Superovulation of ewes immunized against the human recombinant inhibin α subunit associated with increased pre- and postovulatory FSH levels. *Endocrinology* 126:1058–1063.

Rice BF, Hammerstein J, Savard K 1964: Steroid hormone formation in the human ovary. *II.* Action of gonadotropins in vitro in the corpus luteum. *J Clin Endocrinol Metab* 24:606–615.

Rivier C, Vale W 1989: Immunoneutralization of endogenous inhibin modifies hormone secretion and ovulation rate in the rat. *Endocrinology* 125:152–157.

Rossmanith WG, Laughlin GA, Mortola JF, Johnson ML, Veldhuis JD, Yen SSC 1990: Pulsatile cosecretion of estradiol and progesterone by the midluteal corpus luteum: temporal link to LH pulses. *J Clin Endocrinol Metab* 70:990–995.

Thau RB, Yamamoto Y, Sundaram K, Spinola PG 1983: Human chorionic gonadotropin stimulates luteal function in rhesus monkeys immunized against the β-subunit of ovine luteinizing hormone. *Endocrinology* 112:277–283.

Zeleznik AJ 1981: Premature elevation of systemic estradiol reduces serum levels of FSH and lengthens the follicular phase of the menstrual cycle in rhesus monkeys. *Endocrinology* 109:352–355.

Zeleznik AJ, Wildt L, Schuler HM 1980: Characterization of ovarian folliculogenesis during the luteal phase of the menstrual cycle in rhesus monkeys using ^{3}H thymidine autoradiography. *Endocrinology* 107:982–988.

Zeleznik AJ, Schuler HM, Reichert LE 1981: Gonadotropin-binding sites in the rhesus monkey ovary: role of the vasculature in the selective distribution of human chorionic gonadotropin to the preovulatory follicle. *Endocrinology* 109:356–362.

Zeleznik AJ, Hutchison JS, Schuler HM 1985: Interference with the gonadotropin-suppressing actions of estradiol in macaques overrides the selection of a single preovulatory follicle. *Endocrinology* 117:991–999.

Zeleznik AJ, Kubik CJ 1986: Ovarian responses in macaques to pulsatile infusion of FSH and LH: increased sensitivity of the maturing follicle to FSH. *Endocrinology* 119:2025–2032.

Zeleznik AJ, Little-Ihrig LL 1990: Effect of reduced LH concentrations on corpus luteum function during the menstrual cycle of rhesus monkeys. *Endocrinology* 126:2237–2244.

The Feedback Loops

Araki S, Akabori A, Minakami H, Chikazawa K, Tamada T 1980: Further analysis of the positive feedback effect of estrogen on the release of gonadotropin in women. *Endocrinol Jpn* 27:709–716.

Bicsak TA, Cajander SB, Vale W, Hsueh AJW 1988: Inhibin: studies of stored and secreted forms by biosynthetic labeling and immunodetection in cultured rat granulosa cells. *Endocrinology* 122:741–748.

Chappel SC, Resko JA, Norman RL, Spies HG 1981: Studies in rhesus monkeys on the site where estrogen inhibits gonadotropins: delivery of 17β-estradiol to the hypothalamus and pituitary gland. *J Clin Endocrinol Metab* 52:1–8.

Cogen PH, Antunes JL, Louis KM, Dyrenfurth I, Ferin M 1980: The effects of anterior hypothalamic disconnection on gonadotropin secretion in the female rhesus monkey. *Endocrinology* 107:677–683.

Culler MD, Negro-Vilar A 1989: Endogenous inhibin supresses only basal FSH secretion but suppresses all parameters of pulsatile LH secretion in the diestrous female rat. *Endocrinology* 124:2944–2953.

Ferin M, Carmel PW, Zimmerman EA, Warren M, Vande Wiele RL 1974: Location of intrahypothalamic estrogen responsive sites influencing LH secretion in the female rhesus monkey. *Endocrinology* 95:1059–1068.

Ferin M, Dyrenfurth I, Cowchock S, Warren M, Vande Wiele RL 1974: Active immunization to 17β-estradiol and its effects upon the reproductive cycle of the rhesus monkey. *Endocrinology* 94:765–776.

Ferin M, Rosenblatt H, Carmel PW, Antunes JL, Vande Wiele RL 1979: Estrogen-induced gonadotropin surges in female rhesus monkey after pituitary stalk section. *Endocrinology* 104:50–52.

Filicori M, Santoro N, Merriam GR, Crowley WF 1986: Characterization of the physiological pattern of episodic gonadotropin secretion throughout the human menstrual cycle. *J Clin Endocrinol Metab* 62:1136–1144.

Fraser HM, Robertson DM, DeKretser DM 1989: Immunoreactive inhibin concentrations in serum throughout the menstrual cycle of the macaque: suppression of inhibin during the luteal phase after treatment with a LHRH antagonist. *J Endocrinol* 121:R9–R13.

Goodman RL, Karsch FJ 1980: Pulsatile secretion of LH: differential suppression by ovarian steroids. *Endocrinology* 107:1286–1290.

Halasz B 1969: The endocrine effects of isolation of the hypothalamus from the rest of the brain. In: *Frontiers in Neuroendocrinology* (Ganong WF, Martini L eds), Oxford U Press, New York, 307–342.

Helmond FA, Simons PA, Hein PR 1981: Strength and duration characteristics of the facilatory and inhibitory effects of progesterone on the estrogen-induced gonadotropin surges in the female rhesus monkey. *Endocrinology* 108:1837–1842.

Horton RJE, Cummins JT, Clarke IJ 1987: Naloxone evokes large-amplitude GnRH pulses in luteal phase ewes. *J Reprod Fertil* 81:277–286.

Karsch FJ, Weick RF, Butler WR, Dierschke DJ, Krey LC, Weiss G, Hotchkiss J, Yamaji T, Knobil E 1973: Induced LH surges in the rhesus monkey: strength-duration characteristics of the estrogen stimulus. *Endocrinology* 92:1740–1747.

Kaynard AH, Malpaux B, Robinson JE, Wayne NL, Karsch FJ 1988: Importance of pituitary and neural actions of estradiol in induction of the LH surge in the ewe. *Neuroendocrinology* 48:296–303.

Kesner JS, Kaufman JM, Wilson RC, Kurada G, Knobil E 1986: On the short loop feedback regulation of the hypothalamic LHRH pulse generator in the rhesus monkey. *Neuroendocrinology* 42:109–111.

Krey LC, Kamel F 1990: Progesterone modulation of gonadotropin secretion by dispersed rat pituitary cells in culture. *I.* Basal and gonadotropin-releasing hormone-stimulated luteinizing hormone release. *Mol Cell Endocrinol* 68:85–94.

Kyle CV, Griffin J, Jarrett A, Odell WD 1989: Inability to demonstrate an ultrashort loop feedback mechanism for LH in humans. *J Clin Endocrinol Metab* 69:170–176.

Letter to the editor 1988: Inhibin: definition and nomenclature, including related substances. *Endocrinology* 122:1701–1702.

Levine JE, Norman RL, Gliessman PM, Oyama TT, Bangsberg DR, Spies HG 1985: In vivo GnRH release and serum LH measurements in ovariectomized, estrogen treated rhesus macaques. *Endocrinology* 117:711–721.

Liu JH, Yen SSC 1983: Induction of midcycle gonadotropin surge by ovarian steroids in women: a critical evaluation. *J Clin Endocrinol Metab* 57:797–802.

McLachlan RI, Robertson DM, Healy DL, Burger HG, DeKretser DM 1987: Circulating immunoreactive inhibin levels during the normal human menstrual cycle. *J Clin Endocrinol Metab* 65:954–961.

McLachlan RI, Dahl KD, Bremner WJ, Schwall R, Schmelzer CH, Mason AJ, Steiner RA 1989: Recombinant human activin-A stimulates basal FSH and GnRH-stimulated FSH and LH release in the adult male macaque. *Endocrinology* 125:2787–2789.

Moenter SM, Caraty A, Karsch FJ 1990: The estradiol-induced surge of GnRH in the ewe. *Endocrinology* 127:1375–1384.

Moll GW, Rosenfield RL 1984: Direct inhibitory effect of estradiol on pituitary LH responsiveness to LHRH is specific and of rapid onset. *Biol Reprod* 30:59–66.

Monroe S, Jaffe R, Midgley AR 1972: Regulation of human gonadotropins. *XII.* Increase in serum gonadotropins in response to estradiol. *J Clin Endocrinol Metab* 34:342–347.

Naylor AM, Porter DW, Lincoln DW 1989: Inhibitory effect of central LHRH on LH secretion in the ovariectomized ewe. *Neuroendocrinology* 49:531–536.

Nippoldt TB, Reame NE, Kelch RP, Marshall JC 1989: The role of estradiol and progesterone in decreasing LH pulse frequency in the luteal phase of the menstrual cycle. *J Clin Endocrinol Metab* 69:67–76.

Norman RL, Lindstrom SA, Bangsberg D, Ellinwood WE, Gliessman P, Spies HG 1984: Pulsatile secretion of LH during the menstrual cycle of rhesus macaques. *Endocrinology* 115:261–266.

Pau KYF, Gliessman PM, Hess DL, Ronnekleiv OK, Levine JE, Spies HG 1990: Acute administration of estrogen suppresses LH secretion without altering GnRH release in ovariectomized rhesus macaques. *Brain Res* 51:229–235.

Pohl CR, Richardson DW, Marshall G, Knobil E 1982: Mode of action of progesterone in the blockade of gonadotropin surges in the rhesus monkey. *Endocrinology* 110:1454–1455.

Ramirez VD, Park OK 1989: Spontaneous changes in LHRH release during the rat estrous cycle, as measured with repetitive push–pull perfusions of the pituitary gland in the same female rats. *Neuroendocrinology* 50:66–72.

Robertson DM, Tsonis CG, McLachlan RI, Handelsman DJ, Leask R, Baird DT, McNeilly AS, Hayward S, Healy DL, Findlay JK, Burger HG, De Kretser DM 1988: Comparison of inhibin immunological and in vitro biological activities in human serum. *J Clin Endocrinol Metab* 67:438–443.

Rossmanith WG, Yen SSC 1987: Sleep-associated decrease in LH pulse frequency during the early follicular phase of the menstrual cycle: evidence for a opioidergic mechanism. *J Clin Endocrinol Metab* 65:715–718.

Sarkar DK, Mitsugi DK 1990: Correlative changes of the GnRH and GnRH-associated peptide immunoreactivities in the pituitary portal plasma in female rats. *Neuroendocrinology* 52:15–21.

Soules MR, Steiner RA, Clifton DC, Cohen NL, Aksel S, Bremner WJ 1984: Progesterone modulation of pulsatile LH secretion in normal women. *J Clin Endocrinol Metab* 58:378–383.

Stillman RJ, Williams RF, Lynch A, Hodgen GD 1983: Selective inhibition of FSH by porcine follicular fluid extracts in the monkey: effects on midcycle surges and pulsatile secretion. *Fertil Steril* 40:823–828.

Tsonis CG, Messinis IE, Templeton AA, McNeilly AS, Baird DT 1988: Gonadotropic stimulation of inhibin secretion by the human ovary during the follicular and early luteal phase of the cycle. *J Clin Endocrinol Metab* 66:915–921.

Veldhuis JD, Beitins IZ, Johnson ML, Serabian MA, Dufau ML 1984: Biologically active LH is secreted in episodic pulsations that vary in relation to stage of the menstrual cycle. *J Clin Endocrinol Metab* 58:1050–1058.

Weick RF, Pitelka V, Thompson DL 1982: Separate negative feedback effects of estrogen on the pituitary and the central nervous system in the ovariectomized rhesus monkey. *Endocrinology* 112:1862–1864.

Wildt L, Hausler A, Hutchinson JS, Marshall G, Knobil E 1981: Estradiol as a gonadotropin releasing hormone in the rhesus monkey. *Endocrinology* 108:2011–2013.

Wildt L, Hutchinson JS, Marshall G, Pohl CR, Knobil E 1981: On the site of action of progesterone in the blockade of the estradiol-induced gonadotropin discharge in the rhesus monkey. *Endocrinology* 109:1293–1294.

CHAPTER 5. THE GENITAL TRACT

REVIEWS

Brenner RM, West NB 1975: Hormonal regulation of the reproductive tract in female mammals. *Annu Rev Physiol* 37:273–302.
Carson-Jurica MA, Schrader WT, O'Malley BW 1990: Steroid receptor family: structure and function. *Endocr Rev* 11:201–220.
Ferenczy A 1988: The endometrial cycle. In: *Gynecology and Obstetrics* (Sciarra JJ, Speroff L, Simpson JL eds), JB Lippincott Co., Philadelphia, vol. 5, chapter 18, 1–14.
Jansen RPS 1984: Endocrine response in the fallopian tube. *Endocr Rev* 5:525–551.
Noyes RW 1973: Normal phases of the endometrium. In: *The Uterus* (Norris HJ, Hertig AT, Abell NR eds), Williams and Wilkins, Baltimore, 110–135.
Padykula HA 1988: The female reproductive system. In: *Cell and Tissue Biology—A Textbook of Histology* (Weiss L ed), 6th ed., Urban and Schwarzenberg, Baltimore, 853–878.
Partridge WM 1981: Transport of protein-bound hormones into tissues in vivo. *Endocr Rev* 2:103–132.
Walters MR 1985: Steroid hormone receptors and the nucleus. *Endocr Rev* 6:512–543.
Yamamoto KR 1985: Steroid receptor regulated transcription of specific genes and gene networks. *Annu Rev Genet* 19:209–252.

ARTICLES

The Steroid Receptor

Conn PM, McArdle CA, Andrews WV, Huckle WR 1987: The molecular basis of gonadotropin-releasing hormone (GnRH) action in the pituitary gonadotrope. *Biol Reprod* 36:17–35.
Gasc JM, Delahaye F, Baulieu EE 1989: Compared intracellular localization of the glucocorticosteroid and progesterone receptors: an immunocytochemical study. *Exp Cell Res* 181:492–504.
Green S, Kumar V, Theulaz I, Wahli W, Chambon P 1988: The N-terminal DNA-binding "zinc finger" of the oestrogen and glucocorticoid receptors determines target gene specificity. *Embo J* 7:3037–3044.
Green SP, Walter V, Kumar A, Krust JM, Bornert P, Argos M, Chambon P 1986: Human oestrogen receptor cDNA: sequence, expression and homology to v-erb-A. *Nature* 320:134–139.
Huckaby CS, Conneely OM, Beattie WG, Dobson ADW, Tsai MJ, O'Malley BW 1987: Structure of the chromosomal chicken progesterone receptor gene. *Proc Natl Acad Sci USA* 84:8380–8384.
King WJ, Greene GL 1984: Monoclonal antibodies localize oestrogen receptor in the nuclei of target cells. *Nature* 307:745–747.
Kumar V, Green S, Stack G, Berry M, Jin JR, Chambon P 1987: Functional domains of the human estrogen receptor. *Cell* 51:941–951.
Loosfelt H, Atger M, Misrahi M, Guiochon-Mantel A, Merierl C, Logeat F, Benarous R, Milgrom E 1986: Cloning and sequence analysis of rabbit progesterone-receptor complementary DNA. *Proc Natl Acad Sci USA* 83:9045–9049.

McDonnell DP, Mangelsdorf DJ, Pike JW, Haussler MR, O'Malley BW 1987: Molecular cloning of complementary DNA encoding the avian receptor for vitamin D. *Science* 235:1214–1217.

Miller J, McLachlan AD, Klug A 1985: Repetitive-zinc binding domains in the protein transcription factor 111A From Xenopus oocytes. *Embo J* 4:1609–1614.

O'Malley BW 1984: Steroid hormone action in eukaryotic cells. *J Clin Invest* 74:307–312.

Ponglikitmongkol M, Green S, Chambon P 1988: Genomic organization of the human oestrogen receptor gene. *Embo J* 7:3385–3388.

West NB, Bremner RM 1983: Estrogen recepter levels in the oviducts and endometria of cynomolgus macaques during the menstrual cycle. *Biol Reprod* 29:1303–1312.

Cyclic Changes in the Genital Tract

Bensley CM 1951: Cyclic fluctuations in the rate of epithelial mitosis in the endometrium of the rhesus monkey. *Contrib Embryol* 34:87–91.

Brenner RM, Carlisle KS, Hess DL, Sandow BA, West NB 1983: Morphology of the oviducts and endometria of cynomolgus macaques during the menstrual cycle. *Biol Reprod* 29:1289–1302.

Chretien FC 1975: Human cervical mucus during the menstrual cycle and pregnancy in normal and pathological conditions. *J Reprod Med* 14:192–205.

Cornillie FJ, Lauweryns JM, Brosens IA 1985: Normal human endometrium. *Gynecol Obstet Invest* 20:113–129.

Donnez J, Casanas-Roux F, Caprasse J, Ferin J, Thomas K 1985: Cyclic changes in ciliation, cell height, and mitotic activity in human tubal epithelium during reproductive life. *Fertil Steril* 43:554–564.

Ferenczy A 1976: Studies on the cytodynamics of human endometrial regeneration. *Am J Obstet Gynecol* 124:64–74.

Good RG, Moyer DL 1968: Estrogen–progesterone relationships in the development of secretory endometrium. *Fertil Steril* 19:37–49.

Karin SMM 1972: Phsysiological role of prostaglandins in the control of parturition and menstruation. *J Reprod Fertil [Suppl]* 16:105–114.

Markee JE 1940: Menstruation in intraocular endometrial transplants in the rhesus monkey. *Contrib Embryol* 24:223–250.

McClellan M, West NB, Brenner RM 1986: Immunocytochemical localization of estrogen receptors in the macaque endometrium during the luteal-follicular transition. *Endocrinology* 119:2467–2475.

Noyes RW, Hertig AT, Rock J 1950: Dating the endometrial biopsy. *Fertil Steril* 1:3–25.

Padykula HA, Coles LG, McCracken JA, King NW, Longcope C, Kaiserman-Abramof IR 1984: A zonal pattern of cell proliferation and differentiation in the rhesus endometrium during the estrogen surge. *Biol Reprod* 31:1103–1118.

Rock J, Garcia CR, Menkin M 1959: A theory of menstruation. *Ann NY Acad Sci* 75:830–839.

Strinden ST, Shapiro SS 1983: Progesterone-altered secretory proteins from cultured human endometrium. *Endocrinology* 112:862–870.

CHAPTER 6. THE FERTILE MENSTRUAL CYCLE

REVIEWS

Blandau RJ 1969: Gamete transport: Comparative aspects. In: *The Mammalian Oviduct. Comparative Biology and Methodology* (Hafez ESH, Blandau RJ eds), U of Chicago Press, Chicago, 129–162.

Glasser SR, McCormack SA 1981: Cellular and molecular aspects of decidualization and implantation. In: *Proteins and Steroids in Early Pregnancy* (Beier HM, Karlson P eds) Springer-Verlag, NY, 245–310.

Hafez ESE 1973: Gamete transport. In: *Human Reproduction, Conception and Contraception* (Hafez ESE, Evans TN eds), Harper and Row, Hagerstown, MD, 85–118.

Harper MJK 1988: Gamete and zygote transport. In: *The Physiology of Reproduction* (Knobil E, Neill JD eds) Raven Press, NY, 103–126.

Hodgen GD, Itskovitz J 1988: Recognition and maintenance of pregnancy. In: *The Physiology of Reproduction* (Knobil E, Neill JD eds), Raven Press, NY, 1195–2022.

Meyer RK 1972: Chorionic gonadotropin, corpus luteum function and embryo implantation in the rhesus monkey. In: *The Use of Non-Human Primates in Research on Human Reproduction* (Diczfaluszy E, Standley CC eds), WHO, Stockholm, 214–225.

Moore HDM, Bedford JM 1983: The interaction of mammalian gametes in the female. In: *Mechanism and Control of Animal Fertilization* (Hartmann JF ed) Academic Press, NY, 453–497.

Psychoyos A 1973: Endocrine control of egg implantation. In: *Handbook of Physiology* (Greep RD, Astwood EB, Geiger SR eds), American Physiological Society, Bethesda, MD, vol. 2, section 7, part 2, 187–216.

Wassarman PM 1987: Early events in mammalian fertilization. *Ann Rev Cell Biol* 3:109–142.

Wassarman PM, Florman HM, Greve JM 1985: Receptor-mediated sperm–egg interactions in mammals. In: *Fertilization* (Metz CB, Monroy A eds), Academic Press, NY, 341–360.

Yanagimachi R 1988: Mammalian fertilization. In: *The Physiology of Reproduction* (Knobil E, Neill JD eds) Raven Press, NY, 135–172.

ARTICLES

Events at Fertilization

Ahuja KK, Smith W, Tucker M, Craft I 1985: Successful pregnancies from the transfer of pronucleate embryos in an outpatient in vitro fertilization program. *Fertil Steril* 44:181–184.

Austin CR 1951: Observations on the penetration of sperm into the mammalian egg. *Aust J Sci Res* 4:581–596.

Austin CR, Braden WH 1956: Early reaction of the rodent egg to spermatozoa penetration. *J Exp Biol* 33:358–365.

Austin CR, Bishop MWH 1985: Role of the rodent acrosome and perforatorium in fertilization. *Proc R Soc Lond [Biol]* 149:241–248.

Chang MC 1951: Fertilizing capacity of spermatozoa deposited into the fallopian tubes. *Nature* 168:697–698.

Eskin BA, Azarbal S, Sepic R, Slate WG 1973: In vitro responses of the spermatozoa-cervical mucus system treated with prostaglandin $F_{2\alpha}$. *Obstet Gynecol* 41:436–439.

Fox CA, Wulff AS, Baker JA 1970: Measurement of intra-vaginal and intra-uterine pressures during human coitus by radiotelemetry. *J Reprod Fertil* 22:243–251.

Lambert H, Overstreet JW, Morales P, Hanson FW, Yanagimachi R 1985: Sperm capacitation in the female reproductive tract. *Fertil Steril* 43:325–327.

Lundquist F 1949: Aspects of the biochemistry of human semen, viscosimetric determination of hyaluronidase. *Acta Physiol Scand* 17:44–54.

Westrick JC, Boatman DE, Bavister BD 1985: Characteristics of acrosome reaction-inducing factor from hamster cumulus and follicular fluid. *Biol Reprod* 32:352–360.

The First Weeks of Pregnancy

Csapo A, Pulkkinen M 1978: Indispensability of the human corpus luteum in the maintenance of early pregnancy: luteectomy evidence. *Obstet Gynecol Surv* 33:69–81.
Enders AC, Schlaffe 1967: A morphological analysis of the early implantation stages in the rat. *Am J Anat* 120:185–226.
Enders AC, Hendrickx AG, Schlafke S 1983: Implantation in the rhesus monkey: initial penetration of the endometrium. *Am J Anat* 167:275–298.
Enders AC, Welsh AO, Schlafke S 1985: Implantation in the rhesus monkey: endometrial responses. *Am J Anat* 173:147–169.
Hay DL 1985: Discordant and variable production of human chorionic gonadotropin and its free α-and β-subunits in early pregnancy. *J Clin Endocrinol Metab* 61:1195–1200.
Hearn JP 1978: Immunological interference with the maternal recognition of pregnancy in primates. In: *Maternal Recognition of Pregnancy*. Ciba Foundation Symposium Excerpta Medica, Amsterdam, vol. 64, 353–375.
Hearn JP 1986: The embryo-maternal dialogue during early pregnancy in primates. *J Reprod Fertil* 76:809–819.
Herrmann W, Wyss R, Riondel A, Philibert D, Tewtsch G, Sakiz E, Baulieu EE 1982: The effect of an anti-progesterone steroid in women: interuption of the menstrual cycle and early pregnancy. *CR Acad Sci* (III), 294:933–938.
Hodgen GD, 1983: Surrogate embryo transfer combined with estrogen-progesterone therapy in monkeys. Implantation, gestation and delivery without ovaries. *JAMA* 250:2167–2171.
Hodgen GD 1985: Pregnancy prevention by intravaginal delivery of a progesterone antagonist: RU486 tampon for menstrual induction and absorption. *Fertil Steril* 44:263–267.
Hodgen GD, Tullner WW, Vaitukaitis JL, Ward DN, Ross GT 1974: Specific radioimmunoassay of chorionic gonadotropin during implantation in rhesus monkeys. *J Clin Endocrinol Metab* 39:457–464.
Hoos PC, Hoffman LH 1980: Temporal aspects of rabbit uterine vascular and decidual responses to blastocyst stimulation. *J Reprod Fertil* 70:1–6.
Kennedy TG 1983: Embryonic signals and the initiation of blastocyst implantation. *Aust J Biol Sci* 36:531–543.
Lawn AM, Wilson EW, Finn CA 1971: The ultrastructure of human decidual and pre-decidual cells. *J Reprod Fertil* 26:85–90.
O'Shea JD, Fleinfeld RG, Morrow HA 1983: Ultrastructure of decidualization in the pseudopregnant rat. *Am J Anat* 166:271–298.
Shelesnyak MC 1962: Decidualization: the decidua and deciduoma. *Perspect Biol Med* 5:503–518.
Tulchinsky D, Hobel CJ 1973: Plasma human chorionic gonadotropin, estrone, estradiol, estriol, progesterone and 17α-hydroxyprogesterone in human pregnancy. *III.* Early normal pregnancy. *Am J Obstet Gynecol* 117:884–893.
Yoshimi T, Strott CA, Marshall JR, Lipsett MB 1969: Corpus luteum function in early pregnancy. *J Clin Endocrinol Metab* 29:225–230.

CHAPTER 7. THE FIRST MENSTRUAL CYCLE:
ADOLESCENCE AND PUBERTY

REVIEWS

Cutler GB Jr, Cassorla FG, Ross JL, Pescovitz OH, Barnes KM, Comite F, Feuillan PP, Laue L, Foster CM, Kenigsberg D, Caruso-Nicoletti M, Garcia HB, Uriarte M, Hench KD, Skerda MC, Long LM, Loriaux DL 1986: Pubertal growth: physiology and pathophysiology. *Recent Prog Horm Res* 42:443–470.

Delemarre-Vande Waal HA, Plant TM, Van Rees GP, Schoemaker J (eds) 1989: Control of the onset of puberty. *III*. Excerpta Medica International Congress Series 861, Elsevier, Amsterdam.

Grumbach MM, Roth JC, Kaplan SL, Kelch RP 1974: Hypothalamic pituitary regulation of puberty in man: evidence and concepts derived from clinical research. In: *Control of the Onset of Puberty* (Grumbach MM, Grave D, Mayer FF eds), John Wiley and Sons, NY, 115–166.

Lee PA 1988: Neuroendocrinology of puberty. *Semin Reprod Endocrinol* 6:13.

Odell WD 1979: The physiology of puberty: disorders of the pubertal process. In: *Endocrinology* (Degroot LJ ed), Grune and Stratton, NY, vol. 3, 1163–1379.

Ojeda SR, Andrews WW, Advis JP, Smith White S 1980: Recent advances in the endocrinology of puberty. *Endocr Rev* 1:228–257.

Reiter EO, Kulin HE 1972: Sexual maturation in the female—normal development and precocious puberty. *Pediatr Clin North Am* 19:581–603.

Styne DM, Grumbach MM 1978: Puberty in the male and female; its physiology and disorders. In: *Reproductive Endocrinology: Physiology, Pathophysiology and Clinical Management* (Yen SSC and Jaffe RB eds), WB Saunders, Philadelphia, 234–235.

ARTICLES

Mechanisms Controlling The Timing of Puberty

Boyar RM, Finkelstein J, Roffwarg H, Kapen S, Weitzman ED, Hellman L 1972: Synchronization of augmented luteinizing hormone secretion with sleep during puberty. *N Engl J Med* 287:582–586.

Boyar RM, Wu RHK, Roffwarg H, Kapen S, Weitzman ED, Hellman L, Finkelstein JW 1976: Human puberty: 24-hour estradiol patterns in pubertal girls. *J Clin Endocrinol Metab* 43:1418–1421.

Fishman J, Boyar RM, Hellman L 1975: Influence of body weight on estradiol metabolism in young women. *J Clin Endocrinol Metab* 41:989–991.

Fraser MO, Pohl CR, Plant TM 1989: The hypogonadotropic state of the prepubertal male rhesus monkey is not associated with a decrease in hypothalamic GnRH content. *Biol Reprod* 40:972–980.

Frisch RE, Revelle R 1970: Height and weight at menarche and a hypothesis of critical body weights and adolescent events. *Science* 169:397–399.

Frisch RE, McArthur JW 1974: Menstrual cycles: fatness as a determinant of minimum weight for height necessary for their maintenance or onset. *Science* 185:949–951.

Gay VL, Plant TM 1987: N-methyl-DL-aspartate (NMA) elicits hypothalamic GnRH release in prepubertal male rhesus monkeys. *Endocrinology* 120:2289–2296.

Hale PM, Khoury S, Foster CM, Beitins IZ, Hopwood NJ, Marshall JC, Kelch RP 1988: Increased luteinizing hormone pulse frequency during sleep in early to midpubertal boys: effects of testosterone infusion. *J Clin Endocrinol Metab* 66:785–791.

Kapen S, Boyar RM, Finkelstein JW, Hellman L, Weitzman ED 1974: Effect of sleep-wake cycle reversal on luteinizing hormone secretory pattern in puberty. *J Clin Endocrinol Metab* 39:293–299.

Kulin HE, Moore RG, Santner SJ 1976: Circadian rhythm in gonadotropin secretion in prepubertal and pubertal children. *J Clin Endocrinol Metab* 42:770–773.

Levine Ross J, Loriaux DL, Cutler GB Jr 1983: Developmental changes in neuroendocrine regulation of gonadotropin secretion in gonadal dysgenesis. *J Clin Endocrinol Metab* 57:288–293.

Plant TM 1985: A study of the role of the postnatal testes in determining the ontogeny of gonadotropin secretion in the male rhesus monkey. *Endocrinology* 116:1341–1350.

Plant TM 1986: A striking sex difference in the gonadotropin response to gonadectomy during infantile development in the rhesus monkey. *Endocrinology* 119:539–545.

Plant TM, Zorub DS 1984: A study of the role of the adrenal glands in the initiation of the hiatus in gonadotropin secretion during prepubertal development in the male rhesus monkey. *Endocrinology* 114:560–565.

Plant TM, Fraser MO, Medhamurthy R, Gay VL 1989: Somatogenic control of GnRH neuronal synchronization during development in primates: a speculation. *III*. In: *Control of the Onset of Puberty*. (Delemarre-VanDeWaal HA, Plant TM, VanRees GP, Schoemaker J eds), Elsevier, Amsterdam, 111–121.

Schultz NJ, Terasawa E 1988: Posterior hypothalamic lesions advance the time of pubertal changes in LH release in ovariectomized rhesus monkeys. *Endocrinology* 123:445–455.

Waldhauser F, Weissenbacher G, Frisch H, Pollak K 1981: Pulsatile secretion of gonadotropins in early infancy. *Europ J Pediatr* 137:71–74.

Watanabe G, Terasawa E 1989: In vivo release of luteinizing releasing hormone increase with puberty in the female rhesus monkey. *Endocrinology* 125:92–99.

Winter JSD, Faiman C 1973: Pituitary-gonadal relations in female children and adolescents. *Pediatr Res* 7:948–953.

The Physiology of Puberty

Apter D, Viinikka L, Vihko R 1978: Hormonal pattern of adolescent menstrual cycles. *J Clin Endocrinol Metab* 47:944–954.

Comerci GD 1987: Normal pubescent growth and sexual maturation. *Semin Adolesc Med* 3:217–226.

Foster DL, Ryan KD 1979: Endocrine mechanisms governing transition into adulthood: a marked decrease in inhibitory feedback action of estradiol on tonic secretion of LH in the lamb during puberty. *Endocrinology* 105:896–904.

Kulin HE, Grumbach MM, Kaplan SL 1969: Changing sensitivity of pubertal gonadal hypothalamic feedback mechanism in man. *Science* 166:1012–1013.

Marshall WA, Tanner JM 1969: Variations in pattern of pubertal changes in girls. *Arch Dis Child* 44:291–303.

Metcalf MG, Skidmore DS, Lowry GF, Mackenzie JA 1983: Incidence of ovulation in the years after menarche. *J Endocrinol* 77:213–219.

Rapisarda JJ, Bergman KS, Steiner RA, Foster DL 1983: Response to estradiol inhibition of tonic luteinizing hormone secretion decreases during the final stage of puberty in the rhesus monkey. *Endocrinology* 112:1172–1179.

Reiter EO, Fuldauer VG, Root AW 1977: Secretion of the adrenal androgen, dehydroepiandrosterone sulfate, during normal infancy, children with endocrinologic abnormalities. *J Pediatr* 90:766–770.

Resko JA, Goy RW, Robinson JA, Norman RL 1982: The pubescent rhesus monkey: some characteristics of the menstrual cycle. *Biol Reprod* 27:354–361.

Swerdloff RS 1978: Physiological control of puberty. *Med Clin North Am* 62:351–366.

Tanner JM 1973: Trend towards earlier menarche in London, Oslo, Copenhagen, The Netherlands and Hungary. *Nature* 243:95–96.

Tanner JM 1981: Growth and maturation during adolescence. *Nutr Rev* 39:43–55.

Tanner JM, Whitehouse RH, Hughes PCR, Carter BS 1976: Relative importance of growth hormone and sex steroids for the growth at puberty of trunk length, limb length, and muscle width in growth hormone deficient children. *J Pediatr* 89:1000–1008.

Terasawa E, Bridson WE, Nass TE, Noonan JJ, Dierschke DJ 1984: Developmental changes in the LH secretory pattern in peripubertal female rhesus monkeys: comparisons between gonadally intact and ovariectomized animals. *Endocrinology* 115:2233–2246.

Wilson ME, Gordon TP, Collins DC 1986: Ontogeny of LH secretion and first ovulation in seasonal breeding rhesus monkeys. *Endocrinology* 118:293–301.

Winter JSD, Ellsworth L, Fuller G, Hobson WC, Reyes FI, Faiman C 1987: The role of gonadal steroids in feedback regulation of gonadotropin secretion at different stages of primate development. *Acta Endocrinol (Copenh)* 114:257–268.

Zacharias L, Wurtman RJ 1964: Blindness: its relations to age of menarche. *Science* 29:1154–1155.

Zacharias L, Wurtman RJ, Schatzoff M 1970: Sexual maturation in contemporary American girls. *Am J Obstet Gynecol* 108:833–846.

The Pathology of Puberty

Boepple PA, Mansfield MJ, Wierman ME, Rudlin CR, Bode HH, Crigler JF Jr, Crawford JD, Crowley WF Jr 1986: Use of a potent long acting agonist of GnRH in the treatment of precocious puberty. *Endocr Rev* 7:24–33.

Comite F, Schiebinger RJ, Albertson BD, Cassorla FG, VanderVen K, Cullen TF, Loriaux DL, Cutler JB Jr 1984: Isosexual precocious pseudopuberty secondary to a feminizing adrenal tumor. *J Clin Endocrinol Metab* 58:435–440.

Comite F, Cassorla F, Barnes KM, Hench KD, Dwyer A, Skeada MC, Loriaux DL, Cutler GB Jr, Pescovitz OH 1986: Luteinizing hormone releasing hormone analogue therapy for central precocious puberty. Long-term effect on somatic growth, bone maturation, and predicted height. *JAMA* 255:2613–2616.

Crowley W, Hoffman A, Spratt D 1985: Hypogonadotropic hypogonadism and its treatment. In: *Male Sexual Dysfunction* (Santen RH, Swerdloff RS eds), Marcel Dekker, NY, 227–249.

Foster CM, Ross JL, Shawker T, Pescovitz OH, Loriaux DL, Cutler JB Jr, Comite F 1984: Absence of pubertal gonadotropin secretion in girls with McCune-Albright syndrome. *J Clin Endocrinol Metab* 58:1161–1165.

Grumbach MM 1985: True or precocious puberty. In: *Current Therapy in Endocrinology Metabolism* (Krieger DT, Bardin CW eds), BC Decker, Toronto, 4–8.

Judge DM, Kulin HE, Page R, Santen R, Trapukdi S 1977: Hypothalamic hamartoma— a source of luteinizing-hormone-releasing factor in precocious puberty. *N Engl J Med* 296:7–10.

Kauli R, Prager-Lewin R, Laron Z 1978: Pubertal development in the Prader-Labhart-Willi syndrome. *Acta Paediatr Scand* 67:763–767.

Korth-Schutz S, Levine LS, New MI 1976: Serum androgens in normal prepubertal and pubertal children and in children with precocious adrenarche. *J Clin Endocrinol Metab* 42:117–124.

Kosloske AM, Goldthorn JF, Kaufman E, Hayek A 1984: Treatment of precocious pseudopuberty associated with follicular cysts of the ovary. *Am J Dis Child* 138:147–149.

Leiblish JM, Rogol AD, White BJ, Rosen SW 1982: Syndrome of anosmia with hypogonadotropic hypogonadism (Kallmann syndrome). *Am J Med* 73:506–520.

Mansfield MJ, Beardsworth DE, Loughlin JS, Crawford JD, Bode HH, Rivier J, Vale W, Kushner DC, Crigler JF Jr, Crowley WF Jr 1983: Long-term treatment of central precocious puberty with a long-acting analogue of luteinizing hormone-releasing hormone: effects on somatic growth and skeletal maturation. *N Engl J Med* 309:1286–1290.

Mills JL, Stolley PD, Davies J, Moshang T 1981: Premature thelarche. Natural history and etiological investigation. *Am J Dis Child* 135:743–745.

Pang S 1981: Precocious thelarche and premature adrenarche. *Pediatr Ann* 10:340–345.

Pescovitz OH, Cutler GB Jr, Loriaux DL 1985: Management of precocious puberty. *J Pediatr Endocrinol* 1:85–94.

Pescovitz OH, Comite F, Hench K, Barnes K, McNeman A, Foster C, Konigsberg D, Loriaux DL, Cutler GB Jr 1986: The NIH experience with precocious puberty: diagnostic subgroups and response to short-term luteinizing hormone releasing hormone analogue therapy. *J Pediatr* 108:47–54.

Saenz de Rodriguez CA, Bongiovanni AM, Conde de Borrego LC 1985: An epidemic of precocious development in Puerto Rican children. *J Pediatr* 107:393–396.

Styne DM, Kaplan SL 1979: Normal and abnormal puberty in the female. *Pediatr Clin North Am* 26:123–148.

Styne DM, Harris DA, Egli CA, Conte FA, Kaplan SL, Rivier J, Vale W, Grumbach MM 1985: Treatment of true precocious puberty with a potent luteinizing hormone-releasing factor agonist: effect and growth, sexual maturation, pelvic sonography, and the hypothalamic-pituitary gonadal axis. *J Clin Endocrinol Metabol* 61:142–151.

Warren MP 1980: The effects of excercise on pubertal progression and reproductive function in girls. *J Clin Endocrinol Metab* 51:1150–1157.

CHAPTER 8. THE LAST MENSTRUAL CYCLES: THE CLIMACTERIC AND MENOPAUSE

REVIEWS

Lindsay R 1987: The menopause: sex steroids and osteoporosis. *Clin Obstet Gynecol* 30:847–859.

Mishell DR 1989: Interdisciplinary review of estrogen replacement therapy. *Am Obstet Gynecol* 161 (part 2): 1825–1868.

Nelson JF, Felicio LS 1985: Reproductive aging in the female: an etiological perspective. *Rev Biol Res Aging* 2:251–314.

Soules MR, Bremner WJ 1982: The menopause and climacteric: endocrinologic basis and associated symptomatology. *J Am Geriatr Soc* 30:471–486.

Utian WH 1990: Current perspectives in the management of the menopausal and postmenopausal patient. *Obstet Gynecol* 75:1S–83S.

ARTICLES

Physiology and Etiology of Menopause

Longcope C, Franz C, Morello C, Baker R, Johnson CC 1986: Steroid and gonadotropin levels in women during the perimenopausal years. *Maturitas* 8:189–196.

Mattison DR, Evans MI, Schwimmer WB, White BJ, Jensen B, Schulman JD 1948: Familial premature ovarian failure. *Am J Hum Genet* 63:1341–1348.

Metcalf MG, Donald RA, Livesey JA 1981a: Pituitary ovarian function in normal women during the menopausal transition. *Clin Endocrinol (Oxf)* 14:245–255.

Metcalf MG, Donald RA, Livesey JA 1981b: Classification of menstrual cycles in pre-and postmenopausal women. *J Endocrinol* 91:1–10.

Rannevik G, Carlstrom K, Jeppsson S, Bierre B, Suanberg L 1986: A prospective long-term study in women from pre-menopause to post-menopause: changing profiles of gonadotropins, oestrogens and androgens. *Maturitas* 8:297–307.

Richardson S, Senikas V, Nelson SF 1987: Follicular depletion during the menopausal transition: Evidence for accelerated loss and ultimate exhaustion at menopause. *J Clin Endocrinol Metab* 65:1231–1237.

Sherman BM, West JH, Korenman SC 1976: The menopausal transition: analysis of LH, FSH, estradiol and progesterone concentrations during menstrual cycles of older women. *J Clin Endocrinol Metab* 42:629–636.

Spira A 1988: The decline of fecundity with age. *Maturitas* [*Suppl*] 1:15–22.

Stanford JL, Hartge R, Brinton LA, Hoover RN, Brookmeyer R 1987: Factors influencing the age at natural menopause. *J Chronic Dis* 40:995–1002.

Treloar AE 1981: Menstrual cyclicity and the pre-menopause. *Maturitas* 3:249–264.

Utian WH 1987: Overview of menopause. *Am J Obstet Gynecol* 156:1280–1283.

Van Look PFA, Lothian H, Hunter WM, Michie EA, Baird DT 1977: Hypothalamic-pituitary-ovarian function in premenopausal women. *Clin Endocrinol (Oxf)* 7:13–31.

Clinical Symptoms of Menopause

Hällstrom T 1977: Sexuality in the climacteric. *Clin Obstet Gynec* 4:227–239.

Kiel DP, Felson DT, Anderson JJ, Wilson PWF, Morrowitz MA 1987: Hip fracture and the use of estrogens in postmenopausal women. The Framingham study. *N Engl J Med* 317:1170–1175.

Melton LJ, Wahner HW, Richelson LS, O'Fallon WM, Riggs BL 1986: Osteoporosis and the risk of hip fracture. *Am J Epidemiol* 124:254–261.

Ravnikar V 1990: Physiology and treatment of hot flashes. *Obstet Gynecol* 75:3–8.

Rebar RW, Spitzer IB 1987: The physiology and measurement of hot flashes. *Am J Obstet Gynecol* 156:1284–1288.

Riggs LB 1987: Pathogenesis of osteoporosis. *Am J Obstet Gynecol* 1342–1346.

Riggs LB, Wahner HW, Melton LJ, Richelson LS, Judd HL, O'Fallon WM 1987: Dietary calcium intake and rate of bone loss in women. *J Clin Invest* 80:979–82.

Seeman E, Hopper JL, Bach LA, Cooper ME, Parkinson E, McKay J, Jerums G 1989: Reduced bone mass in daughters of women with osteoporosis. *N Engl J Med* 320:554–558.

Sorrel PM 1990: Sexuality and menopause. *Obstet Gynecol* 75:26–30.

Sporrong T, Hellgren M, Samsioe G, Mattson LA 1989: Metabolic effects of continuous estradiol-progestins therapy in postmenopausal women. *Obstet Gynecol* 73:754–758.

Stevenson JC, Whitehead MI, Padwick M, Endacott JA, Sutton C, Banks LM, Freemantle L, Spinks TJ, Hesp R 1988: Dietary intake of calcium and postmenopausal bone loss. *Br Med J* 297:15–17.

Stevenson JC, Lees B, Devenport M, Cust MS, Ganger KF 1989: Determinant of bone density in normal women: risk factors for future osteoporosis? *Br Med J* 298:924–928.

Wickham CA, Walsh K, Cooper C, Barker DJ, Margetts BM, Morris J, Bruce SA 1989: Dietary calcium, physical activity, and the risk of hip fracture: a prospective study. *Br Med J* 299:889–892.

Management of Menopause

Bergkvist L, Adami HO, Persson I, Hoover R, Schairer C 1989: The risk of breast cancer after oestrogen and oestrogen/progestin replacement. *N Engl J Med* 321:293–297.

Bush TL, Barrett-Connor E, Cowan LD, Criqui MH, Wallace RB, Suchindran CM, Tyroler HA, Rifkind BM 1987: Cardiovascular mortality and noncontraceptive use of estrogen in women: results from the Lipid Research Clinics Program Follow-up Study. *Circulation* 75:1102–1109.

Cauley JA, Cummings SR, Black DM, Mascioli SR, Seeley DG 1990: Prevalence and determinants of estrogen replacement therapy in elderly women. *Am J Obstet Gynecol* 163:1438–1444.

Consensus Development Conference 1987: Prophylaxis and treatment of osteoporosis. *Br Med J* 295:914–915.

Cooper C, Barker DJP, Wickham C 1988: Physical activity, muscle strength, and calcium intake in fracture of the proximal femur in Britain. *Br Med J* 297:1443–1446.

Enzelsburger H, Merka M, Heytmanek G, Schurz B, Kurz CH, Kusztrich M 1988: Influence of oral contraceptive use on bone density in climacteric women. *Maturitas* 9:375–378.

Ettinger B, Genant HK, Cann CE 1987: Postmenopausal bone loss is prevented by treatment with low-dosage estrogen with calcium. *Ann Intern Med* 106:40–45.

Farish E, Fletcher CD, Dagen MM, Hart DM, Al-Azzawi F, Parkin DE, Howie CA 1989: Lipoprotein and apolipoprotein levels in postmenopausal women on continuous oestrogen/progestogen therapy. *Br J Obstet Gynecol* 96:358–364.

Gambrell RD 1986: Prevention of endometrial cancer with progestogens. *Maturitas* 8:159–168.

Gambrell RD 1987: Sex steroids and cancer. *Obstet Gynecol Clin North Am* 14:191–206.

Hargrove JT, Maxson WS, Wentz AC, Burnett LS 1989: Menopausal hormone replacement therapy with continuous daily oral micronized estradiol and progesterone. *Obstet Gynecol* 73:606–612.

Hunt K, Vessey MP, MacPherson K, Coleman M 1987: Long-term surveillance of mortality and cancer incidence in women receiving hormone replacement therapy. *Br J Obstet Gynaecol* 94:620–635.

Judd H 1987: Efficacy of transdermal estradiol. *Am J Obstet Gynecol* 156:1326–1331.

Lindsay R 1987: Estrogen therapy in the prevention and management of osteoporosis. *Am J Obstet Gynecol* 156:1347–1351.

Padwick ML, Pryse-Davies J, Whitehead MI 1986: A simple method for determining the optimal dose of progestin in postmenopausal women receiving estrogens. *N Engl J Med* 315:930–934.

Paganini-Hill A, Ross RK, Henderson BE 1989: Endometrial cancer and patterns of use of estrogen replacement therapy: a cohort study. *Br J Cancer* 59:445–447.

Persson I, Adami HO, Bergkvist L, Lindgren A, Petterson B, Hoover R, Scuairer C 1989:

Risk of endometrial cancer after treatment with oestrogens alone or in conjunction with progestogens: results of a prospective study. *Br Med J* [*Clin Res*] 298:147–151.

Prough SG, Aksel S, Wiebe H, Shepherd J 1987: Continuous estrogen/progestin therapy in menopause. *Am J Obstet Gynecol* 157:1440–1453.

Schiff I, Tulchinsky D, Cramer D, Ryan KJ 1980: Oral medroxyprogesterone in the treatment of postmenopausal symptoms. *JAMA* 244:1443–1445.

Shapiro S, Kelly JP, Rosenberg L, Kaufman DW, Helmrich SP, Rosenshein NB, Lewis JL Jr, Knapp RC, Stolly PD, Schottenfell D 1985: Risk of localized and widespread endometrial cancer in relation to recent and discontinued use of conjugated estrogens. *N Engl J Med* 313:969–972.

Sporrong T, Hellgren M, Samsioe G, Mattsson LA 1989: Metabolic effects of continuous estradiol-progestin therapy in postmenopausal women. *Obstet Gynecol* 73:754–758.

Steingold KA, Laufer L, Chetkowski RJ, DeFazio JD, Matt DW, Meldrum DR, Judd HL 1985: Treatment of hot flashes with transdermal estradiol administration. *J Clin Endocrinol Metab* 61:627–632.

Studd J, Savvas M, Waston N, Garnett T, Fogelman I, Cooper D 1990: The relationship between plasma estradiol and the increase in bone density in postmenopausal women after treatment with subcutaneous hormone implants. *Am J Obstet Gynecol* 163:1474–1479.

Weinstein L 1987: Efficacy of a continuous estrogen-progestin regimen in the menopausal patient. *Obstet Gynecol* 69:929–932.

Whitehead MI, Lobo RA 1988: Progestogen use in postmenopausal women consensus conference. *Lancet* 11:1243–1244.

Whitehead MI, Hillerd BM, Crook D 1990: The role and use of progesterone. *Obstet Gynecol* 75:59–76.

Wilson PW, Garrison RJ, Castelli WP 1985: Postmenopausal estrogen use, cigarette smoking and cardiovascular morbidity in women over 50. The Framingham Study. *N Engl J Med* 313:1038–1043.

Wren BG 1989: Dose related response of the endometrium to Provera: interim summary results. *Int Proc J* 1:163–164.

CHAPTER 9. THE ABNORMAL MENSTRUAL CYCLE:
INTRODUCTION

REVIEWS

Archer DF 1987: Current concepts and treatment of hyperprolactinemia. *Obstet Gynecol Clin North Am* 14:979–998.

Leong DA, Frawley S, Neill JD, 1983: Neuroendocrine control of prolactin secretion. *Annu Rev Physiol* 45:109–127.

McNeilly AS 1988: Suckling and the control of gonadotropin secretion. In: *The Physiology of Reproduction* (Knobil E, Neill J, eds) Raven Press, NY, 2323–2349.

Neinstein LS 1985: Menstrual dysfunction in pathophysiologic states. *West J Med* 143:476–484.

ARTICLES

The Ovulatory Menstrual Cycle: An Integrative Description
See previous chapters.

The Initial Clinical Evaluation Process of the Abnormal Cycle

Hull MGR, Glazener CMA, Kelly NJ, Conway DI, Foster PA, Hinton RA, Coulson C, Lambert PA, Wat EM, Desai KM 1985: Population study of causes, treatment, and outcome of infertility. *Br Med J* 91:1693–1697.

Mosher WD 1985: Reproductive impairments in the United States, 1965–1982. Demography. 415–430.

Moghissi KM 1987: Cervical and uterine factors in infertility. *Obstet Gynecol Clin North Am* 14:887–904.

World Health Organization 1988: *Laboratory Manual for Examination of Human Semen and Semen Cervical Mucus Interaction.* Cambridge U Press, Cambridge UK.

CHAPTER 10. INTRODUCTION TO THE
PATHOPHYSIOLOGY OF THE MENSTRUAL CYCLE

REVIEWS

Ben-Jonathan N 1985: Dopamine: a prolactin-inhibitory hormone. *Endocr Rev* 6:564–589.

Halmi KA 1978: Anorexia nervosa: recent investigations. *Annu Rev Med* 29:137–148.

Karsch FJ, Bittman EL, Foster DL, Goodman RL, Legan SJ, Robinson JE 1984: Neuroendocrine basis of seasonal reproduction. *Recent Prog Horm Res* 40:219–240.

MacLeod RM 1976: Regulation of prolactin secretion. In: *Frontiers in Neuroendocrinology* (Martini L, Ganong WF eds), Raven Press, NY, vol. 4, 169–205.

Nicoll CS 1974: Physiological actions of prolactin. In: *Handbook of Physiology* (Greep RO, Astwood EB eds), American Physiological Society, Washington DC, vol. 4, section 7, part 2, 253–292.

Siiteri PK, McDonald PC 1973: Role of extraglandular estrogen in human endocrinology. In: *Handbook of Physiology: Endocrinology* (Greep RO, Astwood E eds), American Physiological Society, Washington DC, vol. 2, 615–650.

ARTICLES

Abnormalities of the GnRH Pulse Generator

Beitins IZ, Barkan A, Klibanski A, Kyung N, Reppert SM, Badger TM, Veldhuis J, McArthur JW 1985: Hormonal responses to short term fasting in postmenopausal women. *J Clin Endocrinol Metab* 60:1120–1126.

Berga SL, Mortola JF, Girton L, Suh B, Laughlin G, Pham P, Yen SSC 1989: Neuroendocrine aberrations in women with functional hypothalamic amenorrhea. *J Clin Endocrinol Metab* 68:301–308.

Beumont PJV, George GC, Pimstone BL, Vinik AL 1976: Body weight and the pituitary response to hypothalamic releasing hormones in patients with anorexia nervosa. *J Clin Endocrinol Metab* 43:487–496.

Boyar RM, Katz J, Finkelstein JW, Kapen S, Weiner H, Weitzman ED, Hellman L 1974: Anorexia nervosa: immaturity of the 24-hour LH secretory pattern. *N Engl J Med* 291:861–865.

Burger CW, Korsen T, Van Kessel H, Van Dop PA, Caron VJM, Schoemaker J 1985: Pulsatile LH patterns in the follicular phase of the menstrual cycle, polycystic ovarian disease (PCOD) and non-PCOD secondary amenorrhea. *J Clin Endocrinol Metab* 61:1126–1132.

Cameron JL, Nosbich C 1991: Suppression of pulsatile LH and testosterone secretion during short term food restriction in the adult male monkey. *Endocrinology* 128:1532–1540.

Gambacciani M, Yen SSC, Rasmussen D 1986: GnRH release from the mediobasal hypothalamus: in vitro inhibition by CRF. *Neuroendocrinology* 43:533–536.

Gindoff PR, Ferin M 1987: Endogenous opioid peptides modulate the effect of CRH on gonadotropin release in the primate. *Endocrinology* 121:837–842.

Guttierez J, Dunn TG, Mos GE 1987: Inanition decreases episodic LH release in ovariectomized ewes. *J Anim Sci* 65 (suppl 1):406–411.

Haresign W 1981: The influence of nutrition on reproduction in the ewe. *I*. Effects on ovulation rate, follicle development and LH release. *Anim Prod* 32:197–201.

Kaye WH, Gwirtsman H, George DT, Ebert MH, Jimmerson DC, Tomai TP, Chrousos GP, Gold PW 1987: Elevated cerebrospinal fluid levels of immunoreactive CRH in anorexia nervosa: relation to state of nutrition, adrenal function, and intensity of depression. *J Clin Endocrinol Metab* 64:203–208.

Khoury SA, Reame NE, Kelch RP, Marshall JC 1987: Diurnal patterns of pulsatile LH secretion in hypothalamic amenorrhea: reproducibility and responses to opiate blockade and an α_2-adrenergic agonist. *J Clin Endocrinol Metab* 64:755–762.

Kile JP, Alexander BM, Moss GE, Hallford DM, Nett TM 1991: Gonadotropin-releasing hormone overrides the negative effect of reduced dietary energy in gonadotropin synthesis and secretion in ewes. *Endocrinology* 128:843–849.

Lachelin GCL, Yen SSC 1978: Hypothalamic chronic anovulation. *Am J Obstet Gynecol* 130:825–831.

Loucks AB, Mortola JF, Girton L, Yen SSC 1989: Alterations in the hypothalamic-pituitary-ovarian and the hypothalamic-pituitary-adrenal axes in athletic women. *J Clin Endocrinol Metab* 68:402–411.

Pohl CR, Richardson DW, Hutchison JJ, Germak JA, Knobil E 1983: Hypophysiotropic signal frequency and the functioning of the pituitary ovarian system in the rhesus monkey. *Endocrinology* 112:2076–2080.

Reame NE, Sauder SE, Case GD, Kelch RP, Marshall JC 1985: Pulsatile gonadotropin secretion in women with hypothalamic amenorrhea: evidence that reduced frequency of GnRH secretion is the mechanism of persistent anovulation. *J Clin Endocrinol Metab* 61:851–858.

Rivier C, Vale W 1984: Influence of CRF on reproductive function in the rat. *Endocrinology* 114:914–921.

Suh BY, Liu JH, Berga SL, Quigley ME, Laughlin GA, Yen SS 1988: Hypercortisolism in patients with functional hypothalamic amenorrhea. *J Clin Endocrinol Metab* 66:733–739.

Veldhuis JD, Evans WS, Demers LM, Thorner MO, Wakat D, Rogol AD 1985: Altered neuroendocrine regulation of gonadotropin secretion in women distance runners. *J Clin Endocrinol Metab* 61:557–563.

Vigersky RA, Anderson AE, Thompson RH, Loriaux DL 1977: Hypothalamic dysfunction in secondary amenorrhea associated with simple weight loss. *N Engl J Med* 297:1141–1145.

Warren MP, Vande Wiele RL 1973: Clinical and metabolic features of anorexia nervosa. *Am J Obstet Gynecol* 117:435–449.

Wildt L, Leyendecker G 1987: Induction of ovulation by the chronic administration of naltrexone in hypothalamic amenorrhea. *J Clin Endocrinol Metab* 64:1334–1335.

Xiao E, Luckhaus J, Niemann W, Ferin M 1989: Acute inhibition of gonadotropin secretion by CRH in the primate: are the adrenal glands involved? *Endocrinology* 124:1632–1637.

Abnormalities in Hypothalamic-Pituitary-Ovarian Communication: Asynchrony

Goodman RL, Bittman EL, Foster DL, Karsch FJ 1982: Alterations in the control of LH pulse frequency underlie the seasonal variation in estradiol negative feedback in the ewe. *Biol Reprod* 27:580–589.

Judd S, Stranks S, Michaizow L 1989: GnRH pacemaker sensitivity to negative feedback inhibition by estradiol in women with hypothalamic amenorrhea. *Fertil Steril* 51:257–262.

Legan SI, Foster DL, Karsch FJ 1977: The endocrine control of seasonal reproductive function in the ewe: a marked change in response to the negative action of estradiol on LH secretion. *Endocrinology* 101:818–824.

Maruca J, Kulin HE, Santen SJ 1983: Perturbation of negative feedback sensitivity in agonadal patients undergoing estrogen replacement therapy. *J Clin Endocrinol Metab* 56:53–59.

Nozaki M, Watanabe G, Taya K 1991: Marked seasonal changes in response to the negative feedback action of estradiol on LH secretion in the female Japanese monkey. *Endocrinology* 128:1291–1297.

Santen RJ, Friend JN, Trojanowsky D, Davis B, Samojlik E, Bardin CW 1978: Prolonged negative feedback suppression after estradiol administration: proposed mechanism of eugonadal secondary amenorrhea. *J Clin Endocrinol Metab* 47:1220–1229.

Sherman BM, Korenman SG 1974: Measurements of plasma LH, FSH, estradiol and progesterone in disorders of the human menstrual cycle: the short luteal phase. *J Clin Endocrinol Metab* 38:89–93.

Soules MR, Clifton DK, Cohen NL, Bremner WJ, Steiner PA 1989: Luteal phase deficiency: abnormal gonadotropin and progesterone secretion patterns. *J Clin Endocrinol Metab* 69:813–820.

Soules MR, McLachlan RI, Ek M, Dahl KD, Cohen NL, Bremner WJ 1989: Luteal phase deficiency: characterization of reproductive hormones over the menstrual cycle. *J Clin Endocrinol Metab* 69:804–812.

Spillar PA, Piacsek BE 1991: Underfeeding alters the effect of low levels of estradiol on LH pulsatility in ovariectomized female rats. *Neuroendocrinology* 53:253–260.

Sprangers SA, Piacsek BE 1988: Increased suppression of LH secretion by chronic and acute estradiol administration in underfed adult female rats. *Biol Reprod* 39:81–87.

Stouffer RL 1990: Corpus luteum function and dysfunction. *Clin Obstet Gynecol* 33:668–689.

Wilks JW, Hodgen GD, Ross GT 1976: Luteal phase defects in the rhesus monkey: the significance of serum FSH:LH ratios. *J Clin Endocrinol Metab* 43:1261–1267.

Hyperprolactinemia

Arbogast LA, Voogt JL 1991: Hyperprolactinemia increases and hypoprolactinemia decreases tyrosine hydroxylase messenger ribonucleic acid levels in the arcuate nuclei, but not the substantia nigra or zona incerta. *Endocrinology* 128:997–1005.

Casper RF, Yen SSC 1981: Simultaneous pulsatile release of prolactin and LH induced by luteinizing hormone releasing factor agonist. *J Clin Endocrinol Metab* 52:934–936.

Demura R, Ono M, Demura H, Shizume K, Oouchi H 1982: Prolactin directly inhibits basal as well as gonadotropin-stimulated secretion of progesterone and 17β-estradiol in the human ovary. *J Clin Endocrinol Metab* 54:1246–1250.

Denef C, Andries M 1983: Evidence for paracrine interaction between gonadotrophs and lactotrophs in pituitary cell aggregates. *Endocrinology* 112:813–822.

Diefenbach WP, Dennison A, Rosenblatt H, Vaughan L, Frantz AG, Ferin M 1980: Effect of estrogen on TRH-induced release of prolactin in intact ovariectomized and stalk sectioned female rhesus monkeys. *Endocrinology* 107:183–186.

Duchen MR, McNeilly AS 1980: Hyperprolactinemia and long term lactational amenorrhea. *Clin Endocrinol (Oxf)* 112:621–627.

Fox SR, Smith MS 1984: The suppression of pulsatile LH secretion during lactation in the rat. *Endocrinology* 115:2045–2051.

Glasier AF, McNeilly AS, Howie PW 1984: Pulsatile secretion of LH in relation to the resumption of ovarian activity postpartum. *Clin Endocrinol (Oxf)* 20:415–426.

Glass MR, Rudd BT, Lynch SS, Butt WR 1981: Oestrogen-gonadotrophin feedback mechanisms in the puerperium. *Clin Endocrinol (Oxf)* 14:257–267.

Gray RH, Campbell OM, Zacur HA, Labbok MH, McRae SL 1987: Postpartum return of ovarian activity in nonbreastfeeding women monitored by urinary assays. *J Clin Endocrinol Metab* 64:645–650.

Gross BA, Eastman CJ 1983: Effect of breast feeding status on prolactin secretion and resumption of menses. *Med J Aust* 1:313–320.

Gross BA, Eastman CJ 1985: Prolactin and the return of ovulation in breast feeding women. *J Biosoc Sci [Suppl]* 9:25–42.

Howie PW, McNeilly AS 1982: Effect of breast-feeding patterns on human birth intervals. *J Reprod Fertil* 65:545–557.

Richardson DW, Goldsmith LT, Pohl CR, Schallenberger E, Knobil E 1985: The role of prolactin in the regulation of the primate corpus luteum. *J Clin Endocrinol Metab* 60:501–504.

Sauder SE, Frager M, Case GD, Kelch RP, Marshall JC 1984: Abnormal patterns of pulsatile LH secretion in women with hyperprolactinemia and amenorrhea: responses to bromocryptine. *J Clin Endocrinol Metab* 59:941–948.

Schallenberger E, Richardson DW, Knobil E 1981: Role of prolactin in the lactational amenorrhea of the rhesus monkey. *Biol Reprod* 25:370–374.

Shome B, Parlow AF 1977: Human pituitary prolactin: the entire linear amino acid sequence. *J Clin Endocrinol Metab* 45:1112–1119.

Smith MS 1981: Site of action of prolactin in the suppression of gonadotropin secretion during lactation in the rat: effect on pituitary responsiveness to LHRH. *Biol Reprod* 24:967–976.

Vaughan L, Carmel PW, Dyrenfurth I, Frantz AG, Antunes JL, Ferin M 1980: Section of the pituitary stalk in the rhesus monkey. *I*. Endocrine Studies. *Neuroendocrinology* 30:70–75.

CHAPTER 11. DIAGNOSIS OF MENSTRUAL CYCLE DYSFUNCTION

ARTICLES

End Organ Dysfunction

Asherman J 1948: Amenorrhea traumatica (atretica). *J Obstet Gynaecol Br Emp* 55:23–27.

Asherman JG 1957: Traumatic intrauterine adhesions and their effects on fertility. *Int J Fertil* 2:49–53.

Bryan AL, Nigro JA, Counseller VS 1949: One hundred cases of congenital absence of vagina. *Surg Gynecol Obstet* 88:79–83.

Cali RW, Pratt JH 1968: Congenital absence of the vagina. *Am J Obstet Gynecol* 100:752–763.

Carson SA, Simpson JL, Malinak LR, Elias S, Gerbie AB, Buttrons VC, Sarto GE 1983: Heritable aspects of uterine anomalies. *II.* Genetic Analysis of Müllerian Aplasia. *Fertil Steril* 40:86–90.

Daly DC, Soto-Albors CE, Aversa MA 1986: Hysteroscopic detection and treatment of adhesions at the tubal ostium/uterine junction in infertile patients. *Fertil Steril* 46:138–140.

Dmowski WP, Greenblatt R 1969: Asherman's syndrome and risk of placenta accreta. *Obstet Gynecol* 34:288–299.

Fore SR, Hammond CB, Parker RT, Anderson EE 1975: Urologic and genital anomalies in patients with congenital absence of the vagina. *Obstet Gynecol* 46:410–416.

Goebelsmann U, Zachmann M, Davajan V, Israel R, Westman JH, Mishell DR 1976: Male pseudohermaphroditism consistent with 17,20-desmolase deficiency. *Gynecol Obstet Invest* 7:138–156.

Griffin JE, Wilson JD 1980: The syndromes of androgen resistance. *N Engl J Med* 302:198–209.

Hamou J, Salat-Baroux J, Siegler AM 1983: Diagnosis and treatment of intrauterine adhesions by microhysteroscopy. *Fertil Steril* 39:321–326.

Jewelewicz R, Khalaf S, Neuwirth RS, Vande Wiele RLV 1976: Obstetric complications after treatment of intrauterine synechiae (Asherman's syndrome). *Obstet Gynecol* 47:701–705.

Jones HW Jr, Wheeless CR 1969: Salvage of the reproductive potential of women with anomalous development of the Müllerian ducts: 1868–1968–2068. *Am J Obstet Gynecol* 104:348–364.

Jones HW Jr, Mermut S 1972: Familial occurrence of congenital absence of the vagina. *Am J Obstet Gynecol* 114:1100–1101.

Jost A, Vigier B, Prépin J, Perchellet JP 1973: Studies on sex differentiation in mammals. *Recent Prog Horm Res* 29:1–41.

Keenan BS, Meyer WJ III, Hadjian AJ, Jones HW Jr, Migeon CJ 1974: Syndrome of androgen insensitivity in man: Absence of 5α-dihydrotestosterone binding protein in skin fibroblasts. *J Clin Endocrinol Metab* 38:1143–1146.

Kershnar AK, Borut D, Kogut MD, Biglieri EG, Schambelan M 1976: Studies in a phenotypic female with 17α-hydroxylase deficiency. *J Pediatr* 89:395–400.

Klein SM, Garcia CR 1973: Asherman's syndrome: a critique and current review. *Fertil Steril* 24:722–735.

Levine LW, Neuwirth RS 1973: Simultaneous laparoscopy and hysteroscopy for intrauterine adhesions. *Obstet Gynecol* 42:441–445.

Mashchak CA, Kletzky OA, Davajan V, Mishell DR 1981: Clinical and laboratory evaluation of patients with primary amenorrhea. *Obstet Gynecol* 57:715–721.

New MI, Dupont B, Pang S, Pollack M, Levine LS 1981: An update of congenital adrenal hyperplasia. *Recent Prog Horm Res* 37:105–181.

Trichopoulos D, Handanos N, Danezis J, Kalandidi A, Kalapothaki V 1976: Induced abortion and secondary infertility. *Br J Obstet Gynaecol* 83:645–650.

Turunen A, Unnerus CE 1967: Spinal changes in patients with congenital aplasia of the vagina. *Acta Obstet Gynecol Scand* 46:99–106.

Wallach EE 1972: The uterine factor in infertility. *Fertil Steril* 23:138–158.

Wilson JD, Harrod MJ, Goldstein JL, Hemsell DL, MacDonald PC 1974: Familial incomplete male pseudohermaphroditism, type 1. Evidence of androgen resistance and variable clinical manifestations in a family with the Reifenstein syndrome. *N Engl J Med* 290:1097–1103.

Winter JSD, Kohn G, Mellman WJ, Wagner S 1968: A familial syndrome of renal, genital and middle ear anomalies. *J Pediatr* 72:88–93.

Ovarian Disorders

Aiman J, Smentek C 1985: Premature ovarian failure. *Obstet Gynecol* 66:9–14.

Coulam CB 1983: Autoimmune ovarian failure. *Semin Reprod Endocrinol* 1:161–167.

Coulam CB, Stringfellow S, Hoefnagel D 1983: Evidence for a genetic factor in the etiology of premature ovarian failure. *Fertil Steril* 40:693–695.

Damewood MD, Grochow LB 1986: Prospects for fertility after chemotherapy or radiation for neoplastic disease. *Fertil Steril* 45:443–459.

DeLange WE, Weeke A, Artz W, Jansen W, Doorenbos H 1973: Primary anenorrhea with hypertension due to 17-hydroxylase deficiency. *Acta Med Scand* 193:565–571.

Dewhurst J 1978: Fertility in 47,XXX and 45,X patients. *J Med Genet* 15:132–135.

Haseltine FP, Ohno S 1981: Mechanism of gonadal differentiation. *Science* 211:1272–1278.

King CR, Magenis E, Bennett S 1978: Pregnancy and the Turner syndrome. *Obstet Gynecol* 52:617–624.

LaBarbera AR, Miller MM, Ober C, Rebar RW 1988: Autoimmune etiology in premature ovarian failure. *Am J Reprod Immunol Microbiol* 16:115–122.

Manuel M, Katayama KP, Jones HW Jr 1976: The age of occurrence of gonadal tumors in intersex patients with a Y chromosome. *Am J Obstet Gynecol* 124:293–300.

McDonough PG, Byrd JR 1977: Gonadal dysgenesis. *Clin Obstet Gynecol* 20:565–579.

Morris J 1975: Gonadal anomalies and dysgenesis. In: *Progress in Infertility* (Behrman SJ, Kistner RW, eds) Little Brown, Boston, 265–279.

Palmer CG, Reichman A 1976: Chromosomal and clinical findings in 110 females with Turner syndrome. *Hum Genet* 34:35–43.

Rebar RW, Erickson GF, Yen SSC 1982: Idiopathic premature ovarian failure: clinical and endocrine characteristics. *Fertil Steril* 37:35–41.

Reyes FI, Koh KS, Faiman C 1976: Fertility in women with gonadal dysgenesis. *Am J Obstet Gynecol* 126:668–670.

Hypothalamic-Pituitary Dysfunction

Abraham SF, Beumont PJV, Fraser IS, LLewellyn-Jones D 1982: Body weight, exercise and menstrual status among ballet dancers in training. *Br J Obstet Gynaecol* 89:507–510.

Avery ME, McAfee JC, Guild HG 1957: The course and prognosis of reticulo-endothelioses, eosinophilic granuloma, Schüller-Christian syndrome and Letterer-Siwe disease. *Am J Med* 22:636–652.

Bailey P 1940: Tumors involving the hypothalamus and their clinical manifestations. In: *The Hypothalamus and Control of Autonomic Functions* (Faulton FF, Ranson SW, Frantz AM eds), Williams & Wilkins, NY, 723–742.

Bauer HG 1954: Endocrine and other clinical manifestations of hypothalamic disease: a survey of 60 cases with autopsies. *J Clin Endocrinol Metab* 14:13–31

Brown E, Barglow P 1971: Pseudocyesis: a paradigm for psychophysiological interactions. *Arch Gen Psychiatry* 24:221–229.

Bullen BA, Skrinar GS, Beitins IZ, Mering GV, Turnbull BA, McArthur JW 1985: Induction of menstrual disorders by strenuous exercise in untrained women. *N Engl J Med* 312:1349–1353.

Christy NP, Warren MP 1989: Other clinical syndromes of the hypothalamus and anterior pituitary, including tumor mass effects. In: *Endocrinology* (DeGroot LJ ed), W.B. Saunders Co Philadelphia, 2d ed., vol. 1, 419–453.

Daneshdoost L, Gennarelli TA, Bashey HM, Savino PJ, Sergott RG, Bosley TM, Snyder PJ 1991: Recognition of gonadotroph adenomas in women. *N Engl J Med* 324:589–594.

Devane GW, Vera MI, Buhi WC, Kalra PS 1985: Opioid peptides in pseudocyesis. *Obstet Gynecol* 65:183–187.

Fichter MM, Pirke KM 1984: Hypothalamic pituitary function in starving healthy subjects. In: *The Psychobiology of Anorexia Nervosa* (Pirke KM, Ploog D eds), Springer-Verlag, Berlin, 124–135.

Garnica A, Netzloff ML, Rosenbloom AL 1980: Clinical manifestations of hypothalamic tumors. *Ann Clin Lab Sci* 10:474–485.

Gharib H, Frey HM, Laws ER Jr, Randall RV, Scheithaver BW 1983: Coexistent primary empty sella syndrome and hyperprolactinemia: report of 11 cases. *Arch Intern Med* 143:1383–1386.

Graham RL, Grimes DL, Gambrele RD Jr 1979: Amenorrhea secondary to voluntary weight loss. *South Med J* 72:1259–1261.

Hall MGR, Murray MAF, Franks S, Jacobs HS 1976: Endocrinopathy of weight recovered anorexia nervosa in women presenting with secondary amenorrhea. *J Endocrinol* 66:43–44.

Hancock KW, Scott JS, Panigrahi NM, Stitch SR 1976: Significance of low body weight in ovulatory dysfunction after stopping oral contraceptives. *Br Med J* 2:399.

Harris RT 1983: Bulimarexia and related serious eating disorders with medical complications. *Ann Intern Med* 99:800–807.

Herzog DB, Copeland PM 1985: Medical progress-eating disorders. *N Engl J Med* 313:295–303.

Holmberg NG, Nylander I 1971: Weight loss in secondary amenorrhea. *Acta Obstet Gynecol Scand* 50:241–246.

Jaffer KA, Obbens EA, EL Gammal TA 1979: "Empty" sella: review of 76 cases. *South Med J* 72:294–296.

Jenkins JS, Gilbert CJ, Ang V 1976: Hypothalamic-pituitary function in patients with craniopharyngiomas. *J Clin Endocrinol Metab* 43:394–399.

Jialal I, Naidoo C, Norman RJ, Rajput MC, Omar AK, Joubert SM 1984: Pituitary function in Sheehan's syndrome. *Obstet Gynecol* 63:15–19.

Kleinberg DL, Noel GL, Frantz AG 1977: Galactorrhea: 235 cases including 48 with pituitary tumors. *N Engl J Med* 296:589–600.

Knuth UA, Hull MGR, Jacobs HS 1977: Amenorrhea and loss of weight. *Br J Obstet Gynaecol* 84:801–807.

Korsgaard O, Lindholm J, Rasmussen P 1976: Endocrine function in patients with suprasellar and hypothalamic tumors. *Acta Endocrinol (Copenh)* 83:1–8.

Loucks AB, Horvath SM 1984: Exercise-induced stress responses of amenorrheic and eumenorrheic runners. *J Clin Endocrinol Metab* 59:1109–1120.

Martin JB, Reichlin S, Brown GM 1977: Neurologic manifestations of hypothalamic disease. In: *Clinical Neuroendocrinology* (Martin J ed), FA Davis Company, Philadelphia, 247–273.

Mecklenburg RS, Loriaux DL, Thompson RH, Andersen AE, Lipsett MB 1974: Hypothalamic dysfunction in patients with anorexia nervosa. *Medicine* 53:147–159.

Molitch ME 1987: Pituitary tumors: diagnosis and management. *Endocrinol Metab Clin North Am* 16:503–528.

Molitch ME 1989: Management of prolactinomas. *Annu Rev Med* 40:225–232.

Moszkowski EF 1973: Postpartum pituitary insufficiency: report of five unusual cases with long-term follow-up. *South Med J* 66:878–882.

Myerson M, Gutin B, Warren MP, May MT, Contento I, Lee M, Pi-Sunyer FX, Pierson RN Jr, Brooks-Gunn J 1991: Resting metabolic rate and energy balance in amenorrheic and eumenorrheic runners. *Med Sci Sports Exerc* 23:15–22.

Pirke KM, Schweiger U, Lemmel W, Krieg JC, Berger M 1985: The influence of dieting on the menstrual cycle of healthy young women. *J Clin Endocrinol Metab* 60:1174–1179.

Pyle RL, Mitchell JE 1981: Bulimia: a report of 34 cases. *J Clin Psychiatry* 42:60–64.

Reid RL 1990: Interactions between lifestyles, environment and the reproductive system. *Semin Reprod Endocrinol* 8:1.

Schwartz AR, Leddy AL 1982: Recognition of diabetes insipidus in postpartum hypopituitarism. *Obstet Gynecol* 59:394–398.

Schwartz B, Cumming DC, Riordan E, Selye M, Yen SSC, Rebar RW 1981: Exercise-associated amenorrhea: a distinct entity? *Am J Obstet Gynecol* 141:662–670.

Shangold MM, Levine HS 1982: The effect of marathon training upon menstrual function. *Am J Obstet Gynecol* 143:862–869.

Speigel AM, Chiro GD, Gorden P, Ommaya AK, Kolins J, Pomeroy TC 1976: Diagnosis of radiosensitive hypothalamic tumors without craniotomy. Endocrine and neuroradiologic studies of intracranial atypical teratomas. *Ann Intern Med* 85:290–293.

Tulandi T, McInnes RA, Lal S 1983: Altered pituitary hormone secretion in patients with pseudocyesis. *Fertil Steril* 40:637–641.

Veldhuis JD, Hammond JM 1980: Endocrine function after spontaneous infarction of the human pituitary: report, review, and reappraisal. *Endocr Rev* 1:100–107.

Vigersky RA, Loriaux DL, Andersen AE, Lipsett MB 1976: Anorexia nervosa: behavioral and hypothalamic aspects. *J Clin Endocrinol Metab* 5:517–535.

Vigersky RA, Andersen AE, Thompson RH, Loriaux DL 1977: Hypothalamic dysfunction in secondary amenorrhea associated with simple weight loss. *N Engl J Med* 297:1141–1145.

Walsh BT 1980: The endocrinology of anorexia nervosa. *Psychiatr Clin North Am* 3:299–319.

Warren MP 1980: The effects of exercise on pubertal progression and reproductive function in girls. *J Clin Endocrinol Metab* 51:1150–1157.

Warren MP 1982: The effects of altered nutritional states, stress and systemic illness on reproduction in women. In: *Clinical Reproductive Neuroendocrinology* (Vaitukaitis J ed), Elsevier, NY, 177–206.

Warren MP 1983: Effects of undernutrition on reproductive function in the human. *Endocr Rev* 4:363–377.

Warren MP 1988: Anorexia nervosa and bulimia. In: *Gynecology and Obstetrics* (Sciarra JJ ed), Harper & Row, Hagerstown, NJ, vol. 5, chapter 26, 1–13.

Warren MP, Vande Wiele RL 1973: Clinical and metabolic features of anorexia nervosa. *Am J Obstet Gynecol* 117:435–449.

Warren MP, Jewelewicz R, Dyrenfurth I, Ans R, Khalaf S, VandeWiele RL 1975: The

References

significance of weight loss in the evaluation of pituitary response to LHRH in women with secondary amenorrhea. *J Clin Endocrinol Metab* 40:601–611.

Yen SSC, Rebar RW, Quesenberry W 1976: Pituitary function in pseudocyesis. *J Clin Endocrinol Metab* 43:132–136.

Zarate A, Canales ES, Soria J, Jacobs LS, Daughaday WH, Kastin AJ, Schally AV 1974: Gonadotropin and prolactin secretion in human pseudocyesis: effect of synthetic luteinizing hormone-releasing hormone (LH-RH) and thyrotropin-releasing hormone (TRH). *Ann Endocrinol (Paris)* 35:445–450.

CHAPTER 12. ALTERATION OF MENSTRUAL CYCLICITY WITH ENHANCED ANDROGEN SECRETION

REVIEWS

Garner PR 1989: The impact of obesity on reproductive function. *Semin Reprod Endocrinol* 8:32.

Gindoff PR, Jewelewicz R 1987: Polycystic ovarian disease. *Obstet Gynecol Clin North Am* 14:931–954.

New MI 1988: Polycystic ovarian disease and congenital and late onset adrenal hyperplasia. *Endocrinol Metab Clin North Am* 17:637–648.

Yen SSC 1980: The polycystic ovary syndrome. *Clin Endocrinol (Oxf)* 12:177–207.

Young RL, Goldzieher JW 1988: Clinical manifestations of polycystic ovarian disease. *Endocrinol Metab Clin North Am* 17:621–635.

ARTICLES

Pathogenesis of PCO

Berger MJ, Taymore ML, Patton WC 1975: Gonadotropin levels and secretory patterns in patients with typical and atypical polycystic ovarian disease. *Fertil Steril* 26:619–626.

Burger CW, Korsen T, Van Kessel H, Vandop PA, Carson FJM, Schoemaker J 1985: Pulsatile LH patterns in the follicular phase of the menstrual cycle, polycystic ovarian disease (PCOD) and non-PCOD secondary amenorrhea. *J Clin Endocrinol Metab* 61:1126–1132.

DeVane GW, Czekala NM, Judd HL, Yen SSC 1975: Circulating gonadotropins, estrogens and androgens in polycystic ovary disease. *Am J Obstet Gynecol* 121:496–506.

Dunaif A 1986: Do androgens directly regulate gonadotropin secretion in PCO syndrome? *J Clin Endocrinol Metab* 63:215–221.

Erickson GF, Magoffin DA, Dyer CA, Hofeditz C 1985: The ovarian androgen producing cells: a review of structure/function relationships. *Endocr Rev* 6:371–399.

Kazer RR, Kessel B, Yen SSC 1987: Circulating LH pulse frequency in women with polycystic ovary syndrome. *J Clin Endocrinol Metab* 65:233–236.

Lachelin GCL, Barnett M, Hopper BR, Brink G, Yen SSC 1979: Adrenal function in normal women and women with the polycystic ovary syndrome. *J Clin Endocrinol Metab* 49:892–898.

Lobo RA, Goebelsmann U, Horton R 1983: Evidence for the importance of peripheral tissue events in the development of hirsutism in polycystic ovary syndrome. *J Clin Endocrinol Metab* 57:393–397.

McKenna TJ, Moore A, Magee F, Cunningham S 1983: Amenorrhea with cryptic hyperandrogenemia. *J Clin Endocrinol Metab* 56:893–896.

Rebar R, Judd HL, Yen SSC, Rakoff J, Vandenberg G, Naftolin F 1976: Characterization of the inappropriate gonadotropin secretion in polycystic ovary syndrome. *J Clin Invest* 57:1320–1329.

Rosenfield RL, Ehrlich EN, Clearly RE 1972: Adrenal and ovarian contributions to the elevated free plasma androgen levels in hirsute women. *J Clin Endocrinol Metab* 34:92–98.

Rosenfield RL, Barnes RB, Cara JF, Lucky AW 1990: Dysregulation of cytochrome P450c17α as the cause of polycycstic ovarian syndrome. *Fertil Steril* 53:785–791.

Waldstreicher J, Santoro NF, Hall JE, Filicori M, Crowley WF Jr 1988: Hyperfunction of the hypothalamic-pituitary axis in women with polycystic ovarian disease: indirect evidence for partial gonadotroph desensitization. *J Clin Endocrinol Metab* 66:165–172.

Zhang YW, Stern B, Rebar RW 1984: Endocrine comparison of obese menstruating and amenorrheic women. *J Clin Endocrinol Metab* 58:1077–1083.

Zumoff B, Freeman R, Coupey S, Saenger P, Markowitz M, Kream J 1983: A chronobiologic abnormality in LH secretion in teenage girls with polycystic ovary syndrome. *N Engl J Med* 309:1206–1209.

Clinical Aspects of PCO

Barnes R, Rosenfield RL 1989: Polycystic ovary syndrome pathogenesis and treatment. *Ann Intern Med* 110:386–399.

Franks S 1989: Polycystic ovary syndrome: a changing perspective. *Clin Endocrinol (Oxf)* 31:87–120.

Goldzieher JW, Axelrod LR 1963: Clinical and biochemical features of polycystic ovarian disease. *Fertil Steril* 14:631–653.

Stein IT, Leventhal ML 1935: Amenorrhea associated with bilateral polycystic ovaries. *Am J Obstet Gynecol* 29:181–189.

Vaitukaitis JL 1983: Polycystic ovary syndrome: what is it? *N Engl J Med* 309:1245–1246.

Specific Aspects in the Treatment of PCO

Araki S, Chikazawa K, Akabori A, Ijima K, Tamada T 1982: Hormonal contributions to the recruitment of follicular development following ovarian wedge resection in PCO syndrome. *Endocrinol Jpn* 29:57–68.

Burger CW, Korsen TJM, Hompes PGA, Van Kessel H, Schoemaker J 1986: Ovulation induction with pulsatile luteinizing releasing hormone in women with clomiphene citrate resistant polycystic ovary-like disease. *Fertil Steril* 46:1045–1054.

Filicori M, Campaniello E, Michelacci L, Pareschi A, Ferrari P, Bolelli G, Flamigni C 1988: GnRH analog suppression renders PCO disease patients more susceptible to ovulation induction with pulsatile GnRH. *J Clin Endocrinol Metab* 66:327–333.

Filicori M, Flamigni C, Campaniello E, Valdiserri A, Ferrari P, Meriggiola MC, Michelacci L, Pareschi A 1989: The abnormal response of PCO disease patients to exogenous GnRH: characterization and management. *J Clin Endocrinol Metab* 69:825–831.

Judd HL, Rigg LA, Anderson DC, Yen SSC 1976: The effects of ovarian wedge resection on circulating gonadotropin and ovarian steroid levels in patients with polycystic ovary syndrome. *J Clin Endocrinol Metab* 43:347–355.

Kelly A, Jewelewicz R 1990: Alternate regimens for ovulation induction in polycystic ovarian disease. *Fertil Steril* 54:195–202.

Steingold K, Deziegler D, Cedars M, Meldrum DR, Lu JK, Judd HL, Chang RJ 1987: Clinical and hormonal effects of chronic GnRH agonist treatment in PCO disease. *J Clin Endocrinol Metab* 65:773–778.

Wang CF, Gemzell C 1980: The use of human gonadotropins for the induction of ovulation in women with polycystic ovarian disease. *Fertil Steril* 33:479–486.

CHAPTER 13. THERAPEUTIC APPROACHES TO
ACYCLICITY

REVIEWS

Huppert LC 1979: Induction of ovulation with clomiphene citrate. *Fertil Steril* 31:1–8.

Pepperell RJ 1983: A rational approach to ovulation induction. *Fertil Steril* 40:1–14.

Reid RL, Fretts R, Van Vugt D 1988: The theory and practice of ovulation induction with gonadotropin-releasing hormone. *Am J Obstet Gynecol* 158:176–185.

Schwartz M, Jewelewicz R 1981: The use of gonadotropins for induction of ovulation. *Fertil Steril* 35:3–12.

Schziock ED, Jaffe RB 1986: Induction of ovulation with gonadotropin releasing hormone. *Obstet Gynecol Surv* 41:414–423.

Wu CH 1978: Monitoring ovulation induction. *Fertil Steril* 30:617–630.

ARTICLES

Management of Menstrual Irregularity

Jaffe SB, Jewelewicz R 1991: Dysfunctional uterine bleeding in the pediatric and adolescent patient. *Adolesc Pediatr Gynecol* 4:62–69.

Van Eijkeren MA, Christiaens GCM, Sixma JJ, Mapels AA 1989: Menorrhagia: a review. *Obstet Gynecol Surv* 44:421–429.

Induction of Ovulation

Adashi EY 1984: Clomiphene citrate: mechanism(s) and site(s) of action-a hypothesis revisited. *Fertil Steril* 42:331–344.

Adreyko JL, Marshall LA, Dumesic DA, Jaffe RB 1987: Therapeutic uses of Gonadotropin-releasing hormone analogs. *Obstet Gynecol Surv* 42:1–21.

Carr JS, Reid RL 1990: Ovulation induction with GnRH. *Semin Reprod Endocrinol* 8:174–185.

Chong L, Lee S 1987: Luteal phase defects. *Obstet Gynecol Surv* 42:267–274.

Diamond MP, Wentz AC 1986: Ovulation induction with human menopausal gonadotropins. *Obstet Gynecol Surv* 41:480–490.

Filicori M, Flamigni C, Meriggiola MC, Cognigni G, Valdiserri A, Ferrari P, Campaniello E 1991: Ovulation induction with pulsatile gonadotropin-releasing hormone: technical modalities and clinical perspectives. *Fertil Steril* 56:1–13.

Golan A, Ron-El R, Herman A, Soffer Y, Weinraub Z, Caspi E 1989: Ovarian hyperstimulation syndrome: an update review. *Obstet Gynecol Surv* 44:430–440.

Hodgen GD 1989: Proceedings from the symposium: current role of GnRH agonists in obstetrics & gynecology. *Obstet Gynecol Surv* 44:293–329.

Jaffe RB, Yen SSC (eds) 1990: Pulsatile GnRH in clinical medecine. *Am J Obstet Gynecol* [Suppl] 163:1719–1770.

Jewelewicz R, Gindoff PR 1989: Induction of ovulation-past, present and future. *Gynecol Obstet Invest* 26:89–103.

Leal JA, Williams RF, Danforth DR, Gordon K, Hodgen GD 1988: Prolonged duration of gonadotropin inhibition by a third generation GnRH antagonist. *J Clin Endocrinol Metab* 67:1325–1327.

Loucopoulos A, Ferin M 1987: The treatment of luteal phase defects with pulsatile infusion of GnRH. *Fertil Steril* 48:933–936.

Martin K, Santoro N, Hall J, Filicori M, Wierman M, Crowley WF 1990: Management of ovulatory disorders with pulsatile GnRH. *J Clin Endocrinol Metab* 71:1081–1086.

Pavlou S, Wakefield G, Schlechter NL, Lindner J, Souza KH, Kamilaris TC, Konidaris S, Rivier JE, Vale WW, Toglia M 1989: Mode of suppression of pituitary and gonadal function after acute or prolonged administration of a LHRH antagonist in normal men. *J Clin Endocrinol Metab* 88:446–454.

Plosker SM, Marshall LA, Martin MC, Jaffe RB 1990: Opioid, catecholamine, and steroid interaction in prolactin and gonadotropin regulation. *Obstet Gynecol Surv* 45:441–453.

Rivier JE, Porter J, Rivier CL, Perrin M, Corrigan A, Hook WA, Siraganian RP, Vale WW 1986: New effective gonadotropin releasing hormone antagonists with minimal potency for histamine release in vitro. *J Med Chem* 29:1846–1851.

Santoro N, Wierman ME, Filicori M, Waldstreicher J, Crowley WF 1986: Intravenous administration of pulsatile GnRH in hypothalamic amenorrhea: effects of dosage. *J Clin Endocrinol Metab* 62:109–116.

Urban RJ, Pavlou SN, Rivier JE, Vale WW, Dufau ML, Veldhuis JD 1990: Suppressive actions of a GnRH antagonist on LH, FSH, and prolactin release in estrogen-deficient postmenopausal women. *Am J Obstet Gynecol* 162:1255–1260.

Wu CH 1984: A rational and practical approach to clomiphene therapy. *Clin Obstet Gynecol* 27:953–960.

Assisted Reproduction

Jones HW, Schrader C 1988: In vitro fertilization and other assisted reproduction. *Ann NY Acad Sci,* vol. 541, 1–292.

In vitro fertilization-embryo transfer (IVF-ET) in the United States 1992: 1990 results from the IVF-ET Registry. *Fertil Steril* 57:15–24.

CHAPTER 14. HORMONAL CONTRACEPTIVES

REVIEWS

Boutaleb Y, Goldzieher JW 1989: Toward a new standard in oral contraception. *Am J Obstet Gynecol* 163:1379–1420.

Derman R 1989: Oral contraceptives: a reassessment. *Obstet Gynecol Surv* 44:662–668.

Elgee NJ 1970: Medical aspects of oral contraceptives. *Ann Intern Med* 72:409–418.

Skouby SV, Jesperson J 1990: Oral contraceptives in the nineties: metabolic aspects—facts and fiction. *Am J Obstet Gynecol* 163:273–446.

Warren MP 1973: Metabolic effects of contraceptive steroids. *Am Rev Med Sci* 264:5–21.

ARTICLES

Chemistry and Mode of Action of Steroid Contraceptives

Back DJ, Bates M, Breckenridge AM, Hall JM, MacIver M, Orme ML, Park BK, Rowe PH 1981: The pharmacokinetics of levonorgestrel and ethynyl estradiol in women—studies with Ovran and Ovranette. *Contraception* 23:229–239.

Brenner PF 1982: The pharmacology of progestogens. *J Reprod Med* 27 (suppl 1):490–497.

Diczfalusy E 1968: Mode of action of contraceptive drugs. *Am J Obstet Gynecol* 100:136–163.

Dorfinger LJ 1985: Relative potency of progestins used in oral contraceptives. *Contraception* 31:557–570.

Goldzieher JW 1989: Pharmacology of contraceptive steroids: a brief review. *Am J Obstet Gynecol* 160:1260–1264.

Grant ECG 1967: Hormone balance of oral contraceptives. *J Obstet Gynaecol Br Commonw* 74:908–918.

Mishell DR Jr, Kletzky OA, Brenner PF, Roy S, Wicoloff J 1977: The effect of contraceptive steroids on hypothalamic-pituitary function. *Am J Obstet Gynecol* 128:60–74.

Newburger J, Goldzieher JW 1985: Pharmacokinetics of ethynyl estradiol: a current view. *Contraception* 32:33–44.

Nilsson S, Nygren KG 1978: Ethinyl estradiol in peripheral plasma after oral administration of 30μg and 50μg to women. *Contraception* 18:469–475.

Orme ML, Back DJ, Breckenridge AM 1983: Clinical pharmacokinetics of oral contraceptive steroids. *Clin Pharmacokinet* 8:95–136.

Scott JZ, Brenner PF, Kletzky OA, Mishell DR Jr 1978: Factors affecting pituitary gonadotropin function in users of oral contraceptive steroids. *Am J Obstet Gynecol* 130:817–821.

Scott JZ, Kletzky OA, Brenner PF, Mishell DR Jr 1978: Comparison of the effects of contraceptive steroid formulations containing two doses of estrogen on pituitary function. *Fertil Steril* 30:141–145.

World Health Organization expanded programme of research, development and research training in human reproduction 1983: Task force on long-acting systemic agents for the regulation of fertility: multinational comparative clinical evaluation of two long-acting injectable contraceptive steroids: norethisterone enanthate and medroxyprogesterone acetate. Final report. *Contraception* 28:1–20.

General Effects of Steroid Contraceptives

Bergkvist L, Adami HO, Persson I, Hoover R, Schairer C 1989: The risk of breast cancer after estrogen and estrogen–progestin replacement. *N Engl J Med* 321:293–297.

Bierman EL 1969: Oral contraceptives, lipoproteins and lipid transport. In: *Metabolic Effects of Contraceptive Steroids* (Salhanick DM, Kipnis DM, Vande Wiele RL eds), Plenum Press, NY, 207–218.

Böttiger LE, Boman G, Eklund G, Westerholm L 1980: Oral contraceptives and thromboembolic disease: effects of lowering oestrogen content. *Lancet* 1:1097–1101.

Briggs MH, Briggs M 1981: A randomized study of metabolic effects of four low-estrogen oral contraceptives. *I*. Results after six cycles. *Contraception* 23:463–471.

Burkman RT 1988: Lipid and lipoprotein changes in relation to oral contraception and hormonal on replacement therapy. *Fertil Steril* 49:39s–50s.

Burkman RT, Robinson JC, Kruszon-Moran D, Kimball AW, Kwiterovich P, Burford RG 1988: Lipid and lipoprotein changes associated with oral contraceptive use: a randomized clinical trial. *Obstet Gynecol* 71:33–38.

Cancer and Steroid Hormone Study of the Centers for Disease Control and The National Institute of Child Health and Human Development 1987a: Combination oral contraceptive use and the risk of endometrial cancer. *JAMA* 257:796–800.

Cancer and Steroid Hormone Study of the Centers for Disease Control and the National Institute of Child Health and Human Development 1987b: The reduction in risk of ovarian cancer associated with oral-contraceptive use. *N Engl J Med* 316:650–655.

Centers for Disease Control and Women's Health Study 1983: Oral contraceptive use and the risk of endometrial cancer. *JAMA* 249:1602–1604.

Centers for Disease Control Cancer and Steroid Hormone Study 1983: Oral contraceptive use and the risk of ovarian cancer. *JAMA* 249:1596–1599.

Crook D, Godsland IF, Wynn V 1988: Oral contraceptives and Coronary heart disease: metabolism of glucose tolerance and plasma lipid risk factors by progestins, prevention and management of cardiovascular risk in women. *Am J Obstet Gynecol* 158:1612–1620.

Gambrell RD 1984: Hormones in the etiology and prevention of breast and endometrial cancer. *South Med J* 77:1509–1511.

Glueck CJ, Levy RI, Fredrickson DJ 1971: Norethindrone acetate, post heparin lipolytic activity and plasma triglycerides in familial types I, III, IV and V hyperlipoproteinemia. *Ann Intern Med* 75:345–352.

Hazzard WR, Spiger MJ, Bierman EL 1969: Studies of the mechanism of hypertriglyceridemia induced by oral contraceptives. In: *Metabolic Effects of Contraceptive Steroids* (Salhanick DM, Kipnis DM, Vande Wiele RL eds), Plenum Press, NY, 232–241.

Inman WH, Vessey MP 1968: Investigation of deaths from pulmonary, coronary and cerebral thrombosis and embolism. *Br Med J* 2:193–199.

Kalkhoff RK 1980: Relative sensitivity of postpartum gestational diabetic women to oral contraceptive agents and other metabolic stress. *Diabetes Care* 3:421–424.

Kaufman DW, Shapiro S, Slone D, Rosenberg L, Miettinen OS, Stolley PD, Knapp RC, Leavitt T Jr, Watring WG, Rosenshein NB, Lewis JL Jr, Schottenfeld D, Engle RL Jr 1980: Decreased risk of endometrial cancer among oral contraceptive users. *N Engl J Med* 303:1045–1047.

Knopp RH, Walden CE, Wahl PW, Hoover JJ, Warnick GR, Albers JJ, Ogilviec JT, Hazzard WR 1981: Oral contraceptive and postmenopausal estrogen effects on lipoprotein triglyceride and cholesterol in an adult female population: relationships to estrogen and progestin potency. *J Clin Endocrinol Metab* 53:1123–1132.

Layde PM, Beral V, Kay CR 1981: Further analyses of mortality in oral contraceptive users: Royal College of General Practitioners study. *Lancet* 1:541–546.

Lipnick RJ, Buring JR, Hennekens CH, Rosner B, Willett W, Bain L, Stampfer MJ, Colditz GA, Peto R, Speizer FE 1986: Oral contraceptives and breast cancer: a prospective cohort study. *JAMA* 255:58–61.

Lipson A, Stoy DB, LaRosa JC, Muesing RA, Cleary RA, Miller VT, Gilbert PR, Stadel B 1986: Progestins and oral contraceptive-induced lipoprotein changes: a prospective study. *Contraception* 34:121–134.

Meade TW 1982: Oral contraceptives, clotting factors, and thrombosis. *Am J Obstet Gynecol* 142:758–761.

Meade TW, Greenberg G, Thompson SG 1980: Progestogens and cardiovascular reactions associated with oral contraceptives and a comparison of the safety of 50-and 30-μg estrogen preparations. *Br Med J* 280:1157–1161.

Radberg T, Gustafson A, Skryten A, Karlsson K 1981: Oral contraception in diabetic women: diabetes control, serum and high density lipoprotein lipids during low-dose progestogen combined oestrogen/progestogen and non-hormonal contraception. *Acta Endocrinol (Copenh)* 98:246–251.

Salmi T 1979: Risk factors in endometrial carcinoma with special reference to the use of estrogens. *Acta Obstet Gynecol Scand* 86:1–119.

Schlesselman JJ, Stadel BV, Murray P, Lai S 1988: Breast cancer in relation to early use of oral contraceptives: no evidence of a latent effect. *JAMA* 259:1828–1833.

Shoupe D, Mishell DR 1989: Norplant: subdermal implant system for long-term contraception. *Am J Obstet Gynecol* 160:1286–1292.

Skouby SO, Molsted-Pedersen L, Kuhl C 1982: Low dosage oral contraception in women with previous gestational diabetes. *Obstet Gynecol* 59:325–328.

Sondheimer S 1981: Metabolic effects of the birth control pill. *Clin Obstet Gynecol* 24:927–941.

Spellacy WN, Buhi W, Birk S 1975: Effects of norethindrone on carbohydrate and lipid metabolism. *Obstet Gynecol* 46:560–563.

Spellacy WN, Buhi WC, Birk SA 1979: Carbohydrate metabolism prospectively studied in women using a low-estrogen oral contraceptive for six months. *Contraception* 20:137–148.

Spellacy WN, Birk SA, Buggie J, Buhi WC 1981: Prospective carbohydrate metabolism studies in women using a low-estrogen oral contraceptive for 1 year. *J Reprod Med* 26:295–298.

Spellacy WN, Buhi W, Birk S 1981: Prospective studies of carbohydrate metabolism in "normal" women using norgestrel for eighteen months. *Fertil Steril* 35:167–171.

Spellacy WN, Kerr DA, White B, Keith GE, Waggoner BL 1984: A family planning risk scoring system for health care providers. *Obstet Gynecol* 63:846–849.

Stadel BV, Rubin GL, Webster LA, Schlesselman JJ, Wingo PA 1985: Oral contraceptives and breast cancer in young women. *Lancet* 2:970–973.

Stokes T, Wynn V 1971: Serum-lipids in women on oral contraceptives. *Lancet* 2: 677–680.

Stolley PD, Tonascia JA, Tockman MS, Sartwell PE, Rutledge AH, Jacobs MP 1975: Thrombosis with low estrogen oral contraceptives. *Am J Epidemiol* 102:197–208.

Vessey MP, Doll R 1969: Investigation of relation between use of oral contraceptives and thromboembolic disease: a further report. *Br Med J* 2:651–657.

Wahl P, Walden C, Knopp R, Hoover J, Wallace R, Heiss G, Rifkind B 1983: Effect of estrogen/progestin potency on lipid/lipoprotein cholesterol. *N Engl J Med* 308:862–867.

Weiss NS, Sayvetz T 1980: Incidence of endometrial cancer in relation to the use of oral contraceptives. *N Engl J Med* 302:551–554.

World Health Organization 1985: A randomized double-blind study of the effects of two low-dose combined oral contraceptives on biochemical aspects. *Contraception* 32:223–236.

World Health Organization Task Force on oral contraceptives 1982: A randomized, double-blind study of two combined and two progestogen-only oral contraceptives. *Contraception* 25:243–252.

Wynn V 1982: Effect of duration of low-dose oral contraceptive administration on carbohydrate metabolism. *Am J Obstet Gynecol* 142:739–746.

Wynn V, Doar JWH 1969: Some effects of oral contraceptives on carbohydrate metabolism. *Lancet* 2:715–719.

Wynn V, Nithyananthan R 1982: The effect of progestins in combined oral contraceptives on serum lipids with special reference to high-density lipoproteins. *Am J Obstet Gynecol* 142:766–772.

Other Hormonal Contraceptives

Bergquist C, Nillius SJ, Wide L 1982: Long-term intranasal luteinizing hormone-releasing hormone agonist treatment for contraception in women. *Fertil Steril* 39:190–193.

Lemay A, Faure N, Labrie F, Fazekas ATA 1985: Inhibition of ovulation during discontinuous intranasal luteinizing hormone-releasing hormone agonist dosing in combination with gestagen-induced bleeding. *Fertil Steril* 43:868–877.
Nillius SJ, Bergquist C, Wide L 1978: Inhibition of ovulation in women by chronic treatment with a stimulatory LRH analogue. A new approach to birth control? *Contraception* 17:537–545.
Silvestre L, DuBois C, Renault M, Rezvani Y, Baulieu EE, Ulmann A 1990: Voluntary interruption of pregnancy with mifepristone (RU 486) and a prostaglandin analogue. *N Engl J Med* 322:645–648.
Ulmann A, Dubois C, Philibert D 1987: Fertility control with RU486. *Horm Res* 28:274–278.

CHAPTER 15. THE PREMENSTRUAL SYNDROME

REVIEWS

Reid RL 1987: Endogenous opiate peptides and premenstrual syndrome. *Semin Reprod Endocrinol* 5:191–197.
Reid RL, Yen SSC 1981: The premenstrual syndrome. *Am J Obstet Gynecol* 139:85–104.
Schachter D, Vaitukaitis J 1987: Diagnosis and management of premenstrual syndrome. *Intern Med Spec* 8:94–116.

ARTICLES

Pathophysiology of PMS

Backstrom CT, Carstensen H 1974: Estrogen and progesterone in plasma in relation to premenstrual tension. *J Steroid Biochem* 5:257–266.
Backstrom CT, Boyle H, Baird DT 1981: Persistence of symptoms of premenstrual tension in hysterectomized women. *Br J Obstet Gynaecol* 88:530–535.
Dennerstein L, Spence-Gardner C, Brunn J 1984: Premenstrual tension-hormonal profiles. *J Psychosom Obstet Gynecol* 3:37–51.
Hammaback S, Backstrom T, Holst J, Von Schoultz B, Lyrenas S 1985: Cyclical mood changes as in premenstrual tension syndrome during sequential estrogen-progestogen postmenopausal replacement therapy. *Acta Obstet Gynecol Scand* 64:393–397.

Clinical Aspects of PMS

Halbreich U, Endicott J, Schacht S, Nee J 1982: The diversity of premenstrual changes as reflected in the Premenstrual Assessment Form. *Acta Psychiatr Scand* 65:46–56.
Halbreich U, Endicott J 1985: Methodological issues in studies of premenstrual changes. *Psychoneuroendocrinology* 10:15–32.
Moos RH 1968: The developmett of a menstrual distress questionnaire. *Psychosom Med* 30:853–867.

Treatment of PMS

Berman M 1990: Vitamin B-6 in premenstrual syndrome. *J Am Diet Assoc* 90:859–861.
Brush M 1988: Pyridoxine in the treatment of premenstrual syndrome. *Br J Clin Prac* 42:448–452.
Casson P, Hahn PM, Van Vugt DA, Reid RL 1990: Lasting response to ovariectomy in severe intractable premenstrual syndrome. *Am J Obstet Gynecol* 162:99–105.
Derzko C 1990: Role of danazol in relieving the premenstrual syndrome. *J Reprod Med* 35:97–102.

References

Freeman E 1990: Ineffectiveness of progesterone suppository treatment for premenstrual syndrome. *Jama* 264:349–353.

Hammarback S 1988: Induced anovulation as treatment of premenstrual tension syndrome. *Acta Obstet Gynecol Scand* 67:159–166.

Harrison W 1990: Treatment of premenstrual dysphoria with alprazolam. *Arc Gen Psychiatry* 47:270–275.

Maddocks MA, Hahn P, Muller F, Reid RL 1986: A double blind placebo controlled trial of progesterone vaginal suppositories in the treatment of premenstrual syndrome. *Am J Obstet Gynecol* 154:573–581.

Magos AL, Brewster E, Singh R, O'Dowd T, Brincat M, Studd JW 1986: The effects of norethisterone in postmenopausal women on oestrogen replacement therapy: a model for the premenstrual syndrome. *Br J Obstet Gynaecol* 93:1290–1296.

Mortola JF, Girton L, Fischer U 1991: Successful treatment of severe premenstrual syndrome by combined use of gonadotropin-releasing hormone agonist and estrogen/progestin. *J Clin Endocrinol Metab* 71:252A–252F.

Muse KN, Cetel NS, Futterman LA, Yen SSC 1984: The premenstrual syndrome: effects of medical ovariectomy. *N Engl J Med* 311:1345–1349.

Rapkin A, Chang LH, Reading AE 1987: Premenstrual syndrome: a double blind placebo controlled study with progesterone vaginal suppositories. *J Obstet Gynecol* 7:217–220.

Robinson G 1990: Problems in the treatment of premenstrual syndrome. *Can J Psychiatry* 35:199–206.

Sander S 1988: Treatment of dysmenorrhoea and premenstrual syndrome with non-steroidal anti-inflammatory drugs. *Drugs* 36:475–490.

Vellacott ID, O'Brien PMS 1987: Effect of spironolactone on premenstrual syndrome symptoms. *J Reprod Med* 32:429–434.

Watts J 1987: A clinical trial using danazol for the treatment of premenstrual tension. *Br J Obstet Gynaecol* 94:30–34.

Wurtman J 1989: Effect of nutrient intake on premenstrual depression. *Am J Obstet Gynecol* 161:1228–1234.

Index

Italic letter *f* indicates a figure; italic letter *t* denotes a table.